Radiologic Gastrointestinal Imaging

Editor

PERRY J. PICKHARDT

GASTROENTEROLOGY CLINICS OF NORTH AMERICA

www.gastro.theclinics.com

Consulting Editor
ALAN L. BUCHMAN

September 2018 • Volume 47 • Number 3

ELSEVIER

1600 John F. Kennedy Boulevard • Suite 1800 • Philadelphia, Pennsylvania, 19103-2899
http://www.theclinics.com

GASTROENTEROLOGY CLINICS OF NORTH AMERICA Volume 47, Number 3
September 2018 ISSN 0889-8553, ISBN-13: 978-0-323-64233-0

Editor: Kerry Holland
Developmental Editor: Sara Watkins

Gastroenterology Clinics of North America (ISSN 0889-8553) is published quarterly by Elsevier Inc., 360 Park Avenue South, New York, NY 10010-1710. Months of issue are March, June, September, and December. Business and Editorial Offices: 1600 John F. Kennedy Blvd., Suite 1800, Philadelphia, PA 19103-2899. Customer Service Office: 6277 Sea Harbor Drive, Orlando, FL 32887-4800. Periodicals postage paid at New York, NY and additional mailing offices. Subscription prices are $350.00 per year (US individuals), $100.00 per year (US students), $659.00 per year (US institutions), $383.00 per year (Canadian individuals), $220.00 per year (Canadian students), $809.00 per year (Canadian institutions), $458.00 per year (international individuals), $220.00 per year (international students), and $809.00 per year (international institutions). Foreign air speed delivery is included in all *Clinics* subscription prices. All prices are subject to change without notice. **POSTMASTER**: Send address changes to *Gastroenterology Clinics of North America*, Elsevier Health Sciences Division, Subscription Customer Service, 3251 Riverport Lane, Maryland Heights, MO 63043. **Telephone: 1-800-654-2452 (U.S. and Canada); 314-447-8871 (outside U.S. and Canada). Fax: 314-447-8029. E-mail: journalscustomerservice-usa@elsevier.com (for print support); journalsonlinesupport-usa@elsevier.com (for online support)**.

Reprints. For copies of 100 or more, of articles in this publication, please contact the Commercial Reprints Department, Elsevier Inc., 360 Park Avenue South, New York, New York 10010-1710. Tel. 212-633-3874, Fax: 212-633-3820, E-mail: reprints@elsevier.com.

Gastroenterology Clinics of North America is also published in Italian by Il Pensiero Scientifico Editore, Rome, Italy; and in Portuguese by Interlivros Edicoes Ltda., Rua Commandante Coelho 1085, 21250 Cordovil, Rio de Janeiro, Brazil.

Gastroenterology Clinics of North America is covered in *MEDLINE/PubMed (Index Medicus)*, *Excerpta Medica*, *Current Contents/Clinical Medicine*, *Science Citation Index*, *ISI/BIOMED*, and *BIOSIS*.

Contributors

CONSULTING EDITOR

ALAN L. BUCHMAN, MD, MSPH, FACP, FACG, FACN, AGAF
Medical Director, Health Care Services Corporation; and Visiting Clinical Professor of Surgery and Medical Director, Intestinal Rehabilitation and Transplant Center, University of Illinois at Chicago, Chicago, Illinois, USA

EDITOR

PERRY J. PICKHARDT, MD
Professor of Radiology, Chief, Gastrointestinal Imaging, Medical Director, Cancer Imaging, University of Wisconsin-Madison School of Medicine and Public Health, Madison, Wisconsin, USA

AUTHORS

EVIE H. CARCHMAN, MD
Assistant Professor, Department of Surgery, University of Wisconsin-Madison School of Medicine and Public Health, Madison, Wisconsin, USA

ANNE M. COVEY, MD
Attending Radiologist, Memorial Sloan Kettering Cancer Center, Professor of Radiology, Weill Cornell Medical Center, New York, New York, USA

AMY R. DEIPOLYI, MD, PhD
Assistant Attending Radiologist, Memorial Sloan Kettering Cancer Center, Assistant Professor of Radiology, Weill Cornell Medical Center, New York, New York, USA

JOEL G. FLETCHER, MD
Department of Radiology, Mayo Clinic, Rochester, Minnesota, USA

KATHRYN J. FOWLER, MD
Associate Professor, Mallinckrodt Institute of Radiology, Washington University School of Medicine, St Louis, Missouri

TYLER J. FRAUM, MD
Clinical Radiology Fellow, Mallinckrodt Institute of Radiology, Washington University School of Medicine, St Louis, Missouri

HELENA GABRIEL, MD
Director, School of Ultrasound, Associate Professor, Department of Radiology, Northwestern Memorial Hospital, Northwestern University Feinberg School of Medicine, Chicago, Illinois, USA

MOHIT GUPTA, MD
Department of Radiology, Northwestern Memorial Hospital, Northwestern University Feinberg School of Medicine, Chicago, Illinois, USA

RICHARD B. HALBERG, PhD
University of Wisconsin-Madison School of Medicine and Public Health, Madison, Wisconsin, USA

CESARE HASSAN, MD
Digestive Endoscopy Unit, Nuovo Regina Margherita Hospital, Rome, Italy

THOMAS A. HOPE, MD
Assistant Professor, Department of Radiology and Biomedical Imaging, University of California, San Francisco, San Francisco, California

DAVID H. KIM, MD
Professor, Department of Radiology, University of Wisconsin-Madison School of Medicine and Public Health, Madison, Wisconsin, USA

GENE KIM, MD
Resident, Department of Radiology, Boston University Medical Center, Boston, Massachusetts, USA

NATHAN Y. KIM, MD
Professor, Department of Radiology, University of Wisconsin-Madison School of Medicine and Public Health, Madison, Wisconsin, USA

TAE YOUNG LEE, MD
Department of Radiology, Research Institute of Radiology, University of Ulsan College of Medicine, Asan Medical Center, Seoul, South Korea

MARC S. LEVINE, MD
Professor, Department of Radiology, Chief of Gastrointestinal Radiology, Hospital of the University of Pennsylvania, Perelman School of Medicine, University of Pennsylvania, Philadelphia, Pennsylvania, USA

MEGHAN G. LUBNER, MD
Associate Professor, Department of Radiology, University of Wisconsin-Madison School of Medicine and Public Health, Madison, Wisconsin, USA

DANIEL R. LUDWIG, MD
Radiology Resident, Mallinckrodt Institute of Radiology, Washington University School of Medicine, St Louis, Missouri

KRISTINA A. MATKOWSKYJ, MD, PhD
University of Wisconsin-Madison School of Medicine and Public Health, Madison, Wisconsin, USA

VINCENT M. MELLNICK, MD
Department of Radiology, Mallinckrodt Institute of Radiology, St Louis, Missouri, USA

CHRISTINE O. MENIAS, MD
Professor of Radiology, Mayo Clinic School of Medicine, Mayo Clinic Hospital, Phoenix, Arizona, USA

FRANK H. MILLER, MD
Lee F. Rogers MD Professor of Medical Education, Chief, Body Imaging Section and Fellowship Program, Medical Director, MRI, Department of Radiology, Northwestern Memorial Hospital, Northwestern University Feinberg School of Medicine, Chicago, Illinois, USA

PARDEEP K. MITTAL, MD
Associate Professor, Department of Radiology and Imaging Sciences, Emory University School of Medicine, Atlanta, Georgia, USA

COURTNEY C. MORENO, MD
Associate Professor, Department of Radiology and Imaging Sciences, Emory University School of Medicine, Atlanta, Georgia, USA

TREVOR MORRISON, MD
Director of Ultrasound, Assistant Professor, Department of Radiology, Boston University Medical Center, Boston, Massachusetts, USA

SEONG HO PARK, MD, PhD
Department of Radiology, Research Institute of Radiology, University of Ulsan College of Medicine, Asan Medical Center, Seoul, South Korea

ROCIO PEREZ-JOHNSTON, MD
Interventional Radiology Fellow, Memorial Sloan Kettering Cancer Center, New York, New York, USA

PERRY J. PICKHARDT, MD
Professor of Radiology, Chief, Gastrointestinal Imaging, Medical Director, Cancer Imaging, University of Wisconsin-Madison School of Medicine and Public Health, Madison, Wisconsin, USA

BRYAN DUSTIN POOLER, MD
Department of Radiology, University of Wisconsin-Madison School of Medicine and Public Health, Madison, Wisconsin, USA

SCOTT B. REEDER, MD, PhD
Departments of Emergency Medicine, Medical Physics, Medicine, Biomedical Engineering and Radiology, University of Wisconsin-Madison School of Medicine and Public Health, Madison, Wisconsin, USA

MICHAEL D. REPPLINGER, MD, PhD
Department of Emergency Medicine, University of Wisconsin-Madison School of Medicine and Public Health, Madison, Wisconsin, USA

JESSICA B. ROBBINS, MD
Associate Professor, Department of Radiology, University of Wisconsin-Madison School of Medicine and Public Health, Madison, Wisconsin, USA

KUMARESAN SANDRASEGARAN, MD
Professor of Radiology, Indiana University School of Medicine, Indianapolis, Indiana, USA

BRETT P. SJOBERG, MD
Department of Radiology, University of Wisconsin-Madison School of Medicine and Public Health, Madison, Wisconsin, USA

JORGE A. SOTO, MD
Chairman, Professor, Department of Radiology, Boston University Medical Center, Boston, Massachusetts, USA

PATRICK S. SULLIVAN, MD
Divisions of Surgical Oncology and Colorectal Surgery, Assistant Professor, Department of Surgery, Emory University School of Medicine, Atlanta, Georgia, USA

ARNOLD WALD, MD
Professor, Department of Medicine, University of Wisconsin-Madison School of Medicine and Public Health, Madison, Wisconsin, USA

BYONG DUK YE, MD, PhD
Department of Gastroenterology, Inflammatory Bowel Disease Center, University of Ulsan College of Medicine, Asan Medical Center, Seoul, South Korea

Contents

abdominal indications. CT metrics are often easily retrospectively obtained without special equipment. Metrics such as liver segmental volume ratio, which quantifies regional hepatic volume changes; splenic volume; and liver surface nodularity scoring show diagnostic performance comparable with elastography techniques for detecting significant and advanced fibrosis. Other emerging CT tools, such as CT texture analysis and fractional extracellular volume, have also shown promise in identifying fibrosis and warrant further study.

The prognosis for hepatocellular carcinoma (HCC) is dependent on tumor stage at diagnosis, with curative treatment options more available to early-detected HCCs. Professional organizations have produced HCC screening guidelines in at-risk groups, with ultrasound imaging the most commonly used screening tool and increased interest in MRI in specific populations. HCC may be diagnosed by imaging features alone and has been universally incorporated into management guidelines. The radiology community has standardized imaging criteria for HCC with the development of the Liver Imaging Reporting and Data System, which has expanded to incorporate computed tomography, MR, and contrast-enhanced ultrasound imaging for diagnostic purposes.

Autoimmune pancreatitis (AIP) is a steroid-responsive fibroinflammatory disorder of the pancreas. There are 2 distinct subtypes of AIP, types 1 and 2. Type 1 is associated with systemic immunoglobulin (Ig)G4 disease and may affect multiple organs in the body. Type 2 is confined to the pancreas and shows an association with ulcerative colitis. This article describes the imaging findings of AIP and IgG4 disease in the liver, bile ducts, kidneys, and retroperitoneal regions. The imaging differentiation of AIP from pancreas cancer is discussed.

Biliary drainage is important in the care of patients with benign and malignant biliary obstruction. Careful preprocedure evaluation of high-quality cross-sectional imaging and inventory of symptoms are necessary to determine whether a percutaneous, endoscopic, or surgical approach is most appropriate. High bile duct obstruction is usually best managed percutaneously; a specific duct can be targeted and enteric contamination of isolated ducts can be avoided. Options for percutaneous biliary intervention include external or internal/external biliary drainage, stent placement, biliary stone retrieval, and bile duct biopsy. Preprocedure evaluation, technique, and indications for percutaneous intervention in benign and malignant diseases are summarized.

GASTROENTEROLOGY
CLINICS OF NORTH AMERICA

THE CLINICS ARE AVAILABLE ONLINE!
Access your subscription at:
www.theclinics.com

Foreword

Diagnostic Imaging: A Peephole into Many of the Body's Dressing Rooms

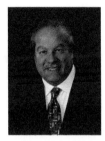

Alan L. Buchman, MD, MSPH, FACP, FACG, FACN, AGAF
Consulting Editor

Diagnostic imaging provides a window in an otherwise cloaked human being. Increasingly, less invasive imaging techniques are replacing direct examination though orifices, regardless of whether natural or manmade. Various imaging techniques can be combined, as in the case of PET/computed tomography or PET/MR, to provide more functional imaging. Today's imaging provides a resolution previously only imagined. In other cases, these evolved imaging techniques serve to complement endoscopic views by revealing what lies beyond the tip or walls of the scope, and in some cases, such techniques as endoscopic ultrasound, radiologic and endoscopic techniques, have been combined. Dr Pickhardt has selected a group of renowned radiologists at the forefront of their fields who discuss recent advancements in gastrointestinal cancer detection and management, as well as the imaging of those organs generally off limits to most endoscopic procedures, including the liver, spleen, and pancreas. The way in which modern imaging techniques, with evolving software, complement endoscopic visualization of the biliary tree, the small intestine, colon and

Gastroenterol Clin N Am 47 (2018) xiii–xiv
https://doi.org/10.1016/j.gtc.2018.04.015
0889-8553/18/© 2018 Published by Elsevier Inc.

rectum, is presented. As pointed out by Dr Pickhardt, the radiologist has evolved from being a competitor to the gastroenterologist in some ways to becoming indispensable to the gastroenterologist in order to provide optimal patient care.

Alan L. Buchman, MD, MSPH, FACP, FACG, FACN, AGAF
Professor of Clinical Surgery
Medical Director, Intestinal Rehabilitation and Transplant Center
University of Illinois at Chicago
Medical Director, Health Care Services Corporation
Chicago, Illinois, USA

959 Oak Drive
Glencoe, IL 60022, USA

E-mail address:
Buchman@uic.edu

Preface

Gastrointestinal Imaging: Rapid Advancements Leading to Improved Patient Care

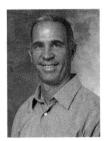

Perry J. Pickhardt, MD
Editor

The field of Gastroenterology has witnessed extraordinary advances over the past decade. Gastrointestinal (GI) imaging has played a central role in this evolution, from both the endoscopic and the radiologic perspective. The classic disciplines of GI Radiology (with fluoroscopy and cross-sectional imaging) and GI endoscopy have become more closely interrelated and complementary. Cross-sectional imaging techniques such as CT and MR provide for advanced visualization techniques such as virtual endoscopy (CT colonography) and noninvasive cholangiopancreatography, whereas endoscopic techniques commonly utilize both fluoroscopy and sonography. In addition, our understanding of many classic GI diseases has substantially deepened (eg, Crohn's disease and colorectal neoplasia), whereas other disease entities have only recently been uncovered (eg, IgG4-related disease and autoimmune pancreatitis). Noninvasive imaging techniques are also being increasingly utilized for screening purposes, including efforts for cancer (hepatocellular carcinoma [HCC] and colorectal cancer) and liver fibrosis.

These overlapping advances in GI imaging underscore the need for mutual understanding and appreciation among Gastroenterologists and Radiologists, in order to optimize both patient care and research strategies. This special issue of *Gastroenterology Clinics of North America* focuses on recent advances in radiologic imaging: the first six articles cover GI tract imaging; the next five articles discuss hepatopancreaticobiliary imaging; and the final two articles focus on advanced imaging techniques for global assessment of the abdomen and pelvis. In detail, the GI tract articles explore the role of fluoroscopy in the workup of dysphagia,[1] the current status of CT and MR enterography in Crohn's disease,[2] the role of radiologic imaging for GI bleeding,[3] the natural history of colorectal polyps,[4] the role of rectal MR for cancer staging and surveillance,[5]

Gastroenterol Clin N Am 47 (2018) xv–xvii
https://doi.org/10.1016/j.gtc.2018.04.014
0889-8553/18/© 2018 Published by Elsevier Inc.

and an overview of the fluoroscopic defecography exam.[6] Two reviews focusing on hepatic imaging explore the use of CT for noninvasive staging of liver fibrosis,[7] and radiologic screening for HCC.[8] Two pancreaticobiliary articles explore autoimmune pancreatitis[9] and radiologic biliary interventions.[10] This is followed by a systematic review of splenomegaly.[11] The final two articles review the current status of MR for assessing the acute nontraumatic abdomen[12] and the current status of PET/MR for oncologic GI imaging.[13]

The rapid pace of change in GI imaging is exciting but also provides challenges for staying abreast of the latest developments. It is hoped this timely update will prove to be valuable to clinicians caring for patients with GI diseases as well as for researchers involved in studying these entities.

Perry J. Pickhardt, MD
Abdominal Imaging Section
Department of Radiology
University of Wisconsin School of Medicine &
Public Health
600 Highland Avenue
Madison, WI 53792, USA

E-mail address:
ppickhardt2@uwhealth.org

REFERENCES

1. Levine MS. Ten questions about Barium esophagography and dysphagia. Gastroenterol Clin N Am 2018;47(3):449–73.
2. Park SH, Ye BD, Lee TY, et al. Computed tomography and magnetic resonance small bowel enterography: current status and future trends focusing on crohn disease. Gastroenterol Clin N Am 2018;47(3):475–99.
3. Kim G, Soto JA, Morrison T. Radiologic Assessment of Gastrointestinal Bleeding. Gastroenterol Clin N Am 2018;47(3):501–14.
4. Pickhardt PJ, Pooler BD, Kim DH, et al. The Natural History of Colorectal Polyps: Overview of Predictive Static and Dynamic Features. Gastroenterol Clin N Am 2018;47(3):515–36.
5. Moreno CC, Sullivan PS, Mittal PK. Rectal MRI for Cancer Staging and Surveillance. Gastroenterol Clin N Am 2018;47(3):537–52.
6. Kim NY, Kim DH, Pickhardt PJ, et al. Defecography: An Overview of Technique, Interpretation, and Impact on Patient Care. Gastroenterol Clin N Am 2018; 47(3):553–68.
7. Lubner MG, Pickhardt PJ. Multidetector Computed Tomography for Retrospective, Noninvasive Staging of Liver Fibrosis. Gastroenterol Clin N Am 2018;47(3): 569–84.
8. Gupta M, Gabriel H, Miller FH. Role of Imaging in Surveillance and Diagnosis of Hepatocellular Carcinoma. Gastroenterol Clin N Am 2018;47(3):585–602.
9. Sandrasegaran K, Menias CO. Imaging in Autoimmune Pancreatitis and Immunoglobulin G4–Related Disease of the Abdomen. Gastroenterol Clin N Am 2018; 47(3):621–37.
10. Perez-Johnston R, Deipolyi AR, Covey AM. Percutaneous Biliary Interventions. Gastroenterol Clin N Am 2018;47(3):639–59.
11. Sjobe RG, Menias CO, Lubner MG, et al. A Combined Clinical and Radiologic Approach to the Differential Diagnosis. Gastroenterol Clin Am 2018;47(3):661–84.

12. Pooler BD, Repplinger MD, Reeder SB, et al. MRI of the Nontraumatic Acute Abdomen: Description of Findings and Multimodality Correlation. Gastroenterol Clin Am 2018;47(3):685–708.
13. Fraum TJ, Ludwig DR, Hope TA, et al. PET/MRI for Gastrointestinal Imaging Current Clinical Status and Future Prospects. Gastroenterol Clin Am 2018;47(3): 709–32.

Ten Questions About Barium Esophagography and Dysphagia

Marc S. Levine, MD

KEYWORDS

- Barium esophagram • Modified esophagram • Technique of examination
- Dysphagia • Odynophagia

KEY POINTS

- The barium esophagram is a global test for patients with dysphagia that can simultaneously detect morphologic abnormalities in the pharynx and esophagus, pharyngeal swallowing dysfunction, esophageal dysmotility, and gastroesophageal reflux.
- The barium esophagram is an inexpensive, noninvasive, and widely available procedure that can serve as the initial diagnostic test for dysphagia and facilitate selection of other diagnostic studies such as endoscopy.
- This article addresses 10 questions about barium esophagography and dysphagia that should help gastroenterologists gain a better perspective about the utility of barium studies in this clinical setting.

INTRODUCTION

Patients with dysphagia may undergo a variety of diagnostic tests to determine the cause of this symptom, including an ear, nose, and throat examination for pharyngeal abnormalities, endoscopy for esophageal abnormalities, high-resolution manometry for esophageal motility disorders, and 24-hour pH esophageal monitoring for gastroesophageal reflux (GER). In contrast, the barium esophagram is a global test that can simultaneously demonstrate morphologic abnormalities in the pharynx and esophagus, pharyngeal swallowing disorders, esophageal dysmotility, and GER.[1] It also is an inexpensive, noninvasive, and widely available procedure that can facilitate selection of other diagnostic studies, such as endoscopy. The esophagram therefore is a cost-effective examination that can serve as the initial diagnostic test for guiding the evaluation and management of patients with dysphagia.

Disclosure: Dr M.S. Levine is a consultant for Bracco Diagnostics, Inc.
Department of Radiology, Hospital of the University of Pennsylvania, Perelman School of Medicine, University of Pennsylvania, 3400 Spruce Street, Philadelphia, PA 19104, USA
E-mail address: marc.levine@uphs.upenn.edu

Gastroenterol Clin N Am 47 (2018) 449–473
https://doi.org/10.1016/j.gtc.2018.04.001
0889-8553/18/© 2018 Elsevier Inc. All rights reserved.
gastro.theclinics.com

This article briefly describes the technique for performing a biphasic esophagram and addresses 10 questions about barium esophagography and dysphagia. The answers to these questions should help gastroenterologists gain a better perspective about the utility of barium studies in the clinical setting of dysphagia.

TECHNIQUE OF EXAMINATION

Barium esophagography usually is performed as a biphasic study that includes both upright double-contrast views and prone single-contrast views of the esophagus.[2] After ingesting an effervescence agent, the patient swallows high-density barium in the upright, left posterior oblique position for double-contrast images of the esophagus. It is important for the patient to swallow barium continuously (although not necessarily rapidly), because repetitive swallowing inhibits peristalsis, so double-contrast images of the esophagus can be obtained while it is adequately distended. The patient is then placed in a recumbent, right-side-down position for a double-contrast image of the gastric cardia, which usually is manifested by 3 or 4 stellate folds radiating to a central point at the gastroesophageal junction, also known as the cardiac rosette (**Fig. 1**).[3]

The patient next takes discrete swallows of thin barium in a prone, right anterior oblique position to evaluate esophageal motility and then continuously swallows thin barium in this position to optimally distend the esophagus and rule out rings, strictures, or other causes of narrowing. The single- and double-contrast phases of the esophagram therefore are complementary, because double-contrast views enable detection of mucosal abnormalities not visible on single-contrast views, whereas single-contrast views enable detection of areas of narrowing not visible on double-contrast views.

TEN QUESTIONS ABOUT BARIUM ESOPHAGOGRAPHY AND DYSPHAGIA
Question 1: How Long Has the Patient Had Dysphagia?

The duration of dysphagia is the single most important clinical parameter for differentiating benign and malignant causes of dysphagia. Benign conditions involving the esophagus evolve slowly over a period of months to years, so these patients usually present with slowly progressive, long-standing (6–12 months or longer) dysphagia

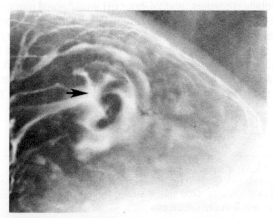

Fig. 1. Normal appearance of gastric cardia. On a right-side-down double-contrast spot image of the gastric fundus, the cardia is characterized by stellate folds radiating to a central point at the gastroesophageal junction (*arrow*), known as the cardiac rosette.

before seeking medical attention.[4] Because of the gradual onset and often intermittent nature of their dysphagia, affected individuals usually have little or no weight loss.[4] In contrast, malignant tumors involving the esophagus are aggressive lesions that progress rapidly over a short period of time, so these patients usually present with recent onset (2–4 months) of worsening dysphagia and weight loss.[5]

Question 2: Is Dysphagia a Common Symptom in Patients with Gastroesophageal Reflux Disease or Its Complications?

Dysphagia is a surprisingly common symptom in patients with gastroesophageal reflux disease (GERD), occurring in 28% to 30% of adults with this condition.[6,7] The pathogenesis of dysphagia in affected individuals is multifactorial. Some patients experience dysphagia (with or without typical reflux symptoms) because of sensitivity to refluxed acid in the esophagus or edema and spasm or esophageal dysmotility associated with reflux esophagitis.[8] Others have dysphagia secondary to swallowing dysfunction caused by nocturnal reflux of acid into the pharynx.[9] Still others have dysphagia secondary to reflux-induced (ie, peptic) strictures, Barrett's strictures, or even infiltrating adenocarcinomas arising in Barrett's esophagus.[10] GERD or one of its complications therefore should be a leading consideration in all patients who undergo barium esophagrams for dysphagia, whether or not they have a known history of reflux disease.

Question 3: Does the Subjective Site of Dysphagia Accurately Localize the Site of Disease or Is Dysphagia Referred Upwards or Downwards? What Are the Implications for Barium Studies Performed on Patients with Dysphagia?

In many if not most patients with dysphagia, the subjective sensation of where food gets stuck does not accurately reflect the site of disease. This discrepancy results from a common clinical phenomenon known as "referred" dysphagia. For reasons that are unclear, dysphagia frequently is referred upwards but never downwards.[11] As a result, patients with abnormalities involving the distal esophagus or even the gastric cardia and fundus often have referred dysphagia, feeling as if food gets stuck at the level of the mid to upper sternum, thoracic inlet, or even the throat, whereas patients with pharyngeal abnormalities have symptoms that are confined to the region of the throat, because dysphagia never is referred downwards.

The phenomenon of referred dysphagia has important ramifications not only for clinical diagnosis but also for the anatomic focus of barium studies performed on these patients. If, for example, a patient presents with subxyphoid dysphagia, the barium study should focus primarily on the lower thoracic esophagus and gastric cardia and fundus, because abnormalities in the pharynx or mid or upper thoracic esophagus never cause dysphagia that is referred downwards to the subxyphoid region. Conversely, if a patient presents with pharyngeal dysphagia, the barium study should include evaluation not only of the pharynx and cervical esophagus but also of the entire thoracic esophagus and even the gastric cardia and fundus, because abnormalities in these locations may cause dysphagia that is referred upwards to the thoracic inlet or throat (**Fig. 2**). The barium study therefore should be tailored based on the patient's subjective site of dysphagia.

Question 4: Is It Necessary to Evaluate the Gastric Cardia and Fundus on Barium Studies in All Patients with Dysphagia?

Over the past 50 years, there has been a slow but steady shift in the distribution of gastric cancer from the antrum and body of the stomach proximally to the cardia and fundus.[12] Carcinoma of the gastric cardia currently is thought to constitute as

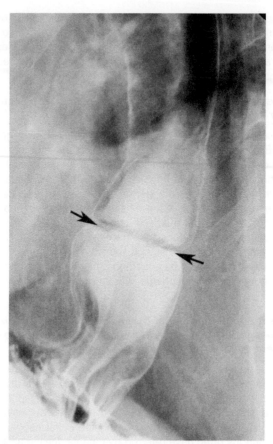

Fig. 2. Schatzki ring. Prone, right anterior oblique spot image from single-contrast esophagram shows a smooth, symmetric ringlike constriction (*arrows*) at the gastroesophageal junction directly above a hiatal hernia. Note how the ring has a vertical height of only 2 to 3 mm. This patient presented with intermittent solid food dysphagia that was referred upwards to the throat.

many as 40% of all gastric cancers.[12] These tumors are 7 times more common in men than in women[13] and are more likely to occur in young patients (ie, <40 years of age) than malignant tumors elsewhere in the gastrointestinal tract,[14] so it is important not to be lulled into a false sense of security about the possibility of malignant tumor because of the patient's age.

Carcinoma of the gastric cardia is notorious for causing referred dysphagia; the cardia and fundus therefore should be carefully evaluated in all patients who undergo esophagrams or endoscopy for dysphagia, regardless of its subjective localization (**Fig. 3**). Because the cardia and fundus are located beneath the rib cage and are not amenable to graded compression, double-contrast technique is particularly important for evaluating this region. Tumor at the cardia may be manifested by distortion, effacement, or obliteration of the cardiac rosette, with irregular areas of mass effect, nodularity, or ulceration in the surrounding gastric fundus and variable extension of tumor into the distal esophagus (see **Fig. 3**).[12] With more advanced disease, barium studies may reveal a large polypoid or ulcerated mass at the cardia or circumferential

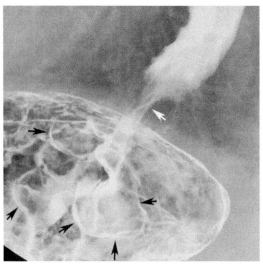

Fig. 3. Carcinoma of the gastric cardia. A right-side-down double-contrast spot image of the gastric fundus shows obliteration of the normal cardiac rosette (shown in **Fig. 1**), with multiple polypoid lesions (*black arrows*) in this region secondary to carcinoma of the gastric cardia. Also note irregular narrowing of the distal esophagus (*white arrow*) secondary to invasion by tumor, with retained barium above the level of narrowing. This patient presented with recent onset of weight loss and dysphagia that was referred upwards to the thoracic inlet.

encasement and narrowing of the fundus by tumor.[12] Whatever the radiographic findings, the gastric cardia and fundus should be carefully evaluated in all patients with dysphagia in order to detect these lesions at the earliest possible stage.

Question 5: Is Double-Contrast Esophagography a Reasonable Test for Esophageal Cancer in Patients with Dysphagia and, if an Esophageal Stricture Is Detected, Can Barium Studies Accurately Differentiate Benign from Malignant Strictures?

Most malignant tumors in the esophagus are squamous cell carcinomas or adenocarcinomas arising in Barrett's mucosa. In general, squamous cell carcinomas tend to be located in the upper or midesophagus, whereas adenocarcinomas predominantly are located in the distal esophagus.[5] The latter tumors have a marked tendency to invade the stomach by direct extension across the gastroesophageal junction, whereas squamous cell carcinomas rarely, if ever, invade the stomach by direct extension.[5]

Some gastroenterologists traditionally have thought that endoscopy is required for all patients with negative esophagrams to detect esophageal tumors missed on barium studies.[15–17] However, double-contrast esophagrams have been shown to have a sensitivity of greater than 95% for detecting esophageal carcinoma.[18–20] In one series of patients with esophageal cancer, the lesion was detected on double-contrast esophagrams in 98% of patients, and malignant tumor was diagnosed or suspected on the basis of the radiographic findings in 96%.[20] An argument could be made that a high sensitivity is achieved in the radiographic diagnosis of esophageal cancer only by exposing an inordinate number of patients to unnecessary endoscopy. In the previous study, however, endoscopy was recommended to rule out malignant tumor in only about 1% of all patients who underwent double-contrast examinations.[20] Endoscopy therefore is not warranted to rule out esophageal cancer when double-contrast barium studies reveal no evidence of tumor.

Some gastroenterologists also think endoscopy and biopsy are needed to rule out malignant tumor in all patients with radiographically diagnosed esophageal strictures because of difficulty differentiating benign strictures from circumferentially infiltrating cancers on barium studies.[21–23] In a large series, however, no patients with unequivocally benign-appearing strictures on double-contrast esophagrams were found to have malignant tumor on endoscopic biopsy specimens,[24] so endoscopy is not needed to rule out esophageal cancer in these patients. Benign strictures typically appear as relatively symmetric segments of narrowing with smooth contours and tapered margins (**Fig. 4**), whereas malignant strictures are more asymmetric and have nodular, irregular, or ulcerated contours and abrupt, shelflike margins (**Fig. 5**).[5,24] If the radiographic findings are equivocal or suspicious for tumor, endoscopy and biopsy specimens are required for a definitive diagnosis.

Question 6: What Is the Best Radiographic Technique for Detecting Schatzki Rings or Peptic Strictures in the Distal Esophagus That Cause Dysphagia? Can Barium Studies Detect Rings or Strictures That Are Missed at Endoscopy?

Lower esophageal rings (ie, Schatzki rings) and peptic strictures are common causes of dysphagia in the distal esophagus (see **Fig. 2**; **Figs. 6** and **7**). When barium studies are performed, these rings and strictures will only be visible if the esophagus above and hiatal hernia below the narrowed segment are distended beyond the caliber of the stenosis. Because single-contrast technique produces greater distention of the distal esophagus than double-contrast technique, single-contrast views should be obtained while thin barium is continuously swallowed in the prone position to visualize rings and strictures that easily are missed on upright double-contrast views secondary to inadequate distention of this region (see **Fig. 6**). As a result, single-contrast technique is more sensitive than double-contrast technique for showing distal esophageal rings and strictures[25] and can even detect subtle areas of narrowing missed at endoscopy.[26,27] It therefore is important to perform a biphasic study that includes prone single-contrast views of the esophagus in all patients with dysphagia in order to optimize detection of these rings and strictures.

At the same time, distal esophageal rings and strictures can be missed with single-contrast technique if overdistention of the esophagus above and hiatal hernia below the narrowing causes these structures to overlap, preventing visualization of the ring or stricture in profile (see **Fig. 7**A).[28] When this "overlap phenomenon" occurs, the patient should swallow the barium more slowly to prevent or minimize overlap between the distal esophagus and adjacent hiatal hernia, often enabling the ring or stricture to be visualized (see **Fig. 7**B). When overlap of the esophagus and hernia persists, however, the patient should swallow a barium tablet of known diameter (12 mm); prolonged retention of the tablet at or just above the segment of overlap suggest a fixed area of narrowing.[28] In such cases, endoscopy should be performed to confirm the presence of a ring or stricture, and, in patients with dysphagia, the narrowed segment can be dilated for amelioration of symptoms. It therefore should be recognized that both underdistention and overdistention may prevent detection of rings or strictures in the distal esophagus, and, depending on the findings, more or less distention may be needed to visualize these areas of narrowing on barium studies.

Question 7: Is Esophagography a Useful Test for Detecting Infectious Esophagitis in Immunocompromised Patients with Dysphagia or Odynophagia?

Patients who are immunocompromised not infrequently present with dysphagia or odynophagia (pain on swallowing) secondary to the development of infectious

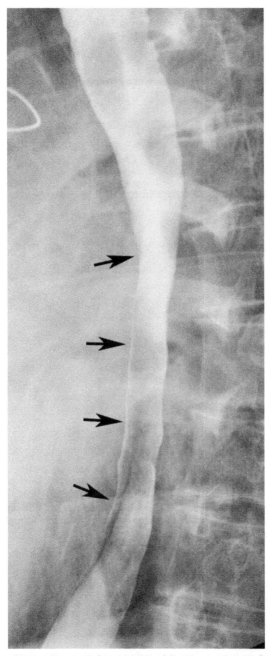

Fig. 4. Radiation stricture. Prone, right anterior oblique spot image from single-contrast esophagram shows a long segment of narrowing with smooth contours and tapered margins (*arrows*) in the midthoracic esophagus. The narrowed segment has the typical radiographic features of a benign stricture. This patient developed dysphagia after undergoing surgery and mediastinal irradiation for a malignant thymoma.

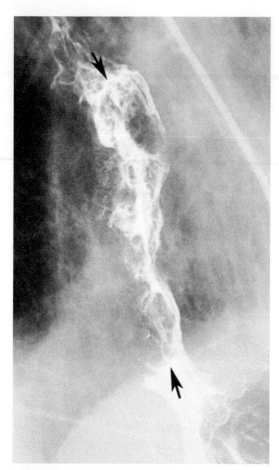

Fig. 5. Esophageal adenocarcinoma. Upright, left posterior oblique spot image from a double-contrast esophagram shows an advanced infiltrating carcinoma in the lower thoracic esophagus, manifested by irregular luminal narrowing, with a nodular, ulcerated contour and shelflike margins (*arrows*). These are typical radiographic features of a malignant tumor. The patient presented with recent onset of dysphagia and weight loss and was found to have an adenocarcinoma arising in Barrett's esophagus.

esophagitis. In some cases, the pain can be so severe that these individuals are unable to swallow their saliva. Although *Candida* esophagitis is by far the most common cause of opportunistic esophagitis, only 50% to 75% of patients with esophageal candidiasis are found to have oropharyngeal candidiasis (ie, thrush), so the absence of oropharyngeal disease in no way excludes this diagnosis.[29] Other causes of infectious esophagitis include the herpes simplex virus, and, in patients with AIDS, cytomegalovirus (CMV) or human immunodeficiency virus (HIV). Such individuals often are treated with an empiric course of fluconazole for presumed *Candida* esophagitis. If empirical therapy fails to alleviate the patient's symptoms, however, a double-contrast esophagram is a useful test for detecting infectious esophagitis and for differentiating the underlying causes.

Candida esophagitis usually is manifested on double-contrast esophagrams by multiple discrete plaquelike lesions that have a linear or irregular configuration

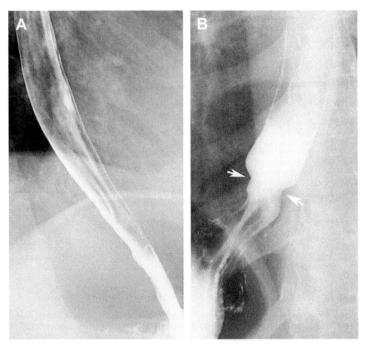

Fig. 6. Importance of prone single-contrast views for detecting strictures in the distal esophagus. (*A*) Upright, left posterior oblique spot image from double-contrast phase of barium study shows no evidence of narrowing in the distal esophagus. (*B*) Prone, right anterior oblique spot image from single-contrast phase of same examination shows a short, tapered peptic stricture (*arrows*) in the distal esophagus above a small hiatal hernia. The stricture was only visualized on single-contrast views because of greater distention of this region.

and are separated by normal intervening mucosa (**Fig. 8**).[29] A more fulminant form of esophageal candidiasis occasionally is encountered in patients with AIDS, who may present with a grossly irregular or so-called shaggy esophagus secondary to innumerable coalescent plaques and pseudomembranes with trapping of barium between these lesions (**Fig. 9**).[30] Although single-contrast esophagrams rarely are able to show the plaquelike lesions of *Candida* esophagitis, double-contrast esophagrams have a sensitivity as high as 90% in detecting this condition in relation to endoscopy, primarily because of the ability to show these mucosal plaques.[31,32] Thus, only mild cases are likely to be missed on double-contrast studies.

Herpes esophagitis, the second most common type of infectious esophagitis, also occurs in immunocompromised patients with dysphagia or odynophagia. Unlike esophageal candidiasis, however, herpes esophagitis usually is manifested on double-contrast esophagrams by multiple small, discrete ulcers that often are surrounded by radiolucent halos of edematous mucosa and predominantly are located in the upper or midesophagus (**Fig. 10**).[33,34] Because esophageal candidiasis almost always is characterized on barium studies by multiple discrete plaquelike lesions or, in advanced disease, a shaggy esophagus, the presence of small discrete esophageal ulcers in the absence of plaques should strongly suggest herpes esophagitis in immunocompromised patients with odynophagia. Such individuals generally have an excellent clinical response to treatment with acyclovir, a relatively innocuous antiviral agent.

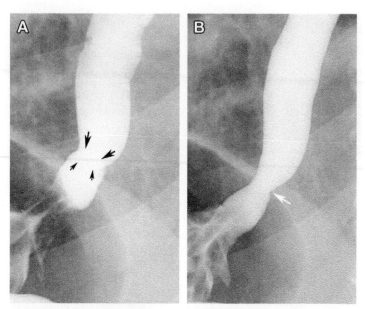

Fig. 7. Inability to visualize peptic stricture because of overlap phenomenon. (*A*) Prone, right anterior oblique spot image from single-contrast esophagram shows a small hiatal hernia without definite narrowing of the distal esophagus. However, there is overlap between the distal end of the esophagus (*small arrows*) and the top of the hernia (*large arrows*), producing a biconvex double density that prevents visualization of the gastroesophageal junction in profile. (*B*) Additional prone, right anterior oblique spot image from the same examination with less distention of the distal esophagus shows a short peptic stricture (*arrow*) that was not visible on the earlier spot image because of this overlap phenomenon.

Herpes esophagitis occasionally may be encountered as an acute, self-limited disease in otherwise healthy patients who have no underlying immunologic problems. This condition usually occurs in young men with a recent history of exposure to sexual partners with oropharyngeal herpes infection.[35] Affected individuals typically present with a clinical prodrome consisting of fever, headaches, myalgias, and upper respiratory infections for a period of 3 to 10 days before the sudden onset of acute odynophagia.[35] Double-contrast esophagrams usually reveal innumerable punctate ulcers clustered together in the midesophagus below the level of the carina.[35] The ulcers are even smaller than those in immunocompromised patients with herpes esophagitis, possibly because these individuals have an intact immune system that can prevent the ulcers from enlarging. Because it is a self-limited condition, herpes esophagitis in otherwise healthy patients usually resolves on conservative treatment with analgesics and sedation. Patients with characteristic clinical and radiographic findings of this disease therefore can be treated medically without need for endoscopy.

In contrast, esophagrams may reveal giant ulcers (defined as ulcers >1 cm in size) in AIDS patients with CMV or HIV esophagitis.[36–38] Unfortunately, it is impossible to differentiate CMV from HIV ulcers on the basis of the radiographic findings.[37,38] Endoscopy with brushings and biopsy specimens therefore are required for a definitive diagnosis. If endoscopy reveals no evidence of CMV, the patient is presumed to have HIV as a diagnosis of exclusion. Differentiation of these infections is important, because patients with CMV esophagitis usually are treated with ganciclovir, a toxic

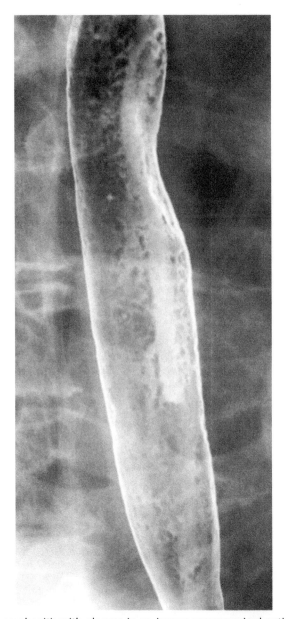

Fig. 8. *Candida* esophagitis with plaques in an immunocompromised patient with odyno-phagia. Upright, left posterior oblique spot image from double-contrast esophagram shows multiple small, discrete plaquelike lesions in the thoracic esophagus. Note how some of the plaques have a linear configuration. These radiographic findings are characteristic of esophageal candidiasis.

antiviral agent that causes bone marrow suppression, whereas patients with HIV esophagitis generally have a marked clinical response to treatment with oral steroids.[37,38] Fortunately, CMV and HIV esophagitis are not often encountered in modern medical practice because of effective therapy for HIV-positive patients.

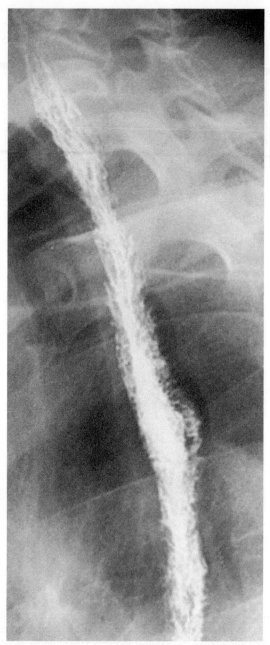

Fig. 9. Advanced *Candida* esophagitis with a shaggy esophagus in a patient with AIDS. Prone, right anterior oblique spot image from single-contrast esophagram shows a grossly irregular or "shaggy" esophagus secondary to innumerable plaques and pseudomembranes, with trapping of barium between the lesions. This appearance is characteristic of fulminant *Candida* esophagitis in AIDS.

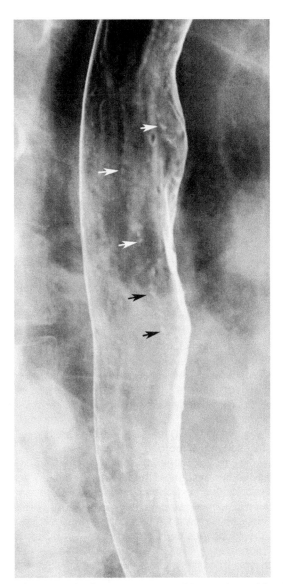

Fig. 10. Herpes esophagitis with ulcers in an HIV-positive patient with odynophagia. Upright, left posterior oblique spot image from double-contrast esophagram shows multiple tiny, discrete ulcers (*arrows*) in the upper and midesophagus (without plaques). In the appropriate clinical setting, this finding should be highly suggestive of herpes esophagitis, because *Candida* esophagitis rarely is associated with ulcers in the absence of plaques.

Question 8: Is a Small-Caliber Esophagus on Esophagography or Endoscopy Diagnostic of Eosinophilic Esophagitis?

Eosinophilic esophagitis (EoE) is a chronic inflammatory disease typically affecting young men with long-standing dysphagia and recurrent food impactions, often associated with an atopic history, asthma, or peripheral eosinophilia.[39] This condition sometimes is associated with the development of a small-caliber esophagus, manifested on barium studies by smooth, long-segment narrowing of the entire or nearly entire thoracic and cervical esophagus (**Fig. 11**).[39] Although this finding is thought to be characteristic of EoE, lichen planus, a chronic inflammatory condition involving the skin, mucus membranes, and esophagus, recently has been recognized as another cause of a small-caliber esophagus indistinguishable from that in EoE (**Fig. 12**).[40] Unlike EoE, however, lichen planus predominantly occurs in elderly women with long-standing dysphagia.[40,41] As many as 50% of patients with lichen planus involving the esophagus present with dysphagia before they develop skin disease,[41] so this condition may not be suspected at the time of clinical presentation. Nevertheless, the age and sex of the patient and the presence or absence of an atopic history, asthma, or peripheral eosinophilia generally enable differentiation of lichen planus from EoE. Both conditions can be definitively diagnosed by characteristic findings on endoscopic biopsy specimens, so appropriate therapy can be instituted.

Question 9: Are Barium Esophagrams Useful for Detecting and Differentiating Various Esophageal Motility Disorders in Patients with Dysphagia?

In a classic study comparing fluoroscopic evaluation of esophageal motility with endoscopy, there was 96% agreement in differentiating normal esophageal motility from esophageal dysmotility when at least 5 separate swallows were assessed at fluoroscopy.[42] Esophagography therefore is an effective technique for detecting major types of esophageal dysmotility associated with dysphagia.

The 2 most common causes of esophageal dysmotility are GERD and aging (formerly known as "presbyesophagus"). In patients with GERD, the dysmotility is manifested on barium studies by weakened or absent primary peristalsis in the mid and lower thoracic esophagus in the absence of nonperistaltic contractions (NPCs) (also known as "tertiary contractions").[43] In contrast, age-related esophageal dysmotility is characterized by intermittently weakened or absent peristalsis associated with multiple NPCs of varying severity.[44] The presence of absence of NPCs therefore is a useful feature for differentiating GERD from age-related esophageal dysmotility as the cause of the patient's esophageal motor dysfunction.

Primary achalasia is an idiopathic condition associated with long-standing dysphagia that mainly occurs in young or middle-aged adults.[44] Achalasia is characterized by absent esophageal peristalsis and incomplete relaxation of the lower esophageal sphincter (LES), manifested on barium studies by a dilated, flaccid esophagus with tapered, beaklike narrowing at the gastroesophageal junction (**Fig. 13**).[44] In advanced disease, the esophagus can become massively dilated and tortuous, producing a "sigmoid" appearance (**Fig. 14**). It previously has been shown that 20% to 33% of patients with typical findings of achalasia on barium studies have normal relaxation of the LES on manometry.[45–47] Nevertheless, such patients have a similar response to endoscopic forms of treatment of achalasia as those with incomplete LES relaxation on manometry.[47] When achalasia is diagnosed on esophagography, treatment therefore can be instituted without need for manometry. However, manometry may still be required for patients with suspected achalasia who have equivocal findings on barium studies.

Unlike primary achalasia, secondary achalasia is caused by other conditions, most commonly malignant tumors that arise at the gastric cardia, destroying the ganglion cells at the gastroesophageal junction.[44] Although secondary achalasia can resemble primary achalasia on barium studies, the length of the narrowed segment often is greater than that in primary achalasia and can be nodular or ulcerated because of underlying tumor in this region (**Fig. 15**).[48] The clinical history also is helpful, because primary achalasia usually occurs in young or middle-age adults with long-standing

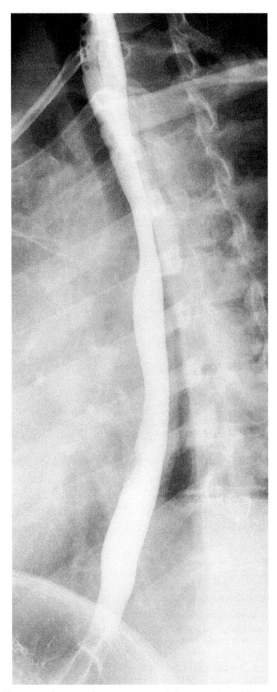

Fig. 11. Small-caliber esophagus of EoE. Prone, right anterior oblique spot image from single-contrast esophagram shows marked loss of caliber of the entire thoracic esophagus. This patient was a young man who presented with long-standing dysphagia, asthma, and an atopic history. The clinical and radiographic findings should be highly suggestive of EoE.

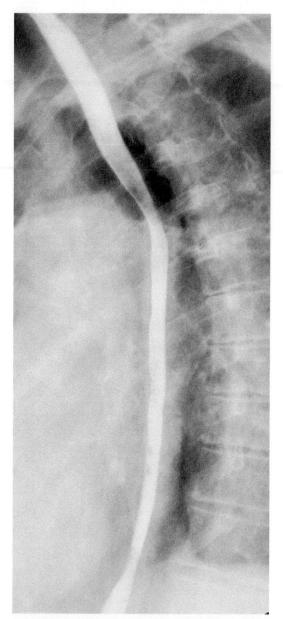

Fig. 12. Small-caliber esophagus of lichen planus. Prone, right anterior oblique spot image from single-contrast esophagram shows smooth narrowing of the entire thoracic esophagus indistinguishable from the small-caliber esophagus of EoE shown in **Fig. 11**. However, this patient was an elderly woman with skin disease, and biopsy specimens from the esophagus revealed lichen planus. The clinical history is essential for differentiating lichen planus from EoE when a small-caliber esophagus is detected on barium studies.

dysphagia and little or no weight loss, whereas secondary achalasia occurs in older patients (>60 years of age) with recent onset of dysphagia (less than 6 months) and greater weight loss.[48] As a result, these conditions usually can be differentiated on the basis of the clinical and radiographic findings.

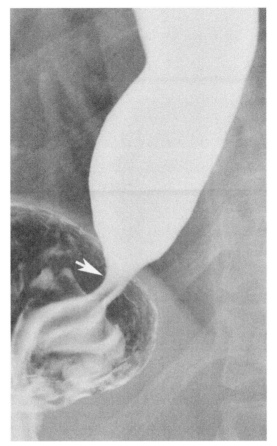

Fig. 13. Primary achalasia. Prone, right anterior oblique spot image from single-contrast esophagram shows a dilated esophagus with a short segment of smooth, tapered narrowing (*arrow*) directly abutting the gastroesophageal junction secondary to incomplete opening of the LES. There was no esophageal peristalsis at fluoroscopy. This patient was a middle-aged man with a 5-year history of dysphagia for but no weight loss. These clinical and radiographic findings are characteristic of primary achalasia.

Diffuse esophageal spasm (DES) is an esophageal motility disorder characterized by intermittently weakened or absent peristalsis associated with multiple NPCs of varying severity.[44] DES is a disease of the elderly. Affected individuals can be asymptomatic or can present with chest pain, dysphagia, or both. DES classically is manifested on barium studies by intermittently absent esophageal peristalsis with lumen-obliterating NPCs that compartmentalize the esophagus, producing a distinctive "corkscrew" appearance (**Fig. 16**).[44] In one study, however, lumen-obliterating NPCs were detected on barium studies in only 14% of patients with DES.[49] Instead, most patients had NPCs of varying magnitude without a classic corkscrew esophagus. In the same study, 64% of patients with DES had impaired opening of the LES, manifested by the beaklike distal esophageal narrowing typically associated with achalasia (**Fig. 17**).[49] DES and achalasia therefore may represent opposite ends of a spectrum of motility disorders.

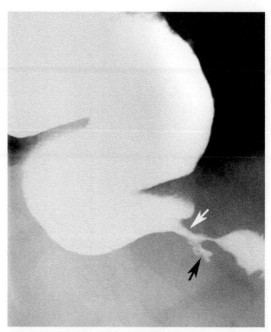

Fig. 14. Advanced achalasia with sigmoid esophagus. Upright, right posterior oblique spot image from single-contrast esophagram shows a markedly dilated thoracic esophagus with a tortuous or "sigmoid" distal configuration and tapered narrowing of the distal-most esophagus (*white arrow*) secondary to LES dysfunction. There was no esophageal peristalsis at fluoroscopy. These findings are characteristic of advanced primary achalasia in a patient with a 30-year history of dysphagia. Also note focal extravasation of barium into a tiny, contained collection (*black arrow*) abutting the inferior aspect of the narrowed segment secondary to a sealed-off perforation occurring after pneumatic dilation of the LES.

Question 10: When Should a Patient with Dysphagia Undergo a Routine Esophagram Versus a Modified Esophagram (ie, Modified Barium Swallow) with Speech Pathology?

A routine esophagram performed by a radiologist technically is a complete *pharyngoesophagram* that includes functional and structural evaluation of the pharynx and esophagus. Nevertheless, most radiologists refer to this examination simply as an *esophagram*, for purposes of brevity. In patients with dysphagia, the study is performed to evaluate for functional or structural abnormalities involving the pharynx, cervical and thoracic esophagus, and gastric cardia and fundus.

In contrast, a modified esophagram in conjunction with a speech pathologist is a focused study for evaluating swallowing function and assessing whether the patient aspirates barium into the larynx or trachea during swallowing. This test frequently is requested for patients with dysphagia who have received radiation therapy to the neck for pharyngeal cancer or who have neurologic conditions, such as strokes, Parkinson disease, multiple sclerosis, and dementia, that predispose to aspiration. When laryngeal penetration or tracheal aspiration is detected, the radiologist and speech pathologist work in tandem to determine whether liquids of higher or lower viscosity (eg, thin, nectar-thick, or honey-thick barium) or various compensatory maneuvers (eg, chin-tuck or forceful swallow) can prevent or minimize aspiration.

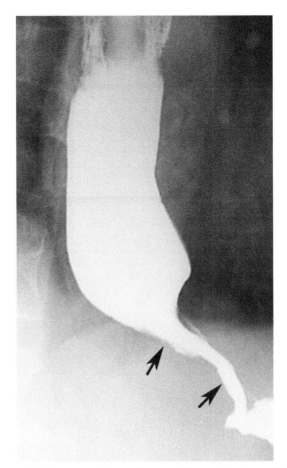

Fig. 15. Secondary achalasia caused by carcinoma of the cardia. An upright, left posterior oblique spot image from a single-contrast esophagram shows a relatively long (3 cm in length) segment of tapered narrowing (*arrows*) in the distal esophagus. There was no esophageal peristalsis at fluoroscopy. This elderly patient presented with recent onset of dysphagia and weight loss, and endoscopic biopsy specimens from the region of the gastro-esophageal junction revealed adenocarcinoma. The clinical and radiographic findings are characteristic of secondary achalasia.

Many patients who undergo a modified esophagram are too old, debilitated, or neurologically impaired to stand beside the fluoroscopy table, so they undergo the examination while seated in a speech therapy chair. In this way, it is possible to evaluate swallowing function even in the most debilitated patients. At the same time, the thoracic esophagus cannot be adequately evaluated because of technical factors related to use of the speech therapy chair. A complete barium study of the esophagus therefore may necessitate physically transferring debilitated patients from the chair onto the fluoroscopy table, so that a limited examination of the thoracic esophagus can be obtained while they swallow barium in a supine, semi-upright position.

Given the time and physical effort needed to transfer a patient from the speech therapy chair onto the fluoroscopy table, some radiologists only evaluate the pharynx and

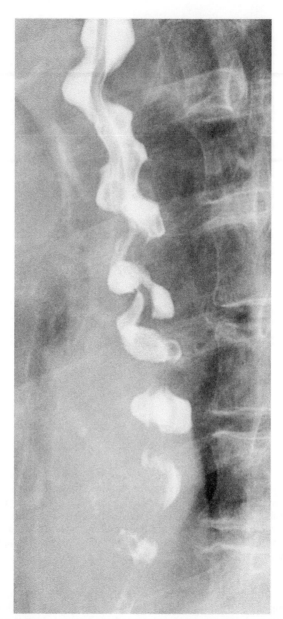

Fig. 16. Diffuse esophageal spasm. Prone, right anterior oblique spot image from single-contrast esophagram shows a "corkscrew" esophagus secondary to multiple lumen-obliterating NPCs, with spiral trapping of barium between these contractions. This finding is classic for diffuse esophageal spasm.

cervical esophagus (in conjunction with a speech pathologist) when a modified esophagram is requested. Is this a reasonable practice? Ultimately, that depends on the indications for the study and the radiographic findings in the pharynx and cervical esophagus. If, for example, a modified esophagram performed on a patient with dysphagia after a recent stroke reveals major swallowing dysfunction with tracheal

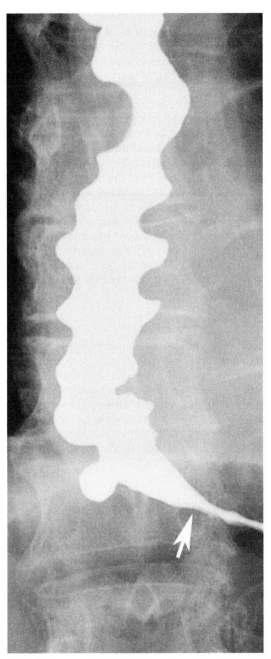

Fig. 17. Diffuse esophageal spasm with LES dysfunction. There are multiple nonperistaltic esophageal contractions of varying severity that are not lumen obliterating (so this patient does not have a corkscrew esophagus). Also note smooth, tapered narrowing (*arrow*) of the distal esophagus secondary to incomplete opening of the LES. Diffuse esophageal spasm is thought to be associated with lower esophageal dysfunction in more than 50% of patients. This patient presented with dysphagia that was relieved by pneumatic dilation of the LES.

aspiration, there is no reason to evaluate the thoracic esophagus, because the explanation for the patient's dysphagia is readily apparent. Moreover, it is not safe to evaluate the thoracic esophagus because of the risk of substantial aspiration when these individuals continuously swallow barium in a supine, semi-upright position.

However, what if a modified esophagram performed on a patient with dysphagia reveals normal swallowing function without an explanation for this symptom? Because dysphagia often is referred upwards, such patients could have abnormalities involving the thoracic esophagus or even the gastric cardia and fundus as the cause of their symptoms. It therefore is incumbent on radiologists to rule out structural (eg, benign or malignant strictures) or functional (eg, achalasia or DES) disease in the thoracic esophagus or proximal stomach when a modified esophagram reveals no explanation for the patient's dysphagia in the pharynx or cervical esophagus.

The need for a complete esophagram becomes even more paramount in patients who have no history of radiation treatment to the neck and no underlying conditions associated with pharyngeal dysphagia. In the end, radiologists must not be satisfied with an incomplete examination simply because the study was ordered as a "modified barium swallow." Even when underlying risk factors for pharyngeal swallowing dysfunction are present, the type of barium study that is performed ultimately depends not only on the clinical setting but also on the findings on the pharyngeal portion of the study.

SUMMARY

The barium esophagram is a global test for patients with dysphagia that can simultaneously detect morphologic abnormalities in the pharynx and esophagus, pharyngeal swallowing dysfunction, esophageal dysmotility, and GER. It also is an inexpensive, noninvasive, and widely available procedure that can serve as the initial diagnostic test for dysphagia and facilitate selection of other diagnostic studies such as endoscopy. This article briefly described the technique for performing biphasic esophagrams and addressed 10 questions about barium esophagography and dysphagia that should help gastroenterologists gain a better perspective about the utility of barium studies in this clinical setting.

REFERENCES

1. Levine MS, Rubesin SE, Laufer I. Barium esophagography: a study for all seasons. Clin Gastroenterol Hepatol 2008;6:11–25.
2. Levine MS. Examination of the esophagus, stomach, and duodenum: techniques and normal anatomy. In: Levine MS, Ramchandani P, Rubesin SE, editors. Practical fluoroscopy of the GI and GU tracts. New York: Cambridge University Press; 2013. p. 23–39.
3. Herlinger H, Grossman R, Laufer I, et al. The gastric cardia in double-contrast study: its dynamic image. AJR Am J Roentgenol 1980;135:21–9.
4. Levine MS. Gastroesophageal reflux disease. In: Gore RM, Levine MS, editors. Textbook of gastrointestinal radiology. 4th edition. Philadelphia: Elsevier; 2015. p. 291–311.
5. Levine MS, Halvorsen RA. Carcinoma of the esophagus. In: Gore RM, Levine MS, editors. Textbook of gastrointestinal radiology. 4th edition. Philadelphia: Elsevier; 2015. p. 366–93.
6. Locke GR 3rd, Talley NJ, Fett SL, et al. Prevalence and clinical spectrum of gastroesophageal reflux: a population-based study in Olmsted Country, Minnesota. Gastroenterology 1997;112:1448–56.

7. Bollschweiler E, Knoppe K, Wolfgarten E, et al. Prevalence of dysphagia in patients with gastroesophageal reflux in Germany. Dysphagia 2008;23:172–6.

8. Kahrilas PJ. Regurgitation in patients with gastroesophageal reflux disease. Gastroenterol Hepatol (NY) 2013;9:37–9.

9. Vaezi MF, Hicks DM, Abelson TI, et al. Laryngeal signs and symptoms and gastroesophageal reflux disease (GERD): a critical assessment of cause and effect association. Clin Gastroenterol Hepatol 2003;1:333–44.

10. Levine MS, Carucci LR, DiSantis DJ, et al. Consensus statement of Society of Abdominal Radiology disease-focused panel on barium esophagography in gastroesophageal reflux disease. AJR Am J Roentgenol 2016;207:1009–15.

11. Levine MS, Rubesin SE. Radiologic investigation of dysphagia. AJR Am J Roentgenol 1990;154:1157–63.

12. Levine MS, Megibow AJ, Kochman ML. Carcinoma of the stomach and duodenum. In: Gore RM, Levine MS, editors. Textbook of gastrointestinal radiology. 4th edition. Philadelphia: Elsevier; 2015. p. 546–70.

13. Morales TG. Adenocarcinoma of the gastric cardia. Dig Dis 1997;15:346–56.

14. Levine MS, Laufer I, Thompson JJ. Carcinoma of the gastric cardia in young people. AJR Am J Roentgenol 1983;140:69–72.

15. Ravich WJ. Esophageal dysphagia. In: Groher ME, editor. Dysphagia: diagnosis and management. 3rd edition. Boston: Butterworth-Heinemann; 1997. p. 107–13.

16. Castell DO, Katz PO. Approach to the patient with dysphagia and odynophagia. In: Yamada T, editor. Textbook of gastroenterology. 3rd edition. Philadelphia: Lippincott Williams & Wilkins; 1999. p. 683–93.

17. O'Connor JB, Richter JE. Esophageal strictures. In: Castell DO, Richter JE, editors. The esophagus. 3rd edition. Philadelphia: Lippincott Williams & Wilkins; 1999. p. 473–83.

18. DiPalma JA, Prechter GC, Brady CE. X-ray-negative dysphagia: is endoscopy necessary? J Clin Gastroenterol 1984;6:409–11.

19. Halpert RD, Feczko PJ, Spichler EM, et al. Radiologic assessment of dysphagia with endoscopy. Radiology 1985;157:599–602.

20. Levine MS, Chu P, Furth EE, et al. Carcinoma of the esophagus and esophagogastric junction: sensitivity of radiographic diagnosis. AJR Am J Roentgenol 1997;168:1423–6.

21. Livstone EM, Skinner DB. Tumors of the esophagus. In: Berk JE, editor. Bockus gastroenterology. 4th edition. Philadelphia: Saunders; 1985. p. 818–40.

22. Goyal RK. Diseases of the esophagus. In: Braunwald E, Isselbacher KJ, Petersdorf RG, et al, editors. Harrison's principles of internal medicine. 11th edition. New York: McGraw-Hill; 1987. p. 1231–8.

23. Aaddad NG, Fleischer DE. Neoplasms of the esophagus. In: Castell DO, editor. The esophagus. 2nd edition. Boston: Little Brown; 1995. p. 269–91.

24. Gupta S, Levine MS, Rubesin SE, et al. Usefulness of barium studies for differentiating benign and malignant strictures of the esophagus. AJR Am J Roentgenol 2003;180:737–44.

25. Chen YM, Ott DJ, Gelfand DW, et al. Multiphasic examination of the esophagogastric region for strictures, rings, and hiatal hernia: evaluation of the individual techniques. Gastrointest Radiol 1985;10:311–6.

26. Ott DJ, Chen YM, Wu WC, et al. Endoscopic sensitivity in the detection of esophageal strictures. J Clin Gastroenterol 1985;7:121–5.

27. Ott DJ, Chen YM, Wu WC, et al. Radiographic and endoscopic sensitivity in detecting lower esophageal mucosal ring. AJR Am J Roentgenol 1986;147:261–5.

28. Hsu WC, Levine MS, Rubesin SE. Overlap phenomenon: a potential pitfall in the radiographic detection of lower esophageal rings. AJR Am J Roentgenol 2003; 180:745–7.

29. Levine MS. Infectious esophagitis. In: Gore RM, Levine MS, editors. Textbook of gastrointestinal radiology. 4th edition. Philadelphia: Elsevier; 2015. p. 312–25.

30. Levine MS, Woldenberg R, Herlinger H, et al. Opportunistic esophagitis in AIDS: radiographic diagnosis. Radiology 1977;165:815–20.

31. Levine MS, Macones AJ, Laufer I. Candida esophagitis: accuracy of radiographic diagnosis. Radiology 1985;154:581–7.

32. Vahey TN, Maglinte DD, Chernish SM. State-of-the-art barium examination in opportunistic esophagitis. Dig Dis Sci 1986;31:1192–5.

33. Levine MS, Laufer I, Kressel HY, et al. Herpes esophagitis. AJR Am J Roentgenol 1981;136:863–6.

34. Levine MS, Loevner LA, Saul SH, et al. Herpes esophagitis: sensitivity of double-contrast esophagography. AJR Am J Roentgenol 1988;151:57–62.

35. Shortsleeve MJ, Levine MS. Herpes esophagitis in otherwise healthy patients: clinical and radiographic findings. Radiology 1992;182:859–61.

36. Balthazar EJ, Megibow AJ, Hulnick DH. Cytomegalovirus esophagitis and gastritis in AIDS. AJR Am J Roentgenol 1985;144:1201–4.

37. Levine MS, Loercher G, Katzka DA, et al. Giant, human immunodeficiency virus-related ulcers in the esophagus. Radiology 1991;180:323–6.

38. Sor S, Levine MS, Kowalski TE, et al. Giant ulcers of the esophagus in patients with human immunodeficiency virus: clinical, radiographic, and pathologic findings. Radiology 1995;194:447–51.

39. White SB, Levine MS, Rubesin SE, et al. The small-caliber esophagus: radiographic sign of idiopathic eosinophilic esophagitis. Radiology 2010;256:127–34.

40. Rauschecker AM, Levine MS, Whitson MJ, et al. Esophageal lichen planus: clinical and radiographic findings in eight patients. AJR Am J Roentgenol 2017;208:101–6.

41. Katzka DA, Smyrk TC, Bruce AJ, et al. Variations in presentations of esophageal involvement in lichen planus. Clin Gastroenterol Hepatol 2010;8:777–82.

42. Ott DJ, Chen YM, Hewson EG, et al. Esophageal motility: assessment with synchronous video tape fluoroscopy and manometry. Radiology 1989;173:419–22.

43. Campbell C, Levine MS, Rubesin SE, et al. Association between esophageal dysmotility and gastroesophageal reflux on barium studies. Eur J Radiol 2006;59:88–92.

44. Ott DJ, Levine MS. Motility disorders of the esophagus. In: Gore RM, Levine MS, editors. Textbook of gastrointestinal radiology. 4th edition. Philadelphia: Elsevier; 2015. p. 279–90.

45. Katz PO, Richter JE, Cowan R, et al. Apparent complete lower esophageal sphincter relaxation in achalasia. Gastroenterology 1986;90:978–83.

46. Ott DJ, Richter JE, Chen YM, et al. Radiographic and manometric correlation in achalasia with apparent relaxation of the lower esophageal sphincter. Gastrointest Radiol 1989;14:1–5.

47. Amaravadi R, Levine MS, Rubesin SE, et al. Achalasia with complete relaxation of lower esophageal sphincter: radiographic-manometric correlation. Radiology 2005;235:886–91.

48. Woodfield CA, Levine MS, Rubesin SE, et al. Diagnosis of primary versus secondary achalasia: reassessment of clinical and radiographic criteria. AJR Am J Roentgenol 2000;175:727–31.

49. Prabhakar A, Levine MS, Rubesin S, et al. Relationship between diffuse esophageal spasm and lower esophageal sphincter dysfunction on barium studies and manometry in 14 patients. AJR Am J Roentgenol 2004;183:409–13.

Computed Tomography and Magnetic Resonance Small Bowel Enterography

Current Status and Future Trends Focusing on Crohn's Disease

Seong Ho Park, MD, PhD[a],*, Byong Duk Ye, MD, PhD[b],
Tae Young Lee, MD[a], Joel G. Fletcher, MD[c]

KEYWORDS

- CT enterography • MR enterography • Small bowel imaging • Crohn's disease
- Update

KEY POINTS

- The Society of Abdominal Radiology (SAR) has recently developed, in collaboration with the American Gastroenterological Association (AGA), recommendations for evaluation and interpretation of computed tomography enterography (CTE) and magnetic resonance enterography (MRE) in patients with Crohn's disease (CD) to help achieve more standardized practice.
- CTE and MRE are useful for monitoring disease-modifying therapy for CD, and we are in the early stages of using CTE and MRE results as endpoints to assess therapeutic outcomes in managing CD patients.
- Radiation dose-reduction techniques for CTE and DWI for MRE are currently well adopted in routine practice, whereas bowel motility and magnetization transfer MR imaging are under further exploration regarding feasibility for clinical use.

 Video content accompanies this article at http://www.gastro.theclinics.com/.

Disclosure Statement: All authors have nothing to disclose.
[a] Department of Radiology, Research Institute of Radiology, University of Ulsan College of Medicine, Asan Medical Center, 88, Olympic-ro 43-gil, Songpa-gu, Seoul 05505, South Korea;
[b] Department of Gastroenterology, Inflammatory Bowel Disease Center, University of Ulsan College of Medicine, Asan Medical Center, 88, Olympic-ro 43-gil, Songpa-gu, Seoul 05505, South Korea; [c] Department of Radiology, Mayo Clinic, 200 First Street, Southwest, Rochester, MN 55905, USA
* Corresponding author.
E-mail address: parksh.radiology@gmail.com

Gastroenterol Clin N Am 47 (2018) 475–499
https://doi.org/10.1016/j.gtc.2018.04.002
0889-8553/18/© 2018 Elsevier Inc. All rights reserved.

Abbreviations	
ADC	Apparent diffusion coefficient
AGA	American Gastroenterological Association
CD	Crohn's disease
CI	Confidence interval
CT	Computed tomography
CTE	Computed tomography enterography
DWI	Diffusion-weighted imaging
MaRIA	Magnetic resonance index of activity
MR	Magnetic resonance
MRE	Magnetic resonance enterography
MRI	Magnetic resonance imaging
ROI	Region of interest
SAR	Society of Abdominal Radiology
TNF	Tumor necrosis factor

INTRODUCTION

Computed tomography enterography (CTE) and magnetic resonance enterography (MRE) are state-of-the-art radiologic tests used to examine the small bowel. These examinations are distinguished from routine abdominopelvic computed tomography (CT) and magnetic resonance imaging (MRI) by the oral administration of a large amount of neutral fluid contrast before scanning to distend the bowel. CTE and MRE are not indicated for every case of suspected small bowel disease. Common clinical settings that require radiologic examination of the small bowel and the preferred techniques are summarized in **Table 1**. Hemodynamically stable suspected small bowel bleeding and Crohn's disease (CD) are the most important indications for CTE and MRE.[1–4] Of these, this article focuses on the use of CTE and MRE for the evaluation of CD. Radiologic assessment of gastrointestinal bleeding is addressed elsewhere in this issue. General reviews regarding the techniques, imaging findings, and utility of CTE and MRE in CD are avoided, because there is now an abundance of excellent review articles on these topics. We explain recent efforts to achieve more standardized interpretation of CTE and MRE for improved care of patients with CD, summarize recent research studies that have investigated the role and impact of CTE and MRE more directly for several specific clinical and research issues beyond general diagnostic accuracy, and provide an update on progress in imaging techniques. We discuss these topics along with some highlights of the areas that need to be further explored in the future.

EFFORTS TO STANDARDIZE INTERPRETATION AND REPORTING OF COMPUTED TOMOGRAPHY ENTEROGRAPHY AND MAGNETIC RESONANCE ENTEROGRAPHY IN CROHN'S DISEASE

CTE and MRE are widely used in the management of CD and are highly accurate for diagnosing bowel inflammation and complications in CD. However, it seems that there is still substantial heterogeneity and inconsistency in how the examinations are interpreted and reported, between different readers within the same institution and across different institutions. Also, standardized criteria for imaging diagnosis of CD are lacking, as are recommendations for the use of these examinations by medical societies. Both quality and consistency in the interpretation and reporting of imaging examinations are crucial for advancing patient care especially for the management of chronic diseases, such as CD. Standardization of the items that should be evaluated on imaging and the nomenclature for describing the imaging findings can help enhance quality and consistency in the communication of CTE and MRE results among different

Table 1
CT and MR techniques in common clinical settings that require examination of the small bowel

Indication	Preferred Techniques	Comment
Suspected small bowel bleeding		
Hemodynamic instability	Nonenterographic abdominopelvic CT	• Unenhanced + dynamic multiphasic contrast-enhanced scans
Hemodynamic stability	CTE (maybe, MRE in limited cases)	• Unenhanced + dynamic multiphasic contrast-enhanced scans • MRE may be used mainly in pediatric patients[103]; however, not much supporting data yet
Crohn's disease		
Initial evaluation of suspected patient	CTE	• Single enteric-phase contrast-enhanced scan • MRE if a history of multiple prior CT examinations
Acutely severely ill patient	CTE or nonenterographic abdominopelvic CT	• In patients who may not be able to hold still for the long acquisition time for MRE • Nonenterographic abdominopelvic CT if unable to tolerate oral contrast
Young age	MRE	• Perhaps, <35 years old[104]
Pregnancy	MRE	• Unenhanced scans only, because MR imaging contrast agents are contraindicated
Therapeutic monitoring	MRE	• As repeated imaging follow-ups are typically required
Suspicion of perianal disease	MRE	• As a separate anal scan can be added to MRE in a single sitting
Suspected bowel obstruction or ischemia	Nonenterographic abdominopelvic CT	• Unenhanced[105] + dynamic multiphasic contrast-enhanced scans if ischemia/strangulation is suspected • Otherwise, single-phase contrast-enhanced scan
Unexplained diarrhea	CTE or MRE	• To evaluate small bowel and pancreas • May obtain axial rather than coronal images, or alter acquisition so that high-resolution, contrast-enhanced coverage of the pancreas is also performed
Malabsorption or celiac sprue	CTE or MRE	• To rule out lymphoma or refractory celiac disease
Polyposis	CTE or MRE	• To define polyp sizes and locations • May consider positive oral contrast at CT, because polyps are intraluminal filling defects

Data from Refs.[1,85,101–105]

disciplines.[3–6] In this regard, the Society of Abdominal Radiology (SAR) CD-focused panel, in collaboration with the American Gastroenterological Association (AGA), has recently developed consensus recommendations for the evaluation and interpretation of CTE and MRE in patients with CD.[3,4] The recommendations list the small bowel imaging findings that should be evaluated and define and describe key imaging findings that relate to the diagnosis, severity, and type of CD involvement on CTE and

MRE. We elaborate on some practical aspects of these recommendations regarding the interpretation of bowel inflammatory severity and strictures in CD. One should directly refer to these recommendations for further details.

Interpretation of Bowel Inflammatory Severity

A decade ago the focus of CTE and MRE was to identify small bowel CD and its immediate complications using an imaging study. As these examinations have been used clinically, it is now recognized that up to 50% of CD with normal ileocolonoscopy results have active inflammatory small bowel CD at CTE or MRE.[7,8] Consequently, CTE and MRE, predominantly the latter because of radiation concerns, are used in follow-up and surveillance of patients with small bowel CD on medical therapy. Thus, the characterization of CD severity and response to treatment is now emerging as an important parameter for radiologists to describe. At this point, radiologists generally describe severity as mild, moderate, and severe and provide an indication of location of disease and extent of involvement. CTE and MRE findings indicating severe small bowel inflammation include mural thickness greater than or equal to 10 mm, intramural edema on T2-weighted images, marked intramural diffusion restriction on diffusion-weighted imaging (DWI), and discernible ulcers (**Fig. 1**).[3,4] There are pitfalls associated with these findings of which readers should be aware. For example, mural thickening is also caused by fibrosis, and false-positive DWI findings are created by multiple factors including poor fluid distention of the bowel. Visibility of an individual ulcer on a cross-sectional image is influenced by the lesion orientation and luminal distention in addition to ulcer size and depth.[3,4,9,10] Therefore, when interpreting MRE, all findings from different sequences should be compared carefully and interpreted collectively instead of relying on any single finding alone. Mural hyperenhancement is a sign of active bowel inflammation. However, the degree of enhancement should not be used as an indicator

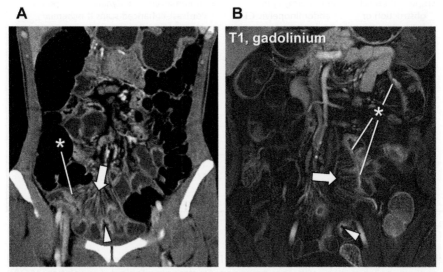

Fig. 1. Individual CD ulcers on coronal CTE and MRE images. (*A*) CTE (35-year-old man) and (*B*) MRE (32-year-old man) images show discrete ulcers (*arrowhead*) in the mesenteric side of ileal segments. Other signs of bowel inflammation, including mural hyperenhancement and thickening (*asterisk*) that preferentially involve the mesenteric border and increased vasa recta (*arrow*), are also noted.

of bowel inflammatory severity unless some internal normalization or quantitative analysis is made, because not only CD itself, but also many physiologic and technical factors can affect the degree of enhancement.[3,4] Mild small bowel inflammation typically displays a 3- to 5-mm mural thickness and the absence of findings of severe inflammation mentioned previously. Moderate small bowel inflammation would be findings in between. Because of patchy and asymmetric inflammation in CD, many involved bowel loops may have different severities of disease in different bowel locations. Using the findings mentioned previously, it is generally straightforward to determine which bowel loop has more severe inflammation than another in relative terms (**Figs. 2** and **3**). Also, apart from specific imaging features, the total length of the inflamed segment is often the most revealing single parameter on whether a patient is responding to therapy. The recent SAR/AGA recommendations introduce the issue of grading inflammatory severity, but state "further refinement of specific imaging criteria that can be readily incorporated into clinical practice for mild, moderate, and severe inflammation will be a subject for future interdisciplinary investigation."[3,4]

There are multiple (semi-)quantitative scoring systems described in the literature to assess bowel inflammatory severity of CD on enterography, especially using MRE.[11,12] The MR index of activity (MaRIA),[13,14] the CD MRI index (either in the form of regression equation or the sum of visual scores),[15,16] the MRE global score,[17,18] and the Nancy score[19] are well-known examples. Details on each scoring system are beyond the scope of this article but are found elsewhere.[11,20,21] However, these scoring methods are mostly used in research studies and have not yet transitioned to routine clinical practice for several reasons.[12] Most notably, there are concerns about the practicality and reproducibility of these scoring systems when used

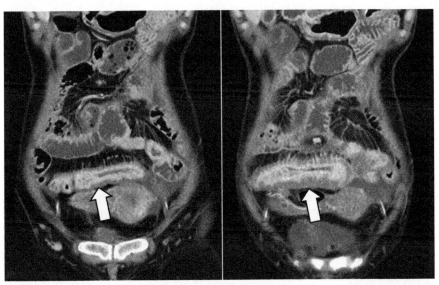

Fig. 2. Comparison of ileal inflammatory severity in a woman with CD during a 2-year follow-up (33–35 year old) using CTE. Compared with the initial CTE (*left*; coronal view), the same ileal segment (*arrow*) shows greater mural thickness at the 2-year follow-up (*right*; coronal view), indicating more severe inflammation. CD activity index and C-reactive protein at the time of the initial CTE were 180 and 1.42 mg/dL, respectively. These were 223 and 4.19 mg/dL at the 2-year follow-up.

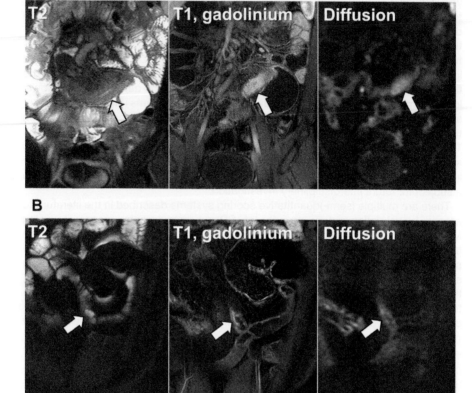

Fig. 3. Comparison of inflammatory severity in ileal segments in two patients with CD. MRE images (coronal view) of patient A (35-year-old man) shows higher T2 signal (*left*), greater mural thickness, and greater diffusion restriction (ie, a brighter signal on DWI; right) compared with patient B (36-year-old man) in the inflamed ileal segments (*arrow*), which indicates more severe inflammation in patient A.

in real-world practice outside research settings, especially for scoring systems that require quantitative measurement in the bowel wall by placing regions of interest (ROIs) instead of using visual cues. Placing measuring cursors in matched ROIs on precontrast and postcontrast images, inserting numeric measurements into an equation to calculate a score, and repeating the whole set of procedures for multiple bowel segments is time-consuming and disruptive for every-day radiology practice.[11] Unlike in large solid organs, such as the liver, the small size of ROIs to be measured in the bowel wall complicates achieving adequate reproducibility between readers.[9,11,22,23] In contrast with endoscopic scores, such as the CD endoscopic index of severity and the simple endoscopic score for CD, enterographic scores, such as the MaRIA,[13,14] the CD MRI index,[15,16] and the Nancy score,[19] are calculated for each ROI and do not consider the extent of bowel inflammation. Therefore, the score values vary according to the selection of exact bowel locations to measure, which may exacerbate the interreader variability particularly given that CD typically involves multiple segments of the bowel. The MRE global score[17,18] considers the extent of bowel involvement. Most of these enterography-based scoring systems have been modeled and validated against endoscopic scoring systems, which may not be methodologically ideal because the validation process inevitably ignores that CTE and MRE assess transmural inflammation and healing, whereas endoscopy mostly evaluates mucosal-side manifestations of the disease alone. In addition, the disease may be more straightforwardly summarized at CTE and MRE with a simple length measurement of continuous regions of inflammation rather than by dividing the bowel into anatomic segments according to endoscopic conventions (ileum, right colon, transverse colon, sigmoid and left colon, and rectum).

Interpretation of Bowel Stricture

Gastroenterologists and radiologists refer to different physical findings when identifying a bowel stricture in CD. Gastroenterologists can directly observe the narrowed luminal diameter to make a call of stricture, which is a smaller than a particular threshold diameter or when the endoscopic passage is impossible, whereas radiologists mainly rely on unequivocal upstream bowel dilatation, defined as greater than 3 cm in diameter in case of the small bowel.[3,4] The radiologic criterion is a specific criterion to avoid false-positive diagnosis. Fixed luminal narrowing without upstream dilation cannot be reliably diagnosed as a stricture on a single image, but SAR/AGA recommendations state that it is appropriate to report a probable stricture when multiple pulse sequences, fluoroscopic/cine imaging, or serial imaging examinations at intervals demonstrate fixed narrowing.[3,4] When a CD stricture is identified, the distinction between inflammatory versus fibrotic strictures is often difficult because most CD strictures have inflammatory and fibrotic components because of repeated inflammation and reparative damage.[24–26] At present, it is recommended to interpret the nature of the stricture from the standpoint of inflammation, that is, whether CTE or MRE findings of inflammation are present within the stricture, rather than from standpoint of the relative contribution of inflammation, muscular hypertrophy, and fibrosis for a few reasons.[3,4,27] First, the presence of inflammation might suggest a possibility, albeit not guaranteed, that the stricture may improve with medical therapy.[3,4,27] Second, there is yet no robust radiologic means to accurately assess the degree of bowel fibrosis in CD, although some MRE findings are related to fibrosis. A recent study compared MRE findings with graded histology in 41 patients who underwent bowel resection, mostly of the small bowel because of intractable CD. Delayed progressive enhancement over 7 minutes was more frequent (87.5% vs 17.9% of the bowels), enhancement gain between 70 seconds and 7 minutes was greater (35% vs 14% enhancement gain), and homogenous mural enhancement instead of layered or mucosa-only enhancement at 7-minute delay was more common (93.8% vs 39.3% of the bowels) in histologic severe fibrosis than in histologic moderate or less fibrosis,[28] suggesting that delayed progressive bowel enhancement might be an imaging marker of bowel fibrosis in CD. By contrast, another recent study treated 97 patients with CD with symptomatic small bowel strictures (Montreal classification B2) with adalimumab and analyzed the factors associated with treatment success, defined as no endoscopic dilatation or surgery needed for the bowel stricture. At 24 weeks, marked enhancement on 8-minute delay was independently associated with treatment success (odds ratio, 5.92),[29] which seems to contradict the aforementioned study,[28] although the two studies may not be directly comparable, because the study populations were different, that is, patients undergoing surgical resection versus medical therapy. The mural signal on T2-weighted image is reported to be helpful for distinguishing predominantly inflammatory (high signal caused by tissue edema) and predominantly fibrotic (dark signal) diseases[30]; however, concurrent inflammation present in fibrotic strictures can often confound the imaging findings (**Fig. 4**).

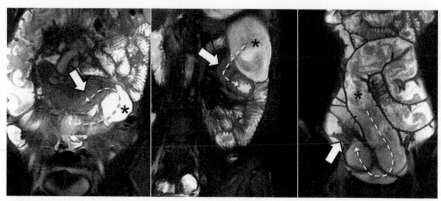

Fig. 4. T2-weighted MRE images (coronal view) in three patients with stricturing CD in the ileum. Course of the bowel (*dotted line with arrowhead*), strictures (*arrow*), and distended bowel (*asterisk*) proximal to the strictures are marked. (*Left*) Patient (35-year-old man; the same patient as in **Fig. 3**A) shows markedly increased mural signals in the stricture segment. Bowel obstruction was resolved after several days with medical therapy, indicating inflammatory nature of the stricture. (*Middle*) Patient (45-year-old man) shows a heterogeneous mixture of dark and high signals in the stricture segment, indicating the presence of fibrosis and inflammation. The patient had to undergo surgery. (*Right*) Patient (24-year-old man) shows fairly high mural signal in the stricture. However, the patient had to undergo surgery because medical management was unsuccessful, which demonstrates the limitation of MRE (ie, obscuration of substantial fibrosis caused by coexisting inflammation).

Other imaging techniques, including ultrasound-based tissue elastography and magnetization transfer MRI, have been used to estimate bowel fibrosis in CD. These techniques are still experimental. Magnetization transfer MRI is explained later in this review. Further details on ultrasound elastography are beyond the scope of this article but are found elsewhere.[31–34]

DEFINING THE ROLE AND IMPACT OF COMPUTED TOMOGRAPHY ENTEROGRAPHY AND MAGNETIC RESONANCE ENTEROGRAPHY BEYOND GENERAL DIAGNOSTIC ACCURACY

Early studies of CTE and MRE in CD largely focused on their general accuracy for diagnosing active inflammation of the bowel; CTE and MRE were reported to have similarly high accuracies.[35,36] According to the most recent meta-analysis, the per-patient sensitivity and specificity for diagnosing small bowel inflammation of CD were 87% (95% confidence interval [CI], 78%–92%) and 91% (95% CI, 84%–95%), respectively, for CTE and 86% (95% CI, 79%–91%) and 93% (95% CI, 84%–97%), respectively, for MRE.[36] More recently, studies aiming at determining the role and impact of CTE and MRE more directly for several specific clinical or research issues beyond general diagnostic accuracy have been reported.

Computed Tomography Enterography and Magnetic Resonance Enterography to Monitor Disease-Modifying Therapy and Computed Tomography Enterography and Magnetic Resonance Enterography Results as Therapeutic End points

The introduction of biologic agents (eg, infliximab, adalimumab, certolizumab pegol, vedolizumab, and ustekinumab) and immunosuppressive therapy (azathioprine, 6-mercaptopurine, and methotrexate) has altered the therapeutic goals in the treatment of CD from symptomatic control to complete mucosal healing of the affected bowel.[37] In particular, anti-tumor necrosis factor (TNF)-α is currently the most important agent used to achieve complete mucosal healing in CD with studies reporting endoscopic complete remission rates of 19% to 30% after 6 months to 1 year of therapy.[38–40]

Accordingly, multiple recent studies have investigated the effect of disease-modifying therapy, especially anti-TNF-α, on CTE and MRE findings (including conventional imaging, dynamic contrast-enhanced imaging, DWI, and cine MRI), and have shown that abnormal imaging findings and measures substantially decrease with treatment response and can normalize (**Figs. 5–7**).[18,41–48] These results support

A

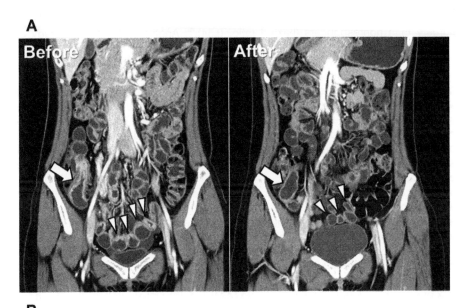

B

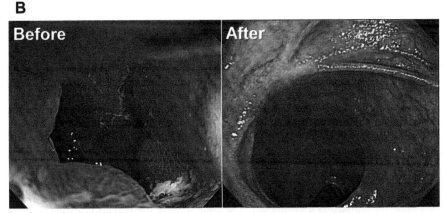

Fig. 5. Complete resolution of CTE abnormalities after the achievement of endoscopic complete remission of CD. (*A*) CTE (coronal view) and (*B*) endoscopic (terminal ileum) images obtained before therapy (*left*) and after the achievement of complete endoscopic remission with a 2-year treatment (*right*) in a woman (29–31 year old) are shown. CTE findings normalized after therapy in the terminal ileum (*arrow*) and in the pelvic ileal segments (*arrowheads*; inaccessible with endoscopy).

the role of CTE and MRE as a tool to monitor therapy. We are in the early stages of using CTE and MRE results as endpoints to assess therapeutic outcomes in the management of CD. However, a few related studies have already been published.[49,50] A recent retrospective study of 150 patients with CD analyzed the associations between treatment response as defined by CTE or MRE and CD-related patient outcomes.[49] The study showed that complete responders (55 patients [37%]), defined as having improvement in all individual bowel lesions (not necessarily complete resolution of inflammatory findings), and partial responders (39 patients [26%]) on CTE or MRE, had significantly decreased risks as compared with nonresponders (56 patients [37%]) in terms of steroid usage (hazard ratios, 0.37 and 0.45, respectively) and hospitalization for active disease (hazard ratios, 0.28 and 0.54, respectively) in the subsequent clinical course.[49] Complete responders also had a significantly reduced risk of CD-related surgery than nonresponders (hazard ratio, 0.34).[49] Another retrospective study of 101 pediatric patients with CD reported that patients who had remission on MRE (36 patients), defined as resolution of bowel abnormalities or recovery of normal T2 signal if residual abnormal mural enhancement and thickening were present, after medical therapy were associated with fewer medication changes (8.3% vs 44.6%) and fewer surgeries (2.8% vs 18.5%) compared with those not showing MRE remission for a subsequent median follow-up of 2.8 years.[50] More studies showing how healing/response defined by radiologic imaging can alter patient outcomes, instead of indirect inferences through correlations with endoscopic findings, will provide a stronger justification for directing treatment of patients with CD toward radiologic endpoints.

Because cross-sectional CTE and MRE provide images of both the bowel lumen and the cross-sectional bowel wall, transmural healing indicated by resolution of imaging findings of inflammation would be thought to represent the cross-sectional therapeutic endpoint, which is likely similar to but not the same as endoscopic mucosal healing. In a prospective study that followed patients with CD with MRE after treatment with corticosteroids or anti-TNF-α, the MRE (MaRIA score <7) showed 85% sensitivity for diagnosing endoscopic mucosal healing defined as CD endoscopic index of severity less than 3.5 (ie, 15% rate of MRE calling inflammation despite endoscopic mucosal healing) and 78% specificity.[43] Consistent with this result, in a recent retrospective study[42] that specifically analyzed CTE findings of 43 bowel sections (18 terminal ileum and 25 colorectum) with complete endoscopic mucosal healing after anti-TNF-α therapy, CTE abnormalities, typically mild mural hyperenhancement or thickening, were present in 26% to 42% according to interpreting readers of the bowel despite endoscopic complete mucosal healing (see **Fig. 7**). These results may indicate that intramural inflammation can exist despite the appearance of a normal mucosa.

The significance of transmural healing or the lack thereof would lie in its predictive power for treatment response and patient outcome. A retrospective study compared patients who had normalization of the bowel on endoscopy and MRE (33 patients, classified as "transmural healing") and those who showed endoscopic healing but findings of inflammation on MRE (52 patients, classified as "mucosal healing") after treatment with immunosuppressive agents or anti-TNF-α and reported significantly better outcomes during subsequent follow-up in the transmural-healing group reporting a need for surgery at 12 months of 0% versus 11.5%, need for hospitalization at 12 months of 3% versus 17.3%, and need for therapy escalation at 12 months of 15.2% versus 36.5%.[51] Conversely, in another smaller study that compared 17 patients who achieved transmural healing as assessed by endoscopy and CTE and 10 patients who achieved endoscopic mucosal healing alone after anti-TNF-α therapy, the two groups did not significantly differ with regards to use of steroids and

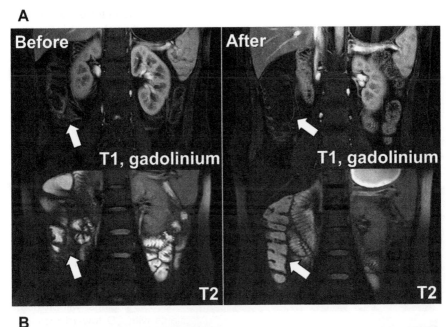

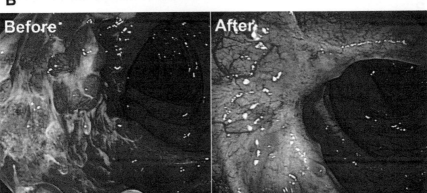

Fig. 6. Complete resolution of MRE abnormalities after achievement of endoscopic complete remission of CD. (*A*) MRE (coronal view) and (*B*) endoscopic images obtained before therapy (*left*) and after the achievement of complete endoscopic remission with a 1-year treatment (*right*) in a woman (19–20 year old) are shown. Mural and pericolic abnormalities in the ascending colon (*arrow*) have normalized on MRE after the therapy.

CD-related hospitalization or surgery for the subsequent follow-up of 15 to 43 months (mean, 28 months).[42] It would be worthwhile to further investigate the clinical significance and implications of residual CTE and MRE abnormalities in the face of endoscopic complete mucosal healing.

Role of Computed Tomography Enterography and Magnetic Resonance Enterography for Screening for Clinical Trial Enrollment

The use of CTE and MRE in the management of patients with CD in clinical practice has been evaluated extensively and CTE and MRE are now widely used as

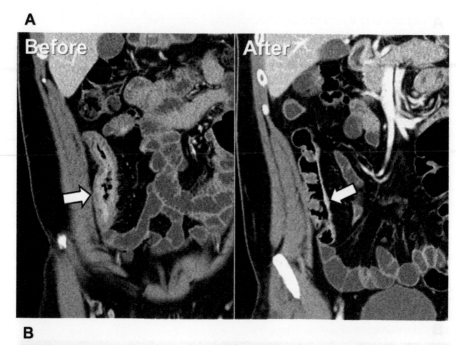

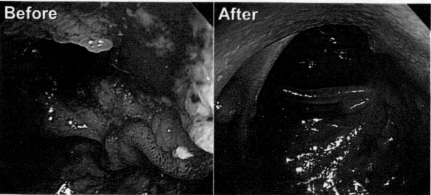

Fig. 7. Residual CTE abnormalities despite endoscopic complete remission of CD in the terminal ileum. (*A*) CTE (coronal view) and (*B*) endoscopic images obtained before therapy (*left*) and after the achievement of complete endoscopic remission with a 4-year treatment (*right*) in a man (34–38 year old) are shown. CTE shows a remarkable decrease in the mural abnormalities and resolution of prominent vasa recta with the achievement of complete endoscopic remission; however, mild mural hyperenhancement and thickening remain in the mesenteric border of the affected terminal ileum (*arrow*) following therapy.

complementary tests to endoscopy in the clinical care of patients with CD.[2] However, it was not until recently that investigators attempted to explicitly define the specific role of CTE and MRE for therapeutic clinical trials.[11,22,52,53] For clinical trials, CTE and MRE could be used to identify patients with appropriate (and similar) disease severity for trial inclusion, to exclude patients unlikely to respond to some medical therapies (eg, stricturing disease or penetrating complications), and to interrogate patients regarding the treatment response and healing after therapy as noninvasive trial endpoints (as discussed in the previous section).[11,52] If patients with penetrating complications need to be excluded from a trial, the role of CTE and MRE is particularly crucial because penetrating complications are frequent in CD and would likely be underdiagnosed without the aid of cross-sectional imaging techniques. According to population-based cohort studies from Europe and the United States, 10% to 14% of patients with CD had penetrating complications at diagnosis[54–56] and, in a retrospective study[57] analyzing the records of 357 previously diagnosed patients with CD who underwent a medically indicated CTE, penetrating disease was identified in 74 patients (20.7%) with the penetrating disease being an unsuspected new clinical feature in 58% of the 74 patients.

Computed Tomography Enterography and Magnetic Resonance Enterography for Early Surveillance of Recurrence After Bowel Resection for Crohn's Disease

Another issue that has recently been raised in the management of CD is routine pre-emptive early postsurgical surveillance for disease recurrence in patients undergoing bowel resection for CD.[58–60] Recurring disease after bowel resection for CD is frequent, especially in the anastomotic region (ie, anastomosis and a short proximal bowel segment), even during the early postsurgical period.[58,59,61] According to a systematic review, the endoscopic recurrence rates (Rutgeerts score $\geq$i2) within 1 year after bowel resection for CD reported in randomized trials were 35% to 85%.[61] Postsurgical recurrence of CD is often clinically silent with more than half of patients who developed recurrence within 1 year of surgery not having any apparent symptoms according to a systematic review.[61] Therefore, examining patients based on symptoms alone may delay the diagnosis of a recurred CD and may pose risks of irreversible bowel damage and additional bowel surgery, which makes preemptive routine postsurgical surveillance important. A recent landmark randomized trial (the POCER trial) has demonstrated the importance of routine early postsurgical surveillance.[62] In this trial,[62] patients with CD who had endoscopically accessible anastomosis after bowel resection were randomly assigned to an active care strategy (n = 122) including routine colonoscopy at 6 months after surgery and stepped-up therapy in case of active disease or to standard care (n = 52) that did not include a colonoscopy at 6 months. At the end of 18 months, 60 of 122 (49%) patients in the active care group had endoscopic recurrence, which was significantly lower than the 67% (35 of 52 patients) in the standard care group.[62] An early routine ileocolonoscopy at 6 to 12 months after bowel resection for CD now seems to be a well-agreed practice.[58–60]

In contrast, CTE and MRE do not seem to have fully achieved recognition for this particular role, although CTE and MRE are already used at some point in clinical practice to examine postsurgical patients with CD. One important reason for the low recognition is likely the paucity of specific evidence to support CTE and MRE for use in early postsurgical surveillance. Multiple published studies have explored the use of CTE or CT enteroclysis[63–66] and MRE or MR enteroclysis[67–69] in the evaluation of postsurgical CD recurrence and have reported a moderate-to-high accuracy of CTE and MRE (79%–100% sensitivity and 60%–100% specificity). Even CTE and MRE scoring systems to grade the severity of anastomotic recurrence adapted from the Rutgeerts score have been proposed.[66,69] Nevertheless, most patients in these studies were symptomatic and underwent examinations after the early surveillance period (ie, after 12 months) and often far beyond this period. A recent retrospective study specifically investigated the use of CTE for early postsurgical surveillance within 12 months after bowel resection for CD.[70] The diagnostic yield of CTE for anastomotic recurrence was similar between asymptomatic (CD activity index <150; 37.3% [19/51]) and symptomatic (CD activity index ≥150; 32.4% [12/37]) patients and the sensitivity and specificity of CTE for anastomotic recurrence (Rutgeerts score ≥i2) in this early period was 84.6% and 83.3%, respectively.[70] These results may suggest the feasibility of CTE and MRE as alternative tools for early postsurgical surveillance (**Figs. 8** and **9**). Additional research to establish the role of CTE and MRE in early postsurgical surveillance is needed and would be helpful for clinical practice for the following reasons. First, adherence to current recommendations for endoscopic surveillance, that is, routine ileocolonoscopy at 6 to 12 months after surgery, may be suboptimal because clinically quiescent patients may refuse to undergo ileocolonoscopy because of its invasiveness.[59,71] Thus, application of CTE and MRE may help improve compliance with early surveillance. Second, CTE and MRE can detect otherwise unsuspected extraluminal complications of CD.[57]

UPDATE ON PROGRESS OF COMPUTED TOMOGRAPHY ENTEROGRAPHY AND MAGNETIC RESONANCE ENTEROGRAPHY TECHNIQUES
Radiation Dose Reduction for Computed Tomography Enterography

According to consensus statements made by academic authorities, the health risks associated with radiation doses less than 50 to 100 mSv are unknown and, if any, are most likely minimal in adults.[72] The radiation dose for a single CTE examination is approximately 10 mSv even without the use of the dedicated dose-reduction techniques described next.[73] Nonetheless, given that patients with CD are mostly young and likely to undergo multiple repeated imaging examinations, and CT accounts for most diagnostic medical radiation that inflammatory bowel disease patients are exposed to,[74] every effort to decrease CTE radiation dose minimizes risk. Multiple studies have demonstrated that the radiation dose for CTE could be substantially reduced by lowering peak kilovoltage or by lowering tube current through the use of automatic exposure controls, with compensation for the increased image noise using iterative reconstruction or other denoising techniques.[75–80] CTE performed with half of the standard radiation dose has been reported to have accuracy that is noninferior to that of a standard-dose examination for diagnosing CD inflammation in the terminal ileum.[75,76] Other studies have experimented on even greater radiation dose reduction down to one-quarter or one-fifth of the routine dose, and have demonstrated the technical feasibility of such approaches, although the effects on diagnostic performance need to be confirmed.[77,78] Various techniques and strategies to reduce CT radiation

A   **B**

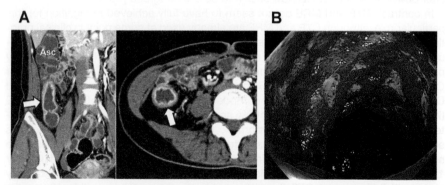

Fig. 8. Postsurgical recurrence of CD in a 41-year-old woman. (*A*) CTE (coronal on the *left* and axial on the *right*) and (*B*) endoscopy images showing recurred CD in the neoterminal ileum (*arrow*) 1 year after ileocecal resection. Asc, ascending colon.

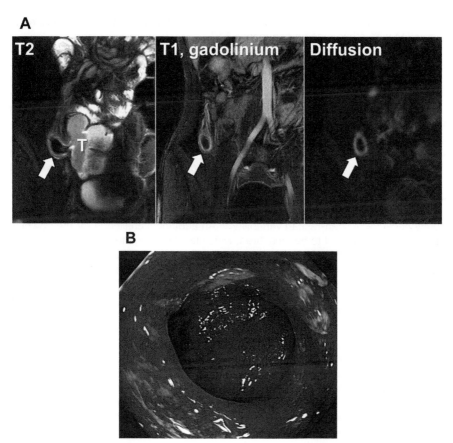

Fig. 9. Postsurgical recurrence of CD in a 29-year-old man. (*A*) MRE (coronal) and (*B*) endoscopy images showing recurred CD in the neoterminal ileum (*arrow*) 1 year after right hemicolectomy. T, transverse colon.

dose are currently available, and efforts should be made to minimize radiation exposure from CTE by the appropriate use of these methods.[81,82]

Diffusion-Weighted Imaging

DWI is an MRI technique that maps the diffusion of water molecules in biologic tissue. Its use has recently been extended to MRE examinations.[9] DWI is a promising tool for the evaluation of bowel inflammation of CD (see **Figs. 3** and **9**) and has advantages because it does not require intravenous contrast and provides a quantitative index, that is apparent diffusion coefficient (ADC) expressed in units of mm^2/s, in addition to images. The correlation between the degree of restricted mural diffusion (ie, decrease in ADC) and bowel inflammatory severity in CD has been demonstrated by numerous studies including single-time correlational studies and longitudinal follow-up studies.[9,47,83] According to a meta-analysis, DWI enterography has moderate sensitivity but low specificity with many factors causing false positives in diagnosing CD inflammation.[3,4,9,84] Indeed, some published studies have seemingly overstated the specificity of DWI. Therefore, the diagnosis of bowel inflammation in

CD should not rely on DWI alone and positive DWI findings should be interpreted in correlation with other imaging sequences.[3,4,9]

DWI may help to avoid perceptive errors and increase reader confidence in interpreting MRE. It may have a role as an alternative for intravenous contrast enhancement in patients who cannot receive gadolinium, such as in patients with decreased renal function, in pregnancy, or in those with contrast allergy.[85,86] Some studies have reported the potential usefulness of ADC as a quantitative parameter to assess bowel inflammatory severity in CD and have even suggested a quantitative score system (ie, the Clermont score[87]). Despite a few promising reports, the use of ADC as a quantitative index of CD inflammation is most likely premature because, unlike visual evaluation of DWI images, which is somewhat crude but robust, quantitative ADC measurement is difficult to standardize and has limited reproducibility as demonstrated in various other abdominal applications.[9,23] For example, according to one study, ADC values measured in the same malignant hepatic tumors differed by 30% merely because of scan-rescan variability.[88] An additional challenge for the bowel is the small size of the ROI to be measured, which is a challenge to be reproducible.[9,23] Therefore, further efforts are needed to standardize DWI techniques and to improve the reproducibility of ADC measurement before ADC is used as a quantitative biomarker of bowel inflammation for CD in clinical practice or clinical trials.

Cine Magnetic Resonance Enterography and Analysis of Bowel Motility

Because MRE does not use ionizing radiation it is safe to acquire multiple images in the same location over time. By rapidly obtaining still images of the bowel in the same position repeatedly at short intervals and then reviewing the images sequentially in a cine loop, one can display the movement of a bowel segment (**Fig. 10**, Video 1). The MRI sequence that is most commonly used for cine imaging is a balanced steady-state free precession. It has a subsecond acquisition time (exact time may vary slightly depending on the vendor, scanner, and specific scan parameters), which makes it ideal for cine imaging among various existing MR sequences. After selecting a plane to scan (typically, a coronal plane with an approximate 1-cm thickness), multiple images are repeatedly obtained in the same position at subsecond intervals (eg, 30 images for 15 seconds at 0.5-s intervals). The same image acquisition is rerun on the next scan position by gradually moving the scan plane through the body. Bowel motility on cine MRE is interpreted visually (see **Fig. 10**) and quantitatively using computerized software programs (**Fig. 11**).[89,90]

There are good data showing that reduced segmental small bowel motility assessed with cine MRE is correlated with CD activity (see **Fig. 10**).[91–94] Recent data also demonstrate that bowel motility evaluated with cine MRE appears in response to treatment with anti-TNFα, possible as early as 12 weeks after treatment initiation.[48,91,95] These results suggest the potential of cine MRE-assessed bowel motility as a biomarker to monitor bowel inflammatory activity in CD. Preliminary data also suggest aberrant motility in an apparently nondiseased small bowel may be correlated to abdominal symptoms in patients with CD.[96] Nevertheless, because decreased bowel motility is not specific to CD bowel inflammation, the finding should be correlated with conventional MRE findings.[93,94] Areas of narrowing on static images are confirmed as true strictures if they persist on cine imaging. Cine MRE is not widely used in clinical practice yet[93] and, in particular, the quantitative analysis of bowel motility is currently limited to the laboratory research level. However, motility imaging has a potential to provide additional useful information that cannot be provided by static images. Further research is needed to improve the technique and to investigate the clinical utility of the method.

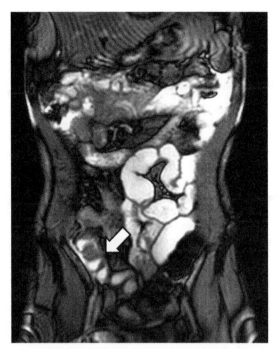

Fig. 10. Cine MRE using a balanced steady-state free precession sequence in a 28-year-old man with CD. In this static image, the terminal ileum (*arrow*) shows pseudosacculation caused by preferential disease involvement and shortening of the mesenteric border. See Video 1 for further details.

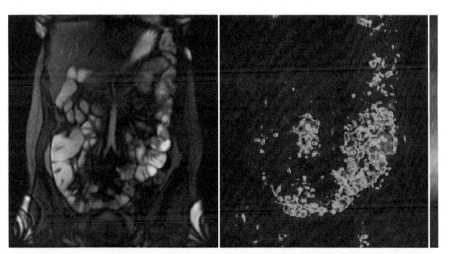

Fig. 11. Quantitative analysis of bowel motility using cine MRE. Single time point from a dynamic series depicting small bowel motility (*left*). This single time point is used as a target to which the other images in the series are registered. A series of deformation fields are generated for each time point by the registration that are summarized in the motility map (*right*). Red represents areas of high motility; blue depicts low motility. (*Courtesy of* Stuart Taylor, MD, London, United Kingdom.)

Magnetization Transfer MRI

Magnetization transfer MRI is a specialized MR technique used to image macromolecules, such as collagen. Therefore, it may have the potential to offer a more direct measurement of bowel wall fibrosis in CD, although it is currently at an experimental stage. In the magnetization transfer MRI technique, the immobile protons bound to macromolecules, which are not imaged by MR, are first selectively saturated with an off-resonance radiofrequency pulse, the saturation is transferred to the mobile protons, which are imaged by MR, in the surrounding water through a process called magnetization transfer.[97] The saturation of mobile protons decreases the MR signal. Therefore, the amount of macromolecules present is estimated by comparing the MRI signals obtained with and without the off-resonance pulse.[97] Experimental studies using rat models of CD have shown a correlation between the degree of magnetization transfer and histologic fibrosis or collagen content in the bowel wall.[98,99] Another study demonstrated that magnetization transfer imaging could to a certain extent distinguish normal bowel segments, segments with fibrotic scarring, and segments with inflammation in patients with CD.[100]

SUMMARY

A decade ago the focus of CTE and MRE was to identify small bowel CD and its immediate complications, and early studies of CTE and MRE in CD mainly focused on their general accuracy for diagnosing active inflammation of the bowel. More recently, in addition to various technical updates, efforts have been made to improve the quality of practice and to identify the role and impact of CTE and MRE more directly for several specific clinical or research issues beyond general diagnostic accuracy. The SAR, in collaboration with the AGA, has developed recommendations for the evaluation and interpretation of CTE and MRE results in patients with CD to help achieve more standardized practice. It is straightforward to describe bowel inflammatory severity of CD in relative terms using CTE and MRE; however, existing (semi-)quantitative CTE or MRE severity scoring systems are rarely used in clinical practice and require further refinement. CTE and MRE criteria for the identification of bowel stricture in CD are rather specific and, when detected, interpreting the stricture from the viewpoint of presence/absence of inflammation considering imaging limitations in assessing fibrosis and frequent coexistence of inflammation and fibrosis is recommended. CTE and MRE are useful for monitoring disease-modifying therapy for CD, and we are in the early stages of using CTE and MRE results as endpoints to assess therapeutic outcomes for managing patients with CD. CTE and MRE are also useful tools for screening patients with CD for clinical trial enrollment and early surveillance of recurrence after bowel resection for CD. Radiation dose-reduction techniques for CTE and DWI for MRE are now routinely adopted in clinical practice, whereas bowel motility imaging and magnetization transfer MRI are under further exploration regarding their feasibility for clinical use.

SUPPLEMENTARY DATA

Supplementary data related to this article can be found online at https://doi.org/10.1016/j.gtc.2018.04.002.

REFERENCES

1. Gerson LB, Fidler JL, Cave DR, et al. ACG clinical guideline: diagnosis and management of small bowel bleeding. Am J Gastroenterol 2015;110(9):1265–87 [quiz: 1288].

2. Panes J, Bouhnik Y, Reinisch W, et al. Imaging techniques for assessment of inflammatory bowel disease: joint ECCO and ESGAR evidence-based consensus guidelines. J Crohns Colitis 2013;7(7):556–85.

3. Bruining DH, Zimmermann EM, Loftus EV, et al. Consensus recommendations for evaluation, interpretation and utilization of computed tomography and magnetic resonance enterography in patients with small bowel Crohn's disease. Radiology 2018;286(3):776–99.

4. Bruining DH, Zimmermann EM, Loftus EV, et al. Consensus recommendations for evaluation, interpretation and utilization of computed tomography and magnetic resonance enterography in patients with small bowel Crohn's disease. Gastroenterology 2018;154(4):1172–94.

5. Wildman-Tobriner B, Allen BC, Bashir MR, et al. Structured reporting of CT enterography for inflammatory bowel disease: effect on key feature reporting, accuracy across training levels, and subjective assessment of disease by referring physicians. Abdom Radiol 2017;42(9):2243–50.

6. Wildman-Tobriner B, Allen BC, Davis JT, et al. Structured reporting of magnetic resonance enterography for pediatric Crohn's disease: effect on key feature reporting and subjective assessment of disease by referring physicians. Curr Probl Diagn Radiol 2017;46(2):110–4.

7. Samuel S, Bruining DH, Loftus EV Jr, et al. Endoscopic skipping of the distal terminal ileum in Crohn's disease can lead to negative results from ileocolonoscopy. Clin Gastroenterol Hepatol 2012;10(11):1253–9.

8. Mansuri I, Fletcher JG, Bruining DH, et al. Endoscopic skipping of the terminal ileum in pediatric Crohn disease. AJR Am J Roentgenol 2017;208(6):W216–W224.

9. Park SH. DWI at MR enterography for evaluating bowel inflammation in Crohn disease. AJR Am J Roentgenol 2016;207(1):40–8.

10. Kim JS, Jang HY, Park SH, et al. MR enterography assessment of bowel inflammation severity in Crohn disease using the MR index of activity score: modifying roles of DWI and effects of contrast phases. AJR Am J Roentgenol 2017;208(5):1022–9.

11. Deepak P, Fletcher JG, Fidler JL, et al. Computed tomography and magnetic resonance enterography in Crohn's disease: assessment of radiologic criteria and endpoints for clinical practice and trials. Inflamm Bowel Dis 2016;22(9):2280–8.

12. Bruining DH, Bhatnagar G, Rimola J, et al. CT and MR enterography in Crohn's disease: current and future applications. Abdom Imaging 2015;40(5):965–74.

13. Rimola J, Ordas I, Rodriguez S, et al. Magnetic resonance imaging for evaluation of Crohn's disease: validation of parameters of severity and quantitative index of activity. Inflamm Bowel Dis 2011;17(8):1759–68.

14. Rimola J, Rodriguez S, Garcia-Bosch O, et al. Magnetic resonance for assessment of disease activity and severity in ileocolonic Crohn's disease. Gut 2009;58(8):1113–20.

15. Steward MJ, Punwani S, Proctor I, et al. Non-perforating small bowel Crohn's disease assessed by MRI enterography: derivation and histopathological validation of an MR-based activity index. Eur J Radiol 2012;81(9):2080–8.

16. Tielbeek JA, Makanyanga JC, Bipat S, et al. Grading Crohn disease activity with MRI: interobserver variability of MRI features, MRI scoring of severity, and correlation with Crohn disease endoscopic index of severity. AJR Am J Roentgenol 2013;201(6):1220–8.

17. Makanyanga JC, Pendse D, Dikaios N, et al. Evaluation of Crohn's disease activity: initial validation of a magnetic resonance enterography global score (MEGS) against faecal calprotectin. Eur Radiol 2014;24(2):277–87.

18. Prezzi D, Bhatnagar G, Vega R, et al. Monitoring Crohn's disease during anti-TNF-alpha therapy: validation of the magnetic resonance enterography global score (MEGS) against a combined clinical reference standard. Eur Radiol 2016;26(7):2107–17.

19. Oussalah A, Laurent V, Bruot O, et al. Diffusion-weighted magnetic resonance without bowel preparation for detecting colonic inflammation in inflammatory bowel disease. Gut 2010;59(8):1056–65.

20. Makanyanga JC, Taylor SA. Current and future role of MR enterography in the management of Crohn disease. AJR Am J Roentgenol 2013;201(1):56–64.

21. Al-Bawardy B, Hansel SL, Fidler JL, et al. Endoscopic and radiographic assessment of Crohn's disease. Gastroenterol Clin North Am 2017;46(3):493–513.

22. Taylor SA. Editorial: can MRI enterography be an efficient tool for patient selection in clinical trials? Aliment Pharmacol Ther 2016;43(5):643–4.

23. Dohan A, Taylor S, Hoeffel C, et al. Diffusion-weighted MRI in Crohn's disease: current status and recommendations. J Magn Reson Imaging 2016;44(6): 1381–96.

24. Adler J, Punglia DR, Dillman JR, et al. Computed tomography enterography findings correlate with tissue inflammation, not fibrosis in resected small bowel Crohn's disease. Inflamm Bowel Dis 2012;18(5):849–56.

25. Zappa M, Stefanescu C, Cazals-Hatem D, et al. Which magnetic resonance imaging findings accurately evaluate inflammation in small bowel Crohn's disease? A retrospective comparison with surgical pathologic analysis. Inflamm Bowel Dis 2011;17(4):984–93.

26. Chiorean MV, Sandrasegaran K, Saxena R, et al. Correlation of CT enteroclysis with surgical pathology in Crohn's disease. Am J Gastroenterol 2007;102(11): 2541–50.

27. Rieder F, Zimmermann EM, Remzi FH, et al. Crohn's disease complicated by strictures: a systematic review. Gut 2013;62(7):1072–84.

28. Rimola J, Planell N, Rodriguez S, et al. Characterization of inflammation and fibrosis in Crohn's disease lesions by magnetic resonance imaging. Am J Gastroenterol 2015;110(3):432–40.

29. Bouhnik Y, Carbonnel F, Laharie D, et al. Efficacy of adalimumab in patients with Crohn's disease and symptomatic small bowel stricture: a multicentre, prospective, observational cohort (CREOLE) study. Gut 2018;67(1):53–60.

30. Maccioni F, Staltari I, Pino AR, et al. Value of T2-weighted magnetic resonance imaging in the assessment of wall inflammation and fibrosis in Crohn's disease. Abdom Imaging 2012;37(6):944–57.

31. Branchi F, Caprioli F, Orlando S, et al. Non-invasive evaluation of intestinal disorders: the role of elastographic techniques. World J Gastroenterol 2017;23(16): 2832–40.

32. Stidham RW, Higgins PD. Imaging of intestinal fibrosis: current challenges and future methods. United European Gastroenterol J 2016;4(4):515–22.

33. Lu C, Gui X, Chen W, et al. Ultrasound shear wave elastography and contrast enhancement: effective biomarkers in Crohn's disease strictures. Inflamm Bowel Dis 2017;23(3):421–30.

34. Orlando S, Fraquelli M, Coletta M, et al. Ultrasound elasticity imaging predicts therapeutic outcomes of patients with Crohn's disease treated with anti-tumour necrosis factor antibodies. J Crohns Colitis 2018;12(1):63–70.

35. Qiu Y, Mao R, Chen BL, et al. Systematic review with meta-analysis: magnetic resonance enterography vs. computed tomography enterography for evaluating disease activity in small bowel Crohn's disease. Aliment Pharmacol Ther 2014; 40(2):134–46.

36. Liu W, Liu J, Xiao W, et al. A diagnostic accuracy meta-analysis of CT and MRI for the evaluation of small bowel Crohn disease. Acad Radiol 2017;24(10): 1216–25.

37. Peyrin-Biroulet L, Sandborn W, Sands BE, et al. Selecting therapeutic targets in inflammatory bowel disease (STRIDE): determining therapeutic goals for treat-to-target. Am J Gastroenterol 2015;110(9):1324–38.

38. Colombel JF, Rutgeerts PJ, Sandborn WJ, et al. Adalimumab induces deep remission in patients with Crohn's disease. Clin Gastroenterol Hepatol 2014; 12(3):414–22.e5.

39. Colombel JF, Sandborn WJ, Reinisch W, et al. Infliximab, azathioprine, or combination therapy for Crohn's disease. N Engl J Med 2010;362(15):1383–95.

40. Rutgeerts P, Van Assche G, Sandborn WJ, et al. Adalimumab induces and maintains mucosal healing in patients with Crohn's disease: data from the EXTEND trial. Gastroenterology 2012;142(5):1102–11.e2.

41. Hashimoto S, Shimizu K, Shibata H, et al. Utility of computed tomographic enteroclysis/enterography for the assessment of mucosal healing in Crohn's disease. Gastroenterol Res Pract 2013;2013:984916.

42. Kim C, Park SH, Yang SK, et al. Endoscopic complete remission of Crohn disease after anti-tumor necrosis factor-alpha therapy: CT enterographic findings and their clinical implications. AJR Am J Roentgenol 2016;206(6):1208–16.

43. Ordas I, Rimola J, Rodriguez S, et al. Accuracy of magnetic resonance enterography in assessing response to therapy and mucosal healing in patients with Crohn's disease. Gastroenterology 2014;146(2):374–82.e1.

44. Van Assche G, Herrmann KA, Louis E, et al. Effects of infliximab therapy on transmural lesions as assessed by magnetic resonance enteroclysis in patients with ileal Crohn's disease. J Crohns Colitis 2013;7(12):950–7.

45. Eder P, Katulska K, Krela-Kazmierczak I, et al. The influence of anti-TNF therapy on the magnetic resonance enterographic parameters of Crohn's disease activity. Abdom Imaging 2015;40(7):2210–8.

46. Stoppino LP, Della Valle N, Rizzi S, et al. Magnetic resonance enterography changes after antibody to tumor necrosis factor (anti-TNF) alpha therapy in Crohn's disease: correlation with SES-CD and clinical-biological markers. BMC Med Imaging 2016;16(1):37.

47. Bhatnagar G, Dikaios N, Prezzi D, et al. Changes in dynamic contrast-enhanced pharmacokinetic and diffusion-weighted imaging parameters reflect response to anti-TNF therapy in Crohn's disease. Br J Radiol 2015;88(1055):20150547.

48. Plumb AA, Menys A, Russo E, et al. Magnetic resonance imaging-quantified small bowel motility is a sensitive marker of response to medical therapy in Crohn's disease. Aliment Pharmacol Ther 2015;42(3):343–55.

49. Deepak P, Fletcher JG, Fidler JL, et al. Radiological response is associated with better long-term outcomes and is a potential treatment target in patients with small bowel Crohn's disease. Am J Gastroenterol 2016;111(7):997–1006.

50. Sauer CG, Middleton JP, McCracken C, et al. Magnetic resonance enterography healing and magnetic resonance enterography remission predicts improved outcome in pediatric Crohn disease. J Pediatr Gastroenterol Nutr 2016;62(3): 378–83.

51. Fernandes SR, Rodrigues RV, Bernardo S, et al. Transmural healing is associated with improved long-term outcomes of patients with Crohn's disease. Inflamm Bowel Dis 2017;23(8):1403–9.

52. Coimbra AJ, Rimola J, O'Byrne S, et al. Magnetic resonance enterography is feasible and reliable in multicenter clinical trials in patients with Crohn's disease, and may help select subjects with active inflammation. Aliment Pharmacol Ther 2016;43(1):61–72.

53. Rimola J, Alvarez-Cofino A, Perez-Jeldres T, et al. Increasing efficiency of MRE for diagnosis of Crohn's disease activity through proper sequence selection: a practical approach for clinical trials. Abdom Radiol 2017;42(12):2783–91.

54. Henriksen M, Jahnsen J, Lygren I, et al. Clinical course in Crohn's disease: results of a five-year population-based follow-up study (the IBSEN study). Scand J Gastroenterol 2007;42(5):602–10.

55. Wolters FL, Russel MG, Sijbrandij J, et al. Phenotype at diagnosis predicts recurrence rates in Crohn's disease. Gut 2006;55(8):1124–30.

56. Thia KT, Sandborn WJ, Harmsen WS, et al. Risk factors associated with progression to intestinal complications of Crohn's disease in a population-based cohort. Gastroenterology 2010;139(4):1147–55.

57. Bruining DH, Siddiki HA, Fletcher JG, et al. Prevalence of penetrating disease and extraintestinal manifestations of Crohn's disease detected with CT enterography. Inflamm Bowel Dis 2008;14(12):1701–6.

58. Hashash JG, Regueiro M. A practical approach to preventing postoperative recurrence in Crohn's disease. Curr Gastroenterol Rep 2016;18(5):25.

59. Yamamoto T. Diagnosis and monitoring of postoperative recurrence in Crohn's disease. Expert Rev Gastroenterol Hepatol 2015;9(1):55–66.

60. Nakase H, Keum B, Ye BD, et al. Treatment of inflammatory bowel disease in Asia: the results of a multinational web-based survey in the 2(nd) Asian Organization of Crohn's and Colitis (AOCC) meeting in Seoul. Intest Res 2016;14(3):231–9.

61. Buisson A, Chevaux JB, Allen PB, et al. Review article: the natural history of postoperative Crohn's disease recurrence. Aliment Pharmacol Ther 2012;35(6):625–33.

62. De Cruz P, Kamm MA, Hamilton AL, et al. Crohn's disease management after intestinal resection: a randomised trial. Lancet 2015;385(9976):1406–17.

63. Mao R, Gao X, Zhu ZH, et al. CT enterography in evaluating postoperative recurrence of Crohn's disease after ileocolic resection: complementary role to endoscopy. Inflamm Bowel Dis 2013;19(5):977–82.

64. Paparo F, Revelli M, Puppo C, et al. Crohn's disease recurrence in patients with ileocolic anastomosis: value of computed tomography enterography with water enema. Eur J Radiol 2013;82(9):e434–40.

65. Soyer P, Boudiaf M, Sirol M, et al. Suspected anastomotic recurrence of Crohn disease after ileocolic resection: evaluation with CT enteroclysis. Radiology 2010;254(3):755–64.

66. Minordi LM, Vecchioli A, Poloni G, et al. Enteroclysis CT and PEG-CT in patients with previous small-bowel surgical resection for Crohn's disease: CT findings and correlation with endoscopy. Eur Radiol 2009;19(10):2432–40.

67. Gallego Ojea JC, Echarri Piudo AI, Porta Vila A. Crohn's disease: the usefulness of MR enterography in the detection of recurrence after surgery. Radiologia 2011;53(6):552–9 [in Spanish].

68. Koilakou S, Sailer J, Peloschek P, et al. Endoscopy and MR enteroclysis: equivalent tools in predicting clinical recurrence in patients with Crohn's disease after ileocolic resection. Inflamm Bowel Dis 2010;16(2):198–203.

69. Sailer J, Peloschek P, Reinisch W, et al. Anastomotic recurrence of Crohn's disease after ileocolic resection: comparison of MR enteroclysis with endoscopy. Eur Radiol 2008;18(11):2512–21.

70. Choi IY, Park SH, Park SH, et al. CT enterography for surveillance of anastomotic recurrence within 12 months of bowel resection in patients with Crohn's disease: an observational study using an 8-year registry. Korean J Radiol 2017;18(6): 906–14.

71. De Cruz P, Bernardi MP, Kamm MA, et al. Postoperative recurrence of Crohn's disease: impact of endoscopic monitoring and treatment step-up. Colorectal Dis 2013;15(2):187–97.

72. Fletcher JG, Kofler JM, Coburn JA, et al. Perspective on radiation risk in CT imaging. Abdom Imaging 2013;38(1):22–31.

73. McCollough CH, Bushberg JT, Fletcher JG, et al. Answers to common questions about the use and safety of CT scans. Mayo Clin Proc 2015;90(10):1380–92.

74. Zakeri N, Pollok RC. Diagnostic imaging and radiation exposure in inflammatory bowel disease. World J Gastroenterol 2016;22(7):2165–78.

75. Gandhi NS, Baker ME, Goenka AH, et al. Diagnostic accuracy of CT enterography for active inflammatory terminal ileal Crohn disease: comparison of full-dose and half-dose images reconstructed with FBP and half-dose images with SAFIRE. Radiology 2016;280(2):436–45.

76. Lee SJ, Park SH, Kim AY, et al. A prospective comparison of standard-dose CT enterography and 50% reduced-dose CT enterography with and without noise reduction for evaluating Crohn disease. AJR Am J Roentgenol 2011;197(1): 50–7.

77. Murphy KP, Crush L, Twomey M, et al. Model-based iterative reconstruction in CT enterography. AJR Am J Roentgenol 2015;205(6):1173–81.

78. Son JH, Kim SH, Cho EY, et al. Comparison of diagnostic performance between 1 millisievert CT enterography and half-standard dose CT enterography for evaluating active inflammation in patients with Crohn's disease. Abdom Radiol 2017. https://doi.org/10.1007/s00261-017-1359-1.

79. Fletcher JG, Hara AK, Fidler JL, et al. Observer performance for adaptive, image-based denoising and filtered back projection compared to scanner-based iterative reconstruction for lower dose CT enterography. Abdom Imaging 2015;40(5):1050–9.

80. Johnson E, Megibow AJ, Wehrli NE, et al. CT enterography at 100 kVp with iterative reconstruction compared to 120 kVp filtered back projection: evaluation of image quality and radiation dose in the same patients. Abdom Imaging 2014; 39(6):1255–60.

81. Lu ZF, Thomas S. Imaging wisely: patient safety in CT. Abdom Radiol 2016; 41(3):452–60.

82. Baker ME, Hara AK, Platt JF, et al. CT enterography for Crohn's disease: optimal technique and imaging issues. Abdom Imaging 2015;40(5):938–52.

83. Huh J, Kim KJ, Park SH, et al. Diffusion-weighted MR enterography to monitor bowel inflammation after medical therapy in Crohn's disease: a prospective longitudinal study. Korean J Radiol 2017;18(1):162–72.

84. Choi SH, Kim KW, Lee JY, et al. Diffusion-weighted magnetic resonance enterography for evaluating bowel inflammation in Crohn's disease: a systematic review and meta-analysis. Inflamm Bowel Dis 2016;22(3):669–79.

85. Grand DJ, Beland M, Harris A. Magnetic resonance enterography. Radiol Clin North Am 2013;51(1):99–112.
86. Seo N, Park SH, Kim KJ, et al. MR enterography for the evaluation of small-bowel inflammation in Crohn disease by using diffusion-weighted imaging without intravenous contrast material: a prospective noninferiority study. Radiology 2016;278(3):762–72.
87. Hordonneau C, Buisson A, Scanzi J, et al. Diffusion-weighted magnetic resonance imaging in ileocolonic Crohn's disease: validation of quantitative index of activity. Am J Gastroenterol 2014;109(1):89–98.
88. Kim SY, Lee SS, Byun JH, et al. Malignant hepatic tumors: short-term reproducibility of apparent diffusion coefficients with breath-hold and respiratory-triggered diffusion-weighted MR imaging. Radiology 2010;255(3):815–23.
89. Odille F, Menys A, Ahmed A, et al. Quantitative assessment of small bowel motility by nonrigid registration of dynamic MR images. Magn Reson Med 2012;68(3):783–93.
90. Bickelhaupt S, Froehlich JM, Cattin R, et al. Software-assisted small bowel motility analysis using free-breathing MRI: feasibility study. J Magn Reson Imaging 2014;39(1):17–23.
91. Menys A, Atkinson D, Odille F, et al. Quantified terminal ileal motility during MR enterography as a potential biomarker of Crohn's disease activity: a preliminary study. Eur Radiol 2012;22(11):2494–501.
92. Hahnemann ML, Nensa F, Kinner S, et al. Quantitative assessment of small bowel motility in patients with Crohn's disease using dynamic MRI. Neurogastroenterol Motil 2015;27(6):841–8.
93. Wnorowski AM, Guglielmo FF, Mitchell DG. How to perform and interpret cine MR enterography. J Magn Reson Imaging 2015;42(5):1180–9.
94. Cullmann JL, Bickelhaupt S, Froehlich JM, et al. MR imaging in Crohn's disease: correlation of MR motility measurement with histopathology in the terminal ileum. Neurogastroenterol Motil 2013;25(9):749-e577.
95. Bickelhaupt S, Pazahr S, Chuck N, et al. Crohn's disease: small bowel motility impairment correlates with inflammatory-related markers C-reactive protein and calprotectin. Neurogastroenterol Motil 2013;25(6):467–73.
96. Menys A, Makanyanga J, Plumb A, et al. Aberrant motility in unaffected small bowel is linked to inflammatory burden and patient symptoms in Crohn's disease. Inflamm Bowel Dis 2016;22(2):424–32.
97. Grossman RI, Gomori JM, Ramer KN, et al. Magnetization transfer: theory and clinical applications in neuroradiology. Radiographics 1994;14(2):279–90.
98. Adler J, Swanson SD, Schmiedlin-Ren P, et al. Magnetization transfer helps detect intestinal fibrosis in an animal model of Crohn disease. Radiology 2011;259(1):127–35.
99. Dillman JR, Swanson SD, Johnson LA, et al. Comparison of noncontrast MRI magnetization transfer and T2 -weighted signal intensity ratios for detection of bowel wall fibrosis in a Crohn's disease animal model. J Magn Reson Imaging 2015;42(3):801–10.
100. Pazahr S, Blume I, Frei P, et al. Magnetization transfer for the assessment of bowel fibrosis in patients with Crohn's disease: initial experience. MAGMA 2013;26(3):291–301.
101. Kim DH, Carucci LR, Baker ME, et al. ACR appropriateness criteria Crohn disease. J Am Coll Radiol 2015;12(10):1048–57.e4.
102. Huprich JE, Fletcher JG. CT enterography: principles, technique and utility in Crohn's disease. Eur J Radiol 2009;69(3):393–7.

103. Casciani E, Nardo GD, Chin S, et al. MR enterography in paediatric patients with obscure gastrointestinal bleeding. Eur J Radiol 2017;93:209–16.

104. Brenner DJ, Hall EJ. Computed tomography: an increasing source of radiation exposure. N Engl J Med 2007;357(22):2277–84.

105. Geffroy Y, Boulay-Coletta I, Julles MC, et al. Increased unenhanced bowel-wall attenuation at multidetector CT is highly specific of ischemia complicating small-bowel obstruction. Radiology 2014;270(1):159–67.

Radiologic Assessment of Gastrointestinal Bleeding

Gene Kim, MD*, Jorge A. Soto, MD, Trevor Morrison, MD

KEYWORDS

- Obscure GI bleeding • Occult GI bleeding • Overt GI bleeding

KEY POINTS

- Gastrointestinal bleeding can be classified into overt, occult, and obscure, depending on clinical presentation, as well as by anatomic location of the source of bleeding.
- The radiologic imaging modalities evaluating overt bleeding are computed tomography (CT) angiography, conventional angiography, and nuclear scintigraphy.
- Imaging workup of occult bleeding mostly involves evaluation of the small bowel with CT enterography, and in some cases, Meckel scan.
- The evaluation of obscure bleeding is variable based on clinical status and provider preference.

Gastrointestinal (GI) bleeding is not a singular disease but a symptom and clinical manifestation of a broad range of diseases of the GI tract. The approach to the treatment and management of GI bleeding is variable and depends on the site and rate of bleeding and the clinical presentation. Patients are categorized based on the location of the source of their bleed and the overall acuity of their symptoms. These distinctions help triage and guide management and treatment strategies and also carry important epidemiologic and prognostic considerations.

When classifying GI bleeding anatomically, patients with upper GI bleeding—a bleed proximal to the ligament of Treitz, which connects the fourth portion of duodenum to the diaphragm—classically present with coffee-ground hematemesis, bright red hematemesis, melena, or even hematochezia when the hemorrhage is brisk and severe. On the other hand, lower GI hemorrhages—bleeds involving the jejunum, ileum, colon, and rectum—typically present with melena or hematochezia. The overlap between upper versus lower GI bleeds who present with melena or hematochezia may further be delineated when considering melena as an indication of intraluminal blood products that have been present within the GI tract for at least 8 hours and is 4 times

Disclosure Statement: The authors have nothing to disclose.
Department of Radiology, Boston University Medical Center, 820 Harrison Avenue FGH Building, 3rd Floor, Boston, MA 02118, USA
* Corresponding author.
E-mail address: Gene.Kim@bmc.org

more likely to arise from an upper GI source; hematochezia, which indicates a brisk severe upper GI bleed or a lower GI bleed, is 6 times more frequent in the setting of a lower GI bleed.[1] In addition, about 75% of patients with acute GI bleeds present with an upper GI source.[2]

Apart from categorizing bleeding with anatomic landmarks, bleeds can also be classified on their clinical presentation. Overt GI bleeding refers to visually apparent bleeding, such as hematemesis and hematochezia, whereas occult GI bleeding alludes to a positive fecal occult blood test (FOBT) and/or iron deficiency anemia without visible evidence of hemorrhage.[3] Furthermore, the term obscure GI bleeding refers to patients with recurrent bleeding of uncertain cause after full diagnostic evaluation of the bowel. In these situations, obscure GI bleed may be overt, when presenting with frank visible blood, or occult.

ACUTE GASTROINTESTINAL BLEEDING

Acute GI bleeding is a common medical emergency with an annual incidence of 40 to 150 episodes per 100,000 people for upper GI bleeds and 20 to 27 episodes per 100,000 people for lower GI bleeds.[4] There is a male predilection with acute GI bleeding being twice as common in men than in women. There is also an increase in incidence with increasing age, with 70% of patients with acute GI bleeding being older than 65 years.[5,6] This important epidemiologic factor lends itself in consideration of localizing the GI bleed. Younger patients are more likely to have upper GI bleeding and older patients are more likely to have lesions in the lower GI tract.[7] Prompt clinical evaluation, hemodynamic stabilization, and treatment are necessary because mortality can be as high as 40% in patients with hemodynamic instability.[8] Hypotension and tachycardia can occur with as little as 500 mL of acute blood loss and hypovolemic shock with as little as 15% of loss of the total circulating blood volume.[9]

CLINICAL APPROACH AND IMAGING CONSIDERATIONS FOR ACUTE GASTROINTESTINAL BLEEDING

Rapid assessment of a patient presenting with symptoms related to a GI bleed is crucial because the clinical status of the patient helps guide the priority and choice of diagnostic and therapeutic management strategies.[4] Hemodynamic instability due to blood loss supersedes the priorities of any diagnostic and therapeutic procedures. Patients who present with a hemoglobin level of less than 7 g/dL should be transfused to maintain hemoglobin levels of 9 g/dL. In addition, patients who are found to be coagulopathic and/or thrombocytopenic should be considered for transfusion with fresh frozen plasma and platelets, respectively.[10] However, if the patient presents with large volume blood loss and is clinically unstable despite resuscitation efforts, urgent exploratory surgery is often indicated to perform, for example, a partial gastrectomy to treat a bleeding gastric ulcer.[11]

Once the patient is clinically stable, efforts to localize the source of the hemorrhage can be undertaken. Traditionally for acute upper GI bleeds, endoscopic procedures, specifically esophagogastroduodenoscopy, provide sensitivity and specificity of 98%.[3] Unfortunately, implementation of endoscopy in an emergent setting poses a variety of logistical challenges, such as availability of anesthesia and gastroenterologists and their support staff. In addition, obscuration of the mucosa due to intraluminal blood and intestinal contents and extent of evaluation of the distal duodenum and small bowel pose technical challenges.[12] Colonoscopy to evaluate for distal lower GI tract lesions is successful in about 13% of cases in some series.[13] The same logistical and technical challenges remain with the added necessity for bowel preparation.

Although limited in the length and extent of bowel that can be evaluated, digital rectal examination and proctoscopy are used to evaluate for anorectal sources of bleeding.[14] In the cases of acute upper GI bleeding, where upper endoscopic evaluation is inconclusive or negative, and in many patients with acute lower GI bleeding, CT angiography (CTA) has rapidly become the preferred method not only to help localize the site of bleeding but also to elucidate the cause. Other options include radionuclide imaging and conventional angiography, often after negative results with endoscopy and CTA.

Computed Tomography Angiography

As a diagnostic tool for the detection and localization of GI bleeding sites, a 2013 meta-analysis reported sensitivity of 85.2% and specificity of 92.1% for the detection of acute GI bleeds.[15] CTA can detect bleeding rates as low as 0.3 mL/min.[16] In addition to the inherent diagnostic quality, the advantages of CTA include high availability, minimally invasive technique, and excellent detection and localization of GI bleeding sites. Along with diagnosis of GI bleeding, CTA also provides further diagnostic information about numerous disease entities, including colitis/enteritis, diverticulosis, bowel ischemia, tumors, as well as vascular anatomy and variants—findings that may help diagnose a cause and guide therapeutic intervention for the GI bleed.

The disadvantages of CTA include the high radiation dose due to the scan being traditionally performed in multiple phases. However, improvements in dose reduction techniques to reduce radiation while providing diagnostic quality procedures have ameliorated these concerns.[17] In addition, CTA requires an injection of iodinated contrast, which is contraindicated in patients with acute renal failure. CTA is usually performed as a triple-phase study. First, a low-dose, noncontrast-enhanced series should be included to identify preexisting hyperdense materials, such as pills and retained barium, which could complicate the interpretation on later phases.[18] Afterward, a minimum contrast dose of 100 cc, which may be adjusted for body weight, is intravenously injected via power injector at a rate of 4 to 5 cc/s.[18] The remainder of the 2 contrast-enhanced image series is acquired in the arterial and portal venous phase.[9,18,19] The arterial phase, typically acquired with the use of an automatic bolus triggering mechanism, is obtained optimally 8 to 10 seconds after the enhancement in the proximal portion of the abdominal aorta reaches 150 Hounsfield units (HU). The additional 8 to 10 seconds allows the contrast to collect within the lumen of the bowel.[20] Then the portal venous phase series is acquired approximately 50 seconds after initiation of the arterial phase.[18] Although not routinely included in most standardized protocols, delayed imaging at 90 to 120 seconds after injection can also be obtained.[20] Of note, neutral enteric contrast is not used because of the extended preparation time in relation to the need for a rapid diagnosis.

The detection and localization of bleeding sites is centered around the finding of active extravasation, evidenced by contrast accumulation within the bowel lumen.[9,18,19] The active extravasation of contrast-enhanced blood typically seems as a "blush" or hyperattenuating focus within the bowel lumen (**Figs. 1** and **2**). The morphology and size of these foci are variable and may seem as a jet of contrast if the source of the bleed is arterial in nature. In the portal venous series, a previously identified focus of contrast extravasation in the arterial phase may be seen moving distally in the bowel tract due to peristalsis. If the bleed is continuous, the amount of contrast extravasation may increase as well (**Figs. 3–6**). In some instances, lower intensity bleeds may become more conspicuous on later portal venous phases because of more accumulation of contrast.[21] If no active bleeding is identified, the presence of hyperdense material in the bowel lumen may represent an intraluminal

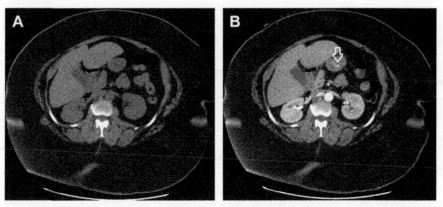

Fig. 1. A 73-year-old woman who presented with melena and light-headedness. (*A*) Noncontrast-enhanced axial slices show no intraluminal hyperdense material within the stomach. (*B*) Axial arterial phase series at the same level show active extravasation within the stomach (*arrow*). Patient ultimately underwent endoscopy, which revealed an ulcer that was clipped.

clot.[18] Differentiating hemorrhage product from other hyperdense materials, such as retained barium or foreign bodies, can be at least partly achieved by measuring the attenuation coefficient. The attenuation coefficient of unclotted blood measures approximately 30 to 45 HU and 40 to 70 HU for clotted blood.[22] The highest attenuation is found at the origin of the bleeding site, the "sentinel clot."[22]

Radionuclide Imaging

In addition to CTA, diagnostic workup for nonemergent intestinal bleeding can include nuclear scintigraphy with radiotracer technetium 99m-labeled autologous red blood cells. The cells are tagged in vitro with approximately 20 to 30 mCi of

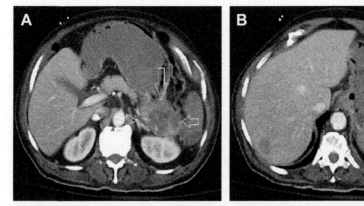

Fig. 2. An 83-year-old man who presented with gross hematemesis. (*A*) Initial CT abdomen and pelvis reveal a heterogeneous mass arising from the posterior wall of the stomach body and fundus invading the splenic hilum and pancreatic tail (*multiple arrows*). (*B*) Active extravasation is seen from the mass into the stomach (*multiple arrows*). A hypoattenuating liver metastasis is incidentally noted. The patient underwent left gastric artery embolization. The patient was subsequently diagnosed with gastric adenocarcinoma.

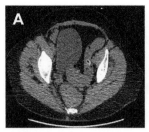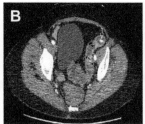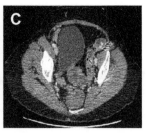

Fig. 3. A 77-year-old woman with known colonic diverticulosis who presented with 4 to 5 episodes of bright red blood per rectum. (*A*) Axial noncontrast-enhanced sequences demonstrate no hyperdense material within the distal descending and sigmoid colon. (*B*) Arterial phase slices at the same level demonstrate active extravasation (*arrow*). (*C*) Delayed sequences demonstrated expansion and propagation of the extravasated blood (both *arrows*).

technetium-99m (^{99m}Tc) and administered as an intravenous bolus. After injection, dynamic scintigraphy of the anterior abdomen are obtained at a rate of approximately 3 seconds per frame for 1 minute to show the flow of abdominal viscera.[23] Static images are then obtained at a rate of every minute for 90 minutes. Whenever there are normal findings, the examination can be discontinued. If, after the examination, there is a concern for an episode of rebleeding, the patient is reimaged with the same tagged bolus for a period up to 24 hours.[23]

Nuclear scintigraphy is the most sensitive imaging modality for detecting GI bleeding, with low-intensity bleeds being detected at a rate of 0.05 cc/min.[24] This, coupled with the ability to imaging over a longer period of time, is beneficial in evaluating intermittent and low-intensity bleeds. Other advantages include the relative ease in preparation, which requires a sample of blood and is noninvasive in nature. Disadvantages include the prolonged time to complete the study, limited access in emergent situations, relative cost compared with CT, and limited ability to localize the site and determine the specific cause of the bleed. Given the static and 2-dimensional planar imaging of the gamma camera, bleeding sites may be localized inaccurately to large or small bowel. In addition, given the noncontinuous rate of imaging acquisition, extravasated radiolabeled blood may represent an origin of bleeding but may also represent the transit from peristalsis at a bleeding site upstream.

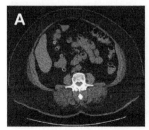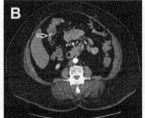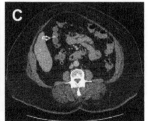

Fig. 4. A 69-year-old woman who presented with hematochezia. (*A*) Axial noncontrast-enhanced images during initial CTA evaluation show diverticulosis of the hepatic flexure. (*B*) Arterial phase images demonstrate active extravasation contained within a diverticula (*arrow*). (*C*) Delayed phase imaging expansion of the contrast indicating active bleeding (*arrow*).

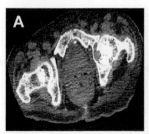
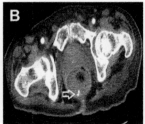
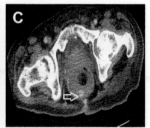

Fig. 5. A 76-year-old man who presented with hematochezia. (*A*) Axial noncontrast-enhanced images before CTA demonstrate no hyperdensity within the rectum. (*B*) Arterial phase images with evidence of active contrast extravasation (*arrow*), which (*C*) increases on delayed imaging (*arrow*). Patient underwent flexible sigmoidoscopy to reveal a single rectal ulcer.

Ideally, a positive ^{99m}Tc-labeled red blood scan will show evidence of increased activity at the site of bleed (**Fig. 7**). During the period of scan, the accumulated radiolabeled blood will show movement along the GI tract due to peristalsis. In order to better localize the source of the bleed, the examination should continue to observe the contour of pathway of the transitioning blood to determine if the bleed is within small or large bowel. After the diagnosis is confirmed, the examination may be discontinued.

Conventional Catheter-Directed Angiography

Conventional mesenteric angiography is generally reserved as a means of providing therapeutic intervention for previously diagnosed bleeding on CTA or nuclear scintigraphy.[25] However, the detection of bleeding is significantly lower than nuclear scintigraphy, with bleeding rates perceptible at 0.5 cc/min.[25] The main advantage of angiography revolves around the implementation of interventions including embolization compared with the purely diagnostic procedures such as CTA and nuclear scintigraphy. Other advantages include the lack of need of bowel preparation.

Disadvantages of conventional angiography include the inherent invasive nature of the procedure and its relative insensitivity when compared with other radiologic imaging studies. When compared with CTA, angiography may not be as readily accessible depending on local expertise and hospital resources. Although angiography may

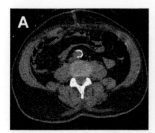
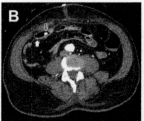
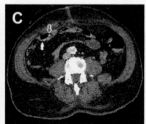

Fig. 6. 76 year old male inpatient with melena and hypotension. (*A*) Axial non-contrast enhanced studies show no hyperdensity within thin the small bowel. (*B*) Arterial phase images reveal an 8 mm polypoid lesion, which demonstrated avid arterial enhancement (*hollow arrow*). There is also active contrast extravasation distal to this lesion (*solid arrow*). (*C*) On delayed imaging, the polypoid lesion decreases in enhancement (*hollow arrow*) with increased pooling of contrast distally (*solid arrow*). These findings were consistent with an actively bleeding small bowel high flow vascular lesion.

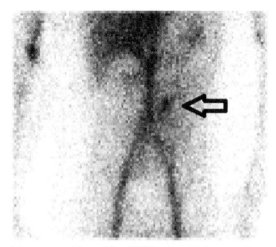

Fig. 7. A 68-year-old woman with positive FOBT and anemia, negative endoscopic workup. Planar image from a 99mTc-labeled red blood cell examination demonstrate radiotracer accumulation in the midabdomen to the left of midline (*arrow*), presumably in the small bowel. Subsequent conventional angiography (not shown) demonstrated bleeding related to an arteriovenous fistula from an ileal branch of the superior mesenteric artery that was coiled.

provide therapeutic intervention, this also can lead to complications, including bowel ischemia. In addition, as is the case with CTA, angiography requires the administration of iodinated contrast necessitating the same considerations in regard to patient renal function. The volume of dose as well as the radiation dose also varies depending on the complexity of the case.

Angiography is typically used for directed therapeutic intervention after diagnosis, therefore dictating which artery is cannulated. A positive result will seem as contrast extravasation outside the normal boundaries of a blood vessel that can increase over time provided the bleed is continuous (**Fig. 8**). After embolization, an angiogram is performed to confirm successful cessation of bleeding.

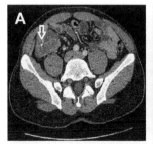
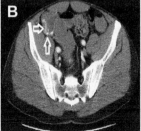
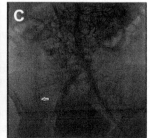

Fig. 8. A 50-year-old man who presented with bright red blood per rectum. A cecal polyp had been removed via colonoscopy 2 weeks before presentation. (*A*) A postpolypectomy CT image in the portal venous phase demonstrates a hyperdense clip within the cecum (*arrow*). (*B*) Axial arterial phase sequences at the time of presentation reveal active extravasation into the cecum (both *arrows*). The clip is also no longer identified. (*C*) Superior mesenteric angiography shows active extravasation within the right lower quadrant (*arrow*). Patient underwent embolization of an ileocolic artery.

CHRONIC (OCCULT) GASTROINTESTINAL BLEEDING

Chronic (occult) GI bleeding (OGIB) is defined as a positive FOBT and/or iron deficiency anemia, with no visible evidence of hemorrhage. In this population, initial investigation necessitates the determination of whether iron deficiency anemia is present. In patients with a positive FOBT and iron deficiency anemia, a colonoscopy and endoscopy should be performed.[26] If no iron deficiency is present, a colonoscopy is only advised unless the patient specifically reports upper GI symptoms.[26] Upper and lower endoscopies reveal a source of bleeding in 29% to 56% and 20% to 30%, respectively. Synchronous upper and lower GI sources are found in 1% to 17%.[27] When upper and lower endoscopy findings are abnormal, the bleeding is presumed to be originating from the small bowel and workup continues with small bowel investigation. Broad approaches to small bowel evaluation include CT enterography (CTE), enteroclysis, double balloon endoscopy (DBE), and video capsule endoscopy (VCE). The development of VCE has allowed for clinicians to evaluate the small bowel mucosa and is used as the first-line approach in 70% to 80% of patients for the evaluation of OGIB.[28] VCE identifies the source of the bleed in 40% to 60% of cases; however, there are several drawbacks, including low specificity, the potential for the capsule to become stuck/retained, incomplete small bowel visualization, as well as limited evaluation of submucosal lesions.[29] In comparison to VCE, CTE also provides information regarding extraluminal disease and can help with interventional planning, in addition to providing causes for OGIBs.[30] CTE may be considered a first-line approach in patients with known or suspected strictures because of risk of capsular retention. CTE and VCE should be considered complementary studies, with an abnormal VCE finding being followed by CTE and vice versa. DBE is a costly and time-consuming study and is typically reserved for patients with abnormal VCE/CTE findings. Patients with a negative workup may also benefit from using a Meckel radionuclide scan to evaluate for a Meckel diverticulum.

The term "obscure GI bleeding" is reserved for patients who have recurrent episodes of hemorrhage but in whom a complete diagnostic evaluation of the bowel does not reveal the source. There is no universal diagnostic algorithm to these patients, and the approach varies based on clinical presentation. In these instances, repeat upper/lower/video endoscopy may be performed to detect lesions that were missed or were otherwise obscured due to intraluminal contents, blood, or otherwise. These patients may additionally benefit from surgical evaluation, iron supplementation, and potentially observation, depending on the clinical preference and presentation.[31]

Computed Tomography Enterography

CTE is one of the most commonly implemented imaging studies to evaluate for OGIB. With hemodynamically stable patients, the goal of CTE revolves around the detection of causes for the bleed than the detection of acute bleeds.[20] To this end, CTE requires distension of small bowel with the ingestion of approximately 1350 to 1500 cc of neutral oral contrast over the course of 1 hour. In regards to intravenous contrast administration and multiphasic imaging, there is no universally agreed upon scanning protocol. Similar to CTA, a noncontrast-enhanced series may be obtained to identify any hyperattenuating materials within the bowel; however, this noncontrast series is optional and not included in most protocols. An arterial phase should be routinely acquired using bolus tracking triggering at the peak of arterial enhancement and that should be followed by with an enteric phase acquired 50 seconds after the injection. Delayed imaging at 90 seconds after injection may also be obtained,[20] but this is not standard in most protocols.

Similar to CTA, the advantages of CTE include the wide availability of the technology and the high spatial resolution. Inherent to the CTE, a wealth of information in regarding the entire length of the GI tract, anatomy, and extraluminal structures are obtained in contrast to direct intraluminal endoscopy. Disadvantages of CTE involve the radiation exposure with multiphasic imaging series.[32] However, advances in dose reduction techniques have lessened this limitation.[33] There is also the potential risk of exposure to iodinated intravenous contrast. In addition, the large amount of oral contrast may not be well tolerated by all patients. CT enteroclysis, which involves the use of a nasoenteric catheter to actively deliver contrast material to distend the small bowel, is an option for patients who do not tolerate the intake of oral contrast and who require a detailed CT examination of the small bowel. However, CT enteroclysis is somewhat invasive and also poorly tolerated by patients.

Findings on CTE are variable based on the cause of the bleeding, which includes vascular lesions, polyps, neoplasms, inflammation as seen in Crohn's disease, and heterotopic pancreatic/gastric tissue, among others.

Vascular abnormalities are categorized into angioectasias, arterial lesions, and all other lesions.[34] Of these lesions, the most common are angioectasias, which consist of thin tortuous veins that lack an internal elastic layer and classically appear with an arborizing pattern.[35] On CTE, angioectasias enhance on enteric phase and fade on delayed series. Their detection requires a close evaluation of intramural veins throughout the small bowel because nodular or elliptical terminal ends suggest angioectasias.[20] Although common in occurrence, they are typically multifocal and do not tend to bleed.[34] Arterial lesions, which include Dieulafoy lesions, arteriovenous malformations (AVM), and arteriovenous fistulas (AVF), are potentially life threatening because of their inherent high-flow nature.[36] Dieulafoy lesions are arterial vessels that protrude through a mucosal defect.[20] They are essentially normal vessels in an abnormal location and most commonly occur in the stomach, but approximately 16% can be found in the small bowel.[36] AVM and AVF result when there is an abnormal communication between a feeding artery and vein. Enlarged feeding artery and early draining vein suggest these abnormalities (**Fig. 9**). On CTE, arterial lesions will avidly enhance during the arterial phase and may become undetectable on enteric and delayed sequences[36] (see **Fig. 9**).

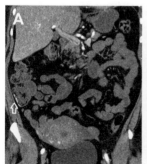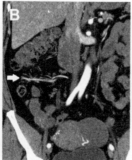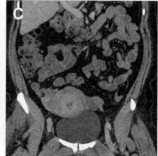

Fig. 9. A 45-year-old woman with iron deficiency anemia. (*A*) Coronal arterial phase image demonstrates nodular hyperenhancement foci in the wall of the cecum (*open arrow*). (*B*) Coronal arterial phase image shows an early draining vein (*solid arrow*). (*C*) Coronal enteric phase image demonstrates fading of the initial mural nodular enhancement. Findings strongly suggest an arteriovenous malformation.

Neoplasms in the small bowel include neuroendocrine tumors (NET), adenocarcinomas, lymphoma, GI stromal tumors (GIST), and metastasis, among others. The most common lesions are the NET, often times multifocal, which have a typical imaging appearance of a hyperenhancing mural nodule. Because of small size and typical plaquelike morphology, they can be difficult to detect on CTE.[37] Small bowel adenocarcinoma typically presents as a polypoid or constricting, hypoenhancing mass. Small bowel lymphoma can have a similar appearance, however may have aneurysmal dilation of the bowel. GIST has a variable imaging appearance and may be well circumscribed and enhancing when small. They start as a mural lesion and may extend endoluminally or exophytically as they grow[37] (**Fig. 10**). Small bowel metastasis most commonly occurs from intraperitoneal seeding; however, it also occurs from hematogenous or lymphatic spread. Imaging appearance is variable, and metastasis should always be considered in patients with small bowel mass with history of malignancy (**Fig. 11**).

Meckel Scan

A specific cause of occult bleed to consider, Meckel diverticulum, occurs in approximately 1% to 3% of the population.[38] Although most of them are asymptomatic, 38% of symptomatic patients present with bleeding as the most common presentation.[39] In addition, 50% of diverticula contain ectopic gastric tissue or ectopic pancreatic tissue.[40] The ^{99m}Tc pertechnetate scan (Meckel scan) is a radionuclide imaging study that exploits the ectopic gastric mucosa within a diverticulum. The study has been shown to have a sensitivity of 85% to 90% in the pediatric population and 62% in patients who are of 16 years of age and older.[40] However, a false-negative result may occur if the diverticulum contains only ectopic pancreatic tissue and is without ectopic gastric mucosa, because technetium pertechnetate does not demonstrate increased uptake within pancreatic tissue. In addition, false-positive results may occur when the scan detects ectopic gastric mucosa in another location, such as duplication cyst, gastrogenic cyst, or enteric duplication cyst.[41] Another advantage of a Meckel scan is the relative ease of execution.

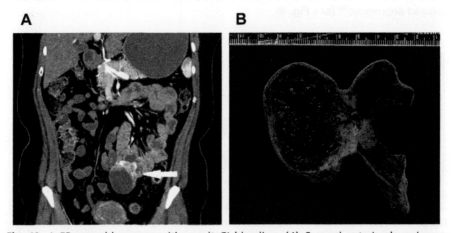

Fig. 10. A 53-year-old woman with occult GI bleeding. (*A*) Coronal enteric phase image demonstrates an exophytic mass extending from the jejunum (*arrow*) with mural hyperenhancement and central hypoenhancement (necrosis). (*B*) Pathology specimen demonstrates exophytic mass with central necrosis. Final diagnosis was a GIST.

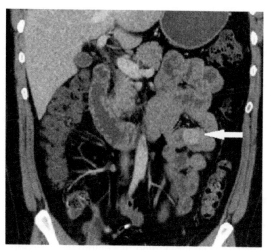

Fig. 11. Coronal enteric phase CT image demonstrates a hyperenhancing mass within the jejunum (*arrow*) in a 70-year-old man with known metastatic lung cancer. CTE was performed as part of a workup for recurrent abdominal pain.

Approximately 1.85 Mbq/kg of ^{99m}Tc pertechnetate is administered with images acquired dynamically at a frame rate of 1 static image per 30 to 60 seconds for a minimum of 30 minutes. The examination may be extended to 60 minutes if the clinically suspicion is high but initial images within the 30 minute examination are negative.[41] A normal scan result is identified by a focus of increased activity within the upper pelvis or lower abdominal region that appears at the same time the normal gastric mucosa becomes visible[41] (**Fig. 12**).

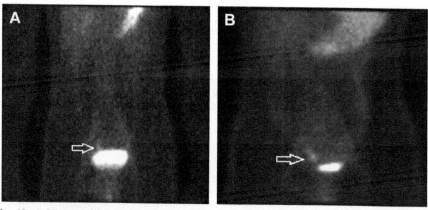

Fig. 12. A 26-year-old man who presented with multiple episodes of bright red blood per rectum. Initial CTA finding was normal for an active GI bleed. Esophagogastroduodenoscopy and colonoscopy also did not reveal a source of bleeding. The small bowel was thought to be the likely culprit. (*A*) Meckel scan shows increased pertechnetate uptake along the right lateral, superior dome of the bladder (*arrow*). (*B*) Postvoid imaging demonstrates a more clear focus of uptake, positive for a Meckel diverticulum (*arrow*). Note the similar intensity of radiotracer uptake in the diverticulum and stomach.

SUMMARY

GI bleeding can be broken up into overt, occult, and obscure types based on the clinical presentation and further categorized as upper or lower based on the location of the bleed. Imaging workup for overt bleeding is centered around CTA, conventional angiography, and nuclear scintigraphy. The main imaging tool for occult bleeding is CTE, with Meckel scan being a complementary tool in cases of abnormal CTE findings. Workup of obscure bleeding continues to be controversial, with a variable workup based on clinical status and provider preference.

REFERENCES

1. Peura DA, Lanza FL, Gostout CJ, et al. The American College of Gastroenterology Bleeding Registry: preliminary findings. Am J Gastroenterol 1997;92(6): 924–8.
2. Ernst AA, Haynes ML, Nick TG, et al. Usefulness of the blood urea nitrogen/creatinine ratio in gastrointestinal bleeding. Am J Emerg Med 1999;17(1):70–2.
3. Rockey DC. Gastrointestinal bleeding. In: Feldman M, Friedman LS, Brandt LJ, editors. Sleigenger and Fordtran's gastrointestinal and liver disease. 8th edition. Philadelphia: Saunders; 2006. p. 255–99.
4. Manning-Dimmitt LL, Dimmitt SG, Wilson GR. Diagnosis of gastrointestinal bleeding in adults. Am Fam Physician 2005;71(7):1339–46.
5. Zimmerman HM, Curfman K. Acute gastrointestinal bleeding. AACN Clin Issues 1997;8(3):449–58.
6. Lee EW, Laberge JM. Differential diagnosis of gastrointestinal bleeding. Tech Vasc Interv Radiol 2004;7(3):112–22.
7. Strate LL, Naumann CR. The role of colonoscopy and radiological procedures in the management of acute lower intestinal bleeding. Clin Gastroenterol Hepatol 2010;8(4):333–43 [quiz: e44].
8. Walsh RM, Anain P, Geisinger M, et al. Role of angiography and embolization for massive gastroduodenal hemorrhage. J Gastrointest Surg 1999;3(1):61–5 [discussion: 66].
9. Laing CJ, Tobias T, Rosenblum DI, et al. Acute gastrointestinal bleeding: emerging role of multidetector CT angiography and review of current imaging techniques. RadioGraphics 2007;27(4):1055–70.
10. Barkun AN, Bardou M, Kuipers EJ, et al. International consensus recommendations on the management of patients with nonvariceal upper gastrointestinal bleeding. Ann Intern Med 2010;152(2):101–13.
11. Palmer K. Non-variceal upper gastrointestinal haemorrhage: guidelines. Gut 2002;51(Suppl 4):iv1–6.
12. Frattaroli FM, Casciani E, Spoletini D, et al. Prospective study comparing multidetector row CT and endoscopy in acute gastrointestinal bleeding. World J Surg 2009;33(10):2209–17.
13. Lee SS, Oh TS, Kim HJ, et al. Obscure gastrointestinal bleeding: diagnostic performance of multidetector CT enterography. Radiology 2011;259(3):739–48.
14. Kerr SF, Puppala S. Acute g1astrointestinal haemorrhage: the role of the radiologist. Postgrad Med J 2011;87(1027):362.
15. García-Blázquez V, Vicente-Bártulos A, Olavarria-Delgado A, et al. Accuracy of CT angiography in the diagnosis of acute gastrointestinal bleeding: systematic review and meta-analysis. Eur Radiol 2013;23(5):1181–90.
16. Kuhle WG, Sheiman RG. Detection of active colonic hemorrhage with use of helical CT: findings in a Swine model. Radiology 2003;228(3):743–52.

17. Mayo-Smith WW, Hara AK, Mahesh M, et al. How i do it: managing radiation dose in CT. Radiology 2014;273(3):657–72.
18. Artigas JM, Martí M, Soto JA, et al. Multidetector CT angiography for acute gastrointestinal bleeding: technique and findings. RadioGraphics 2013;33(5): 1453–70.
19. Martí M, Artigas JM, Garzón G, et al. Acute lower intestinal bleeding: feasibility and diagnostic performance of CT angiography. Radiology 2012; 262(1):109–16.
20. Soto JA, Park SH, Fletcher JG, et al. Gastrointestinal hemorrhage: evaluation with MDCT. Abdom Imaging 2015;40(5):993–1009.
21. Kirchhof K, Welzel T, Mecke C, et al. Differentiation of white, mixed, and red thrombi: value of CT in estimation of the prognosis of thrombolysis—phantom study. Radiology 2003;228(1):126–30.
22. Hamilton JD, Kumaravel M, Censullo ML, et al. Multidetector CT evaluation of active extravasation in blunt abdominal and pelvic trauma patients. RadioGraphics 2008;28(6):1603–16.
23. Zuckier LS. Acute gastrointestinal bleeding. Semin Nucl Med 2003;33(4): 297–311.
24. Howarth DM. The role of nuclear medicine in the detection of acute gastrointestinal bleeding. Semin Nucl Med 2006;36(2):133–46.
25. Laine L. Acute and chronic gastrointestinal bleeding. Gastrointestinal and liver disease: pathophysiology, diagnosis, and management. Philadelphia: WB Saunders; 1998. p. 198–218.
26. Raju GS, Gerson L, Das A, et al. American Gastroenterological Association (AGA) Institute medical position statement on obscure gastrointestinal bleeding. Gastroenterology 2007;133(5):1694–6.
27. Zuckerman GR, Prakash C, Askin MP, et al. AGA technical review on the evaluation and management of occult and obscure gastrointestinal bleeding. Gastroenterology 2000;118(1):201–21.
28. Tatar EL, Shen EH, Palance AL, et al. Clinical utility of wireless capsule endoscopy: experience with 200 cases. J Clin Gastroenterol 2006;40(2):140–4.
29. Gerson LB, Fidler JL, Cave DR, et al. ACG clinical guideline: diagnosis and management of small bowel bleeding. Am J Gastroenterol 2015;110(9):1265–87 [quiz: 1288].
30. Huprich JE, Fletcher JG, Alexander JA, et al. Obscure gastrointestinal bleeding: evaluation with 64-section multiphase CT enterography—initial experience. Radiology 2008;246(2):562–71.
31. Gerson LB. Small bowel bleeding: updated algorithm and outcomes. Gastrointest Endosc Clin N Am 2017;27(1):171–80.
32. Huprich JE, Fletcher JG, Fidler JL, et al. Prospective blinded comparison of wireless capsule endoscopy and multiphase CT enterography in obscure gastrointestinal bleeding. Radiology 2011;260(3):744–51.
33. Baker ME, Hara AK, Platt JF, et al. CT enterography for Crohn's disease: optimal technique and imaging issues. Abdom Imaging 2015;40(5):938–52.
34. Yano T, Yamamoto H, Sunada K, et al. Endoscopic classification of vascular lesions of the small intestine. Gastrointest Endosc 2008;67:169–72.
35. Raju GS, Gerson L, Das A, et al. American Gastroenterological Association (AGA) institute technical review on obscure gastrointestinal bleeding. Gastroenterology 2007;133:1697–717.
36. Huprich JE, Barlow JM, Hansel SL, et al. Multiphase CT enterography evaluation of small-bowel vascular lesions. Am J Roentgenol 2013;201(1):65–72.

37. McLaughlin PD, Maher MM. Primary malignant diseases of the small intestine. Am J Roentgenol 2013;201(1):W9–14.
38. Turgeon DK, Barnett JL. Meckel's diverticulum. Am J Gastroenterol 1990;85(7): 777–81.
39. Park JJ, Wolff BG, Tollefson MK, et al. Meckel diverticulum: the mayo clinic experience with 1476 patients (1950–2002). Ann Surg 2005;241(3):529–33.
40. Lin S, Suhocki P, Ludwig K, et al. Gastrointestinal bleeding in adult patients with Meckel's diverticulum: the role of technetium 99m pertechnetate scan. South Med J 2002;95(11):1338–41.
41. Grady E. Gastrointestinal bleeding scintigraphy in the early 21st century. J Nucl Med 2016;57(2):252–9.

The Natural History of Colorectal Polyps

Overview of Predictive Static and Dynamic Features

Perry J. Pickhardt, MD[a,b],*, Bryan Dustin Pooler, MD[b],
David H. Kim, MD[b], Cesare Hassan, MD[b],
Kristina A. Matkowskyj, MD, PhD[b], Richard B. Halberg, PhD[b]

KEYWORDS

- Colorectal cancer • Colorectal polyps • CT colonography • Virtual colonoscopy
- Optical colonoscopy

KEY POINTS

- Subcentimeter colorectal polyps are highly prevalent in adults.
- Subcentimeter colorectal polyps are invariably benign, and the vast majority will never develop into cancer.
- Polyp size is an important determinant of clinical relevance and management.
- Polyp growth rates provide further insight into natural history and clinical significance.
- CT colonography is unique among screening tools by allowing for accurate assessment of volumetric growth rates, which are likely tied to underlying genetic and epigenetic alterations.

INTRODUCTION

It is widely accepted that colorectal cancers (CRC) generally derive from once benign dysplastic colorectal polyps. However, it is also true that colorectal polyps are a highly prevalent human condition, affecting most of the adults according to recent

Disclosures: Dr P.J. Pickhardt is the co-founder of VirtuoCTC; advisor to Check-Cap and Bracco; and shareholder in SHINE, Elucent, and Cellectar Biosciences; Dr D.H. Kim is the co-founder of VirtuoCTC and shareholder in Elucent and Cellectar Biosciences. This work was supported in part by NIH NCI grant 1R01 CA220004-01.
[a] University of Wisconsin School of Medicine & Public Health, 600 Highland Avenue, Madison, WI, 53793 USA; [b] Digestive Endoscopy Unit, Nuovo Regina Margherita Hospital, Via Emilio Morosini 30, 00153, Rome, Italy
* Corresponding author. University of Wisconsin School of Medicine & Public Health, 600 Highland Avenue, Madison, WI, 53793 USA.
E-mail address: ppickhardt2@uwhealth.org

Gastroenterol Clin N Am 47 (2018) 515–536
https://doi.org/10.1016/j.gtc.2018.04.004
0889-8553/18/© 2018 Elsevier Inc. All rights reserved.

endoscopic screening data. As such, the most of the colorectal polyps behave in a benign fashion and will of course never develop into cancer. Furthermore, although the precise timing and sequence of events for progression to cancer have not yet been fully elucidated, the typical dwell time for this infrequent transformation is likely a decade or more, whether via the classic adenocarcinoma sequence or the serrated polyp pathway. When taking all these factors into consideration, CRC can clearly be effectively prevented through the detection and removal of benign dysplastic colorectal polyps, but also a strategy of universal polypectomy is an inefficient approach, leading to excessive resource utilization, costs, and complications. At the other end of the spectrum, tests that primarily target cancer detection ignore the larger benefit of cancer prevention. Between these 2 extremes, a more rational CRC screening approach that targets large and/or growing polyps and early cancers likely represents a more clinically efficacious and cost-effective strategy.

A large and ever-growing volume of data exist surrounding static cross-sectional features of colorectal polyps, such as lesion size, morphology, and location, and their relationship to underlying histologic features. Much of these data come from large colonoscopic databases, where detected polyps are removed without any knowledge of their preceding growth rates. With the emergence of computed tomography colonography (CTC) as an attractive CRC screening tool, the authors have the ability to follow polyps longitudinally before resection. This dynamic in vivo investigation also provides unique opportunities for studying the natural history of polyps, such as correlating growth rates with underlying polyp histology and genetic alterations. These insights could ultimately inform future strategies for screening and surveillance, as well as fuel novel theories on tumor evolution.

CROSS-SECTIONAL (STATIC) POLYP DATA: SIZE, MORPHOLOGY, AND LOCATION

Static polyp features, including lesion size, morphology, and anatomic location, have long served as the major determinants of clinical significance. Of these, polyp size is likely the single most important consideration, because it directly correlates with important histologic features such as high-grade dysplasia (HGD) and invasive cancer.[1,2] However, polyp morphology and segmental location can both further enhance classification and risk stratification, as discussed later after polyp size considerations. Implicit in this discussion on static polyp features is ensuring sensitive detection by both CTC and optical colonoscopy (OC), because this represents the only means for preventing polyp progression.

Given the extremely high prevalence of subcentimeter (sub-cm) colorectal polyps and their potential influence on screening algorithms, it is critical to first focus attention on this subset. Sub-cm polyps are further subdivided into diminutive ($\leq$5 mm) and small (6–9 mm) size categories. Although abundant prior cumulative evidence has demonstrated very low rates of HGD and exceedingly low (or even nonexistent) rates of cancer among sub-cm polyps,[1–3] a recent study by Ponugoti and colleagues[4] has further crystallized these findings. This report on greater than 40,000 sub-cm colorectal polyps resected at OC has substantially increased our cumulative experience. From prior observational series, rates of HGD and invasive cancer typically ranged from 0.5% to 0.8% and 0% to 0.5%, respectively for small polyps, and would be even lower for diminutive lesions.[2] The large study by Ponugoti and colleagues[4] essentially doubles the cumulative data on sub-cm polyps. In this study, rates of HGD and invasive cancer among diminutive conventional adenomas and small conventional adenomas were 0.3% and 0% and 0.8% and 0%, respectively. Reported rates of advanced histology (villous component, HGD, or invasive cancer) are somewhat higher, typically around 0.3% to 1.2% for diminutive adenomas and 2.9% to 5.3% for small adenomas. However, as witnessed by the very low rates of HGD and cancer, sub-cm advanced adenomas are therefore almost exclusively determined by a prominent villous component, which is of more debatable immediate clinical relevance. The actual prevalence of advanced diminutive and small polyps (as the largest advanced lesion) has been estimated at 0.1% to 0.3% and 0.3% to 0.6%, respectively.[5]

From the preceding discussion, it can be concluded that colorectal polyps less than 10 mm in size can be considered to behave in a benign fashion—but what about larger polyps? According to more recent data, including our own experience with CTC, large polyps measuring 1 to 2 cm harbor invasive cancer is only about 1% of cases (or less).[1,2] This percentage is considerably lower than the traditional quote of 5% to 10% cancer risk that was based on older surgical literature. For colorectal masses (3 cm or larger), rates of HGD and invasive cancer increase precipitously with lesion size. However, in our CTC screening experience, approximately 50% of OC-confirmed and resected colorectal lesions greater than or equal to 3 cm prove to not be invasive cancers, most often tubulovillous adenomas, villous adenomas, and serrated polyps (sessile serrated and traditional subtypes). Carpet lesions (flat superficially spreading tumors) comprise a substantial proportion of these benign but potentially premalignant "masses", because their large linear size belies their limited tumor bulk in terms of volume (**Fig. 1**).[6] This has been indirectly supported by a large OC database of large superficial colorectal lesions (mean size, 3.7 cm), where the rate of submucosal invasion was only 7.6%.[7]

Beyond polyp size, lesion morphology has also long been recognized as an important static determinant of clinical significance. For example, pedunculated polyps tend to be larger in size relative to sessile polyps, on average, and more often have tubulovillous or villous architecture at histologic evaluation. For flat (nonpolypoid) lesions, however, controversy and confusion exist in terms of their clinical relevance and rate of growth. To clarify, "flat" is somewhat of a misnomer because these lesions are typically raised slightly at the edges in a plaquelike manor and only rarely truly flush with the surrounding mucosa.[8–10] At colonoscopy, most of the so-called aggressive flat lesions are mixed lateral spreading tumors characterized by a typically large sessile nodular component emerging from a flatter carpetlike lesion. Because the invasive cancer component tends to be associated with the polypoid portion, these lesions would be readily identified at CTC as sessile lesions in the first place. Furthermore, because a very small subset of these flat lesions might be more aggressive in nature, especially those with a central depression, some have assumed that all flat lesions are therefore more aggressive in general. However, our experience has been quite the opposite, with flat lesions acting more benign and indolent in nature (especially for their typically large linear size, as noted earlier) compared with their polypoid counterparts.[6,10] Because flat lesions are less conspicuous at both OC and CTC, they are more likely to be missed on initial evaluation, leading to the appearance of a rapidly growing new lesion as opposed to the true case. As discussed in the later dynamic section, large flat lesions missed at initial evaluation often show little or no progression at follow-up CTC examinations. Increased awareness and improved techniques at both CTC and OC are leading to the detection of more and more flat colorectal lesions, many of which are right-sided serrated lesions.[11,12]

Given the recent strides in the awareness and understanding of serrated polyps and their associated alternative pathway to cancer,[11–14] these lesions deserve separate consideration. Sessile serrated polyps (SSPs; also referred to as "sessile serrated adenomas" or SSP/As), previously mischaracterized as hyperplastic polyps without

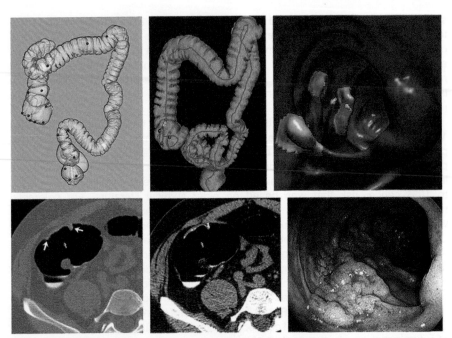

Fig. 1. Carpet lesions (flat superficially spreading tumors). Three-dimensional (3D) CTC map (*upper row, left*) shows anatomic locations (1 *red dot* for each patient) of colorectal carpet lesions detected at CTC in the authors' experience. Except for 2 cases, all carpet lesions were located in the proximal right colon or rectosigmoid colon. The remaining images are from a cecal carpet lesion detected at CTC screening in a 50-year-old man. Three-dimensional colon map (*upper row, middle*) and 3D endoluminal CTC view (*upper row, right*) show 3 CAD marks in the cecum (*yellow dots* and *blue regions* with *arrows*, respectively), which identify focal areas of a broad 3.5-cm carpet lesion. The lesion is located across from the normal-appearing ileocecal. Transverse 2D images in polyp window (*lower row, left*) and soft-tissue window (*lower row, middle*) confirm a flat soft-tissue lesion (*arrows*). Note the etching of positive oral contrast material on the surface of the lesion, which is better seen on soft tissue windowing. The lesion was confirmed at same-day colonoscopy (*lower row, right*) and proved to be a tubulovillous adenoma without HGD after laparoscopic right hemicolectomy. (*From* Pickhardt PJ, Lam VP, Weiss JM, et al. Carpet lesions detected at CT colonography: clinical, imaging, and pathologic features. Radiology 2014;270:435–43; with permission.)

malignant potential, may ultimately account for up to 20% to 25% of sporadic CRC.[14] The serrated pathway of carcinogenesis is characterized by mutations in BRAF and epigenetic methylation that silence mismatch repair genes and lead to cancers with microsatellite instability.[11,14] The time course for this transformation is many years, possibly longer than that of the adenocarcinoma sequence (natural history behavior at CTC is discussed later). This is supported by a recent colonoscopy series of large SSPs (mean size, 2.9 cm), where the rate of invasive cancer was only 3.9%; another 3.3% showed high-grade cytologic dysplasia without invasive cancer.[15] SSPs tend to be right-sided in location and flat in morphology and were likely a common cause of screen failures at OC (and CTC) owing to their often subtle appearance.[16,17] Fortunately, many of these SSP lesions exhibit a mucus cap on their surface, which allows for improved detection at both OC and CTC (**Fig. 2**). Luminal contrast agents (particularly barium), however, are needed to leverage this advantage at CTC by

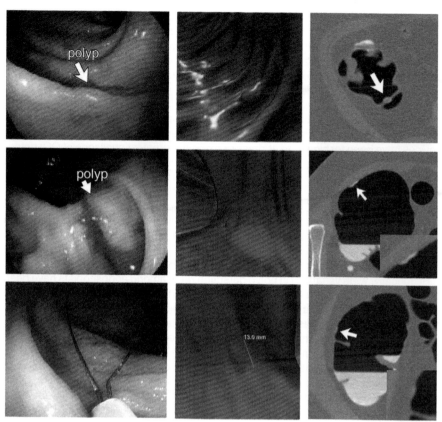

Fig. 2. SSPs detected at screening CTC. Three different patients with right-sided SSPs (each row corresponds to one patient) detected at screening CTC. OC images (*left images* in each row) depict the flat, subtle nature of these large right-sided polyps. CTC 3D endoluminal images show the corresponding appearance that led to detection and same-day referral for polypectomy at colonoscopy. Notice that the polyps are slightly more prominent and protruding at CTC compared with the OC. Transverse 2D CTC images (*right images*) demonstrate how the 3D appearance represents a combination of the flat polyp and the overlying adherent tagging contrast agent (*arrows*). Magnified images (*insets* on lower 2 rows) better depict the subtle soft-tissue thickening underneath the overlying contrast cap. (*From* Kim DH, Matkowskyj KA, Lubner MG, et al. Serrated polyps at CT colonography: prevalence and characteristics of the serrated polyp spectrum. Radiology 2016;280:455–63; with permission.)

preferentially coating the lesional surface.[11,12] This contrast surface coating phenomenon at CTC is critical for improved detection of flat lesions in general, whether serrated or adenomatous (see **Fig. 1**).[18,19] Lack of barium tagging (and possibly also lack of reader awareness) in a recent Dutch trial[20] might account for the decreased detection of SSPs relative to OC. Our experience in CTC detection of SSPs (and the less common traditional serrated adenoma) seems to be different.[11] Previous OC studies have also described markedly variable rates in SSP detection.[17] In general, simple awareness of the subtle nature of SSPs is the first critical step in their detection at either OC or CTC. In addition, it has been recently shown that cytologic dysplasia in large SSP/As is usually associated with a sessile polypoid component that would be readily identifiable at CTC.[15]

A wide variety of novel OC techniques and approaches are also provided for improved detection and clinical management of colorectal polyps.[21] Improvements in bowel preparation, such as split regimen dosing of the cathartic agent, may seem mundane, but 1 randomized trial showed a 35% increase in advanced adenoma detection with the split regimen.[22] Endoscopist factors include scope withdrawal time and retraining in newer techniques.[21,23] Most advances relate to improvements in endoscope technology and technique.[21] Wider lens angles and, more recently, lenses that are lateral to the tip of the scope (full spectrum endoscopy) help to close the gap on the mucosal coverage advantage enjoyed by CTC.[24] Several OC add-on devices have been fashioned to address perhaps the greatest challenge at OC: detection of right-sided lesions, especially those behind folds (**Fig. 3**).[25,26] These devices include a variety of fitted caps, cuffs, or rings on the scope tip to flatten folds, as well retrograde camera angles to image behind folds. Finally, several approaches aim to improve OC detection of flat lesions, especially those in the right colon.[21] Dye-spraying chromoendoscopy can improve detection of subtle flat lesions, but is generally considered too cumbersome to perform on a routine basis for screening. Electronic processing of white light, as with narrow band imaging, provides a form of virtual chromoendoscopy, but its additive value for polyp detection is less clear.

Historically, wide variations in polyp detection rates among endoscopists have been associated with OC,[23] particularly when compared with CTC performance.[27] The aforementioned measures for improving OC have presumably helped close this gap. Considerable emphasis has recently been placed on the adenoma detection rate (ADR) by endoscopists, which can be considered a proxy measure for examination quality.[28] However, a more relevant measure would be the advanced ADR, because most of the OC-detected adenomas will be diminutive in size and of doubtful clinical significance. Although higher ADRs at screening OC are associated with a reduction in CRC risk,[29] excessive focus on this statistic alone might shift attention away from clinically relevant lesions to those of little or no importance. Finally, resect

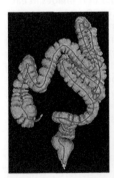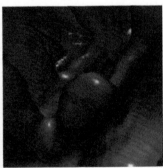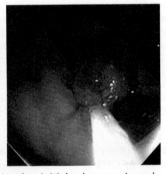

Fig. 3. Malignant right-sided polyp in ascending colon missed at initial colonoscopic evaluation. Three-dimensional colon map (*right*) shows the location of a large polyp in the ascending colon at CTC; 3D endoluminal CTC view shows the large polypoid lesion on or adjacent to a fold. This patient was enrolled in the DoD CTC screening trial. This polyp was not found at initial colonoscopy immediately following CTC. However, after segmental unblinding of the CTC results, the polyp was eventually found after several attempts to reposition the instrument because of repeated slippage in this region. Invasive adenocarcinoma was confirmed at surgery. (*From* Pickhardt PJ, Nugent PA, Mysliwiec PA, et al. Location of adenomas missed by optical colonoscopy. Ann Intern Med 2004;141:352–9; with permission.)

and discard strategies may help alleviate some of the cost burden related to diminutive lesions.[30] However, molecular analysis of even these diminutive lesions may identify patients at increased risk for ultimately developing CRC and consequently this analysis could affect individualized screening intervals.

LONGITUDINAL (DYNAMIC) POLYP DATA: GROWTH RATES AND NATURAL HISTORY

Despite the wealth of data on static polyp features that correlate with increased risk, the fate of resected polyps had they been left in place cannot be inferred. Although it is clear from the existing cross-sectional data that sub-cm polyps behave in an overwhelmingly benign fashion, in vivo longitudinal follow-up with at least 2 time points is required to actually determine growth rates and progression.

The natural history of colorectal polyps, especially those less than 10 mm in size, has become a highly relevant clinical issue. Although largely missed and ignored by stool-based tests and generally removed when detected by OC, the situation is quite different for CTC, which allows for the opportunity of selective referral for polyp removal.[31] This important filtering function minimizes unnecessary resource utilization and complications related to removal of pseudodisease.[32] Overall screen detection rates of nondiminutive polyps (≥6 mm) have been shown to be similar in prospective CTC-OC trials.[32,33] In contrast, performance drops off for CTC detection of diminutive lesions. Although it is undoubtedly highly efficacious and cost-effective to refer all large CTC-detected polyps to OC, isolated diminutive lesions (≤5 mm) are actually intentionally ignored at CTC, given the absence of cancer and low rates of HGD, as discussed earlier.[34,35] For small polyps (6–9 mm) detected at CTC, however, the appropriate management is less certain, and may depend on several factors, including patient preference and health condition. Although we know from the preceding static data that these small polyps are invariably benign, the likelihood of ultimate progression to cancer is quite low, but certainly not zero. Based on both clinical and economic modeling, one could make a plausible argument for either immediate polypectomy or CTC surveillance,[34–36] choices that were reflected in the first major guidelines governing CTC.[37] As such, the CTC practice of in vivo surveillance of unresected lesions is providing new insights into the natural history of colorectal polyps. However, before delving into this unique CTC experience, a brief review of the cumulative data on polyp growth rates based on older colorectal modalities is warranted.

Before CTC surveillance, several older endoscopy and barium enema studies reported on experiences with small unresected polyps. Although these studies were limited in their ability to precisely localize and measure polyps, a fair amount of preliminary data on polyp natural history exists from these older longitudinal trials. Some of these studies were published over 50 years ago. When considered together as a group, all of these longitudinal studies have repeatedly shown the benign, indolent nature of unresected sub-cm colorectal polyps.

In a longitudinal study using barium enemas to follow unresected colorectal polyps, Welin and colleagues[38] showed exceedingly slow growth rates by studying 375 unresected polyps over a mean interval of 30 months. In Norway, Hofstad and colleagues[39] performed serial colonoscopy on unresected 189 sub-cm polyps, finding that only one (0.5%) lesion eclipsed the 10-mm threshold after a 1-year time interval. At the 3-year follow-up mark, most polyps in this study remained stable or even regressed in size, with an overall tendency to net regression amongst small (5–9 mm) polyps.[40] The investigators of this endoscopic trial concluded that following unresected 5 to 9 mm polyps for 3 years was a safe practice. Other longitudinal studies using flexible sigmoidoscopy have also demonstrated the stability of small polyps over time.[41–43]

In one study that used serial sigmoidoscopy to follow polyps measuring up to 15 mm in size over a 3 to 5 year period, Knoernschild[41] reported a significant increase in polyp size in only 4% of patients. In a classic study by Stryker and colleagues[44] using barium enema for surveillance, the cumulative 5-year and 10-year risks of cancer related to large colorectal polyps ($\geq$10 mm) left in place were less than 3% and 10%, respectively. Although routine polypectomy remains indicated for large colorectal lesions, the indolent nature suggested by this study matches the static data for 1- to 2-cm polyps discussed earlier. In the National Polyp Study, the high observed ADRs noted at surveillance, in conjunction with the low observed CRC incidence, was thought to be explainable (indirectly) only by the regression of adenomas.[45] More recently, a longitudinal colonoscopy study by Togashi and colleagues[46] followed 412 diminutive polyps over an average interval of 3.6 years in patients who had previously undergone CRC resection. At the final OC examination, 74% were stable or decreased in size, 15% were increased in size, and 11% could not be identified. Of 88 resected polyps, histology showed neither HGD nor cancer in any case.

Although these longitudinal endoscopic and barium enema studies provide some reassurance of the benign course of sub-cm polyps, detail is lacking regarding polyp growth rates and clinical implications. These shortcomings are largely addressed by CTC surveillance. CTC is an ideal tool for polyp monitoring, because it allows for both precise localization and size assessment. Confirming whether a detected polyp is in the exact same location over serial studies is difficult with endoscopy but rather straightforward with CTC, where confident determination of specific localization is possible. Beyond improved linear size measurement, CTC also has the distinct advantage of volumetric assessment, which greatly amplifies interval changes in polyp size compared with linear measurement.[47] Because the initial standard of care was to refer all CTC-detected polyps measuring greater than or equal to 6 mm to OC for polypectomy, the authors undertook a prospective natural history trial to follow small (6–9 mm) polyps at CTC.[48]

This ongoing polyp natural history trial was initiated at the University of Wisconsin (UW) in 2004, with the National Naval Medical Center (NNMC) in Bethesda, MD joining soon after. Complementary protocols provided histology-rich data in the NNMC arm, whereby all polyps were resected after 1-year CTC surveillance, and longer follow-up intervals in the UW arm, where only progressing polyps were typically referred for polypectomy. Consenting patients with only small polyps (6–9 mm in size, 1–2 in number) detected at initial CTC screening were enrolled for in vivo CTC surveillance. Progression, stability, and regression of polyps at follow-up CTC were based on a 20% volumetric change per year from baseline (ie, 20% or more growth for progression; −20% or more reduction for regression; and stability when annual change is <20% in either direction). Results from the initial 8-year period of investigation involved 243 adults (mean age, 57.4 years; 106 [37%] women) with 306 small colorectal polyps. The mean surveillance interval was 2.3 ± 1.4 years (range 1–7 years). In total, 68 (22%) of the 306 polyps progressed by the volumetric criteria discussed earlier (**Fig. 4**), 153 (50%) were stable, and 85 (28%) regressed, including an apparent total resolution of the polyp in 32 (10%) cases (**Fig. 5**).

At the time of submission, polyp histology had been established in 131 lesions that were confirmed and removed at colonoscopy. Of the 23 proven advanced adenomas, 21 (91%) progressed in size; the other 2 advanced adenomas both had positive growth rates (8%/year) but were less than the +20%/year defining threshold. In comparison, 31 (37%) of 84 proven nonadvanced adenomas progressed in size, and only 15 (8%) of 198 other resected lesions ($P < .0001$) progress. Of note, serrated polyps represented a major subset of this the "other" category, but these lesions were not

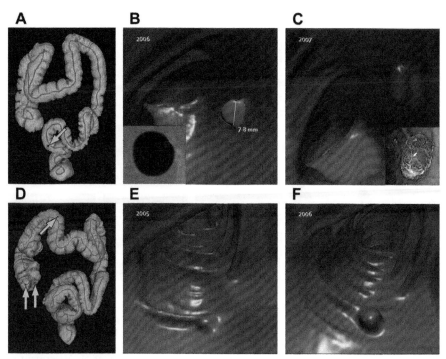

Fig. 4. Interval progression of small colorectal polyps in 2 patients undergoing CTC surveillance. 3D colon map from CTC (*A*) showing the location of a small sigmoid polyp (*arrow, red dot*), which measured 7.8 mm at the index screening examination (*B*). Polyp segmentation for volume measurement is shown on both 3D and 2D (*inset*) views of B. At follow-up CTC 1 year later (*C*), the polyp grew only 0.8 mm in linear size but showed a 50% increase in volume (to 205 mm^3). The lesion proved to be a tubulovillous adenoma after polypectomy at same-day colonoscopy (*inset*). 3D colon map (*D*) in a second patient showing the location of 3 small polyps in the right colon (*arrows, red dots*). 3D images from the index CTC (*E*) and surveillance CTC 16 months later (*F*) show a small sessile polyp in the proximal transverse colon that increased from 6.0 mm to 8.0 mm, but increased in volume by 203% (153% per year). Similar growth was seen with the 2 cecal polyps (not shown). The polyp in the transverse colon was a tubular adenoma, whereas the cecal lesions were both tubulovillous adenomas. (*From* Pickhardt PJ, Kim DH, Pooler BD, et al. Assessment of volumetric growth rates of small colorectal polyps with CT colonography: a longitudinal study of natural history. Lancet Oncol 2013;14:711–20; with permission.)

yet recognized as such. The odds ratio for a growing polyp at CTC surveillance to become an advanced adenoma was 15.6 (95% CI: 7.6–31.7) compared with 6 to 9 mm polyps detected and removed at initial CTC screening (without surveillance). Polyp volume showed a mean 77% annual increase for the 23 proven advanced adenomas, compared with a 16% annual increase for 84 proven nonadvanced adenomas, and a 13% annual *decrease* for all other polyps, including serrated, nonneoplastic, and unresected polyps ($P<.0001$) (**Fig. 6**). An absolute polyp volume of more than 180 mm^3 at surveillance CTC was predictive of advanced neoplasia with a sensitivity of 92% (22 of 24 polyps), specificity of 94% (266 of 282 polyps), positive-predictive value of 58% (22 of 38 polyps), and negative-predictive value of 99% (266 of 268 polyps).

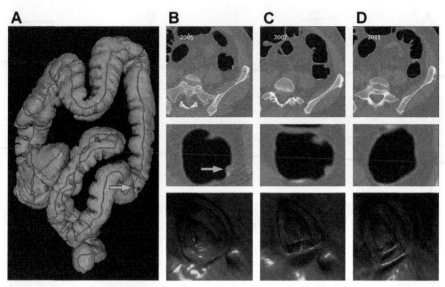

Fig. 5. Polyp regression at CTC surveillance. 3D colon map (*A*) showing the location of a 6.2 mm polyp in the descending colon (*arrows, red dot*) detected at screening CTC (*B*). Surveillance CTC 2 years later (*C*) showed no interval change in size. By the time of continued surveillance (*D*), 6.4 years after the initial CTC, the polyp had completely resolved. Detection of the small polyp on the intermediate CTC in 2007 essentially excludes the possibility of a false-positive interpretation. (*From* Pickhardt PJ, Kim DH, Pooler BD, et al. Assessment of volumetric growth rates of small colorectal polyps with CT colonography: a longitudinal study of natural history. Lancet Oncol 2013;14:711–20; with permission.)

Changes in linear size of polyps also correlated with histology in this trial, albeit the magnitude of these changes was blunted relative to the amplified volumetric changes (see **Fig. 4**). In general, linear measurement leads to an increased proportion of lesions categorized as stable. For example, the percentage of advanced adenomas categorized as stable by the 3 different linear size criteria (changes of <1 mm per year, <10% per year, and <25% total) ranged from 38% to 58%, compared with only 8% to 12% categorized as stable for 3 volumetric criteria (changes of <20% per year, <15 mm^3 per year, and <30% total). Only 5% of all 6 to 9 mm polyps exceeded 10 mm in size at final CTC follow-up. Lesion morphology also correlated with future growth pattern, with 45% of pedunculated polyps showing growth, compared with 21% of sessile polyps and 8% of flat lesions (*P* < .0001). Again, our experience with flat lesions argues against a more aggressive nature.

A second longitudinal study of small colorectal polyps using CTC surveillance was published 2 years later by a Dutch group.[49] A total of 70 patients with one or two 6 to 9 mm colorectal polyps identified at the index CTC underwent surveillance a mean 3.3 years later. Of these, 57 patients underwent subsequent colonoscopy with polypectomy of 68 polyps. Defining progression as a greater than or equal to 30% increase in polyp volume, the investigators found that after 3 years, 35% of polyps progressed in size, 38% remained stable, and 27% regressed, with apparent resolution in 14%. Advanced histology was present in 47% of the progressing polyps, 21% of stable polyps, and none of the regressing polyps. None of the resected polyps harbored HGD or CRC. Overall, these results are in concert with our natural history trial.[48]

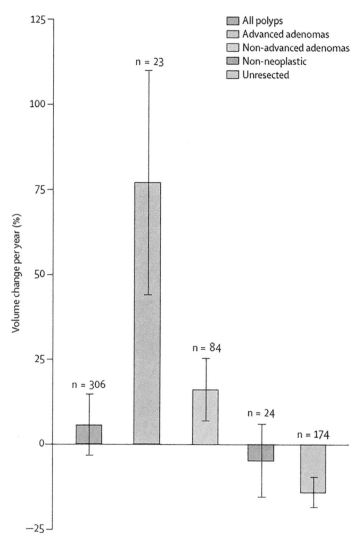

Fig. 6. Polyp growth according to histologic subgroup. Polyp growth categories are shown according to the definition 20% volume change per year as progression or regression. Note overall mean growth in adenomas, especially those that are advanced. (*From* Pickhardt PJ, Kim DH, Pooler BD, et al. Assessment of volumetric growth rates of small colorectal polyps with CT colonography: a longitudinal study of natural history. Lancet Oncol 2013;14:711–20; with permission.)

Little longitudinal work has focused on diminutive colorectal lesions (≤5 mm) in size. This reality is due in part to the difficulty of confidently identifying these lesions on index and follow-up studies, but also if small (6–9 mm) polyps are safe to follow, diminutive lesions would be as well. The Japanese colonoscopic surveillance by Togashi and colleagues[46] described earlier showed that, even in patients with high-risk CRC, diminutive lesions are of little or no immediate concern. In reviewing our own experience with routine 5- to 10-year CTC screening after initial negative screening in 1429 adults,[16] the authors were able to indirectly assess the natural history of diminutive lesions. Because potential isolated diminutive lesions (ie, without associated polyps ≥6 mm) constitute a negative CTC screening examination, the 5-year CTC routine screening follow-up effectively represents a surveillance study for these highly prevalent diminutive lesions. Given the acceptably low rate of positive nondiminutive findings at follow-up screening (lower than the initial round of CTC screening), this study provided further evidence that nonreporting of isolated diminutive lesions at CTC screening is a valid clinical approach. Not surprisingly, the authors were able to identify some diminutive lesions that progressed to nondiminutive polyps (**Fig. 7**). Of the nondiminutive lesions missed at initial CTC screening but detected at follow-up, many were large, flat, right-sided serrated lesions. The natural history of serrated lesions has not been well established and has been the source of ongoing debate. In our CTC experience to date, these flat serrated lesions tend to show an indolent course, with little or no growth seen in most cases, even at 5 or more years (**Fig. 8**). In general, flat lesions seem to portend a lower risk for future advanced neoplasia, an observation noted by the Pathologist from the National Polyp Study.[50] Given our ever-expanding experience with serrated lesions at CTC, the authors specifically intend to study their natural history in the near future.

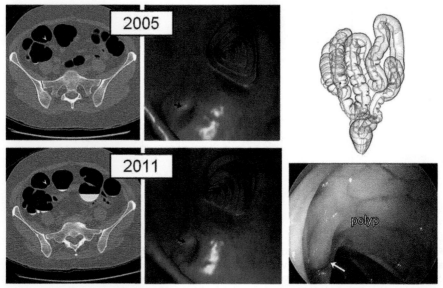

Fig. 7. Diminutive polyp at initial CTC screening that grew into small size at follow-up screening 6 years later in an asymptomatic woman (61 years old at initial screening). Top: 2D (*left*) and 3D (*middle*) images from the initial CTC screening in 2005 show a diminutive lesion (*arrowhead* for 2D, *arrow* for 3D) measuring less than 5 mm in the proximal transverse colon. The specific colonic location is indicated on the colon map (*right*) by the red dot. We do not report isolated diminutive lesions at CTC screening. Bottom: 2D (*left*) and 3D (*middle*) images from repeat CTC screening in 2011 show that the sessile polyp has grown in the intervening 6 years, now measuring 7 mm (*arrowhead* for 2D, *arrow* for 3D). The polyp was confirmed (*arrow*) and removed at same-day colonoscopy (*right*) and proved to be a tubular adenoma at pathologic evaluation. Most of the diminutive lesions do not progress to nondiminutive size. (*From* Pickhardt PJ, Pooler BD, Mbah I, et al. Colorectal findings at repeat CT colonography screening after initial CT colonography screening negative for polyps larger than 5 mm. Radiology 2017;282:139–48; with permission.)

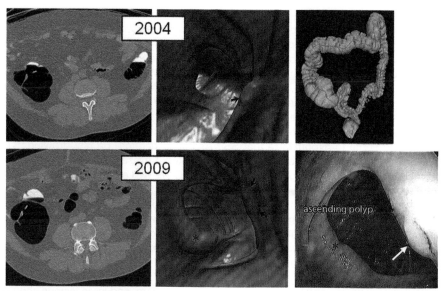

Fig. 8. Large right-sided flat serrated lesion missed at initial CTC screening that was detected at follow-up screening 5 years later in an asymptomatic man (50 years old at initial screening). Top: 2D (*left*) and 3D (*middle*) images from the initial CTC screening in 2004 show a subtle flat lesion (*arrows*) was missed in the ascending colon just distal to the ileocecal valve (*asterisks*). The specific colonic location is indicated on the colon map (*right*) by the red dot. Little or no contrast material coating of the polyp surface is seen. Bottom: 2D (*left*) and 3D (*middle*) images from repeat CTC screening in 2009 show the same flat lesion (*arrows*), which measured 12 mm without significant change in size from 2004. The lesion now demonstrates subtle contrast coating, which increases conspicuity and reader confidence. The polyp was confirmed (*arrow*) and removed at same-day colonoscopy (*right*) and proved to be a sessile serrate polyp at pathologic evaluation. The asterisk indicates ileocecal valve. (*From* Pickhardt PJ, Pooler BD, Mbah I, et al. Colorectal findings at repeat CT colonography screening after initial CT colonography screening negative for polyps larger than 5 mm. Radiology 2017;282:139–48; with permission.)

The authors have also assessed the theoretic cost-effectiveness of immediate polypectomy versus 3-year CTC surveillance for small and diminutive polyps detected at CTC screening.[34,36] If all detected diminutive lesions at CTC screening were referred for OC polypectomy, an estimated 2352 lesions would need to be resected to prevent one cancer over 10 years, at a cost of $464,407 per life-year gained. Without any intervention, the authors estimated that the 5-year CRC death rate for patients with unresected 6 to 9 mm polyps was 0.08%, which already represents a seven-fold decrease from the 0.56% 5-year CRC death rate in the general screening population, most of whom do not harbor nondiminutive polyps. Therefore, for patients with 6 to 9 mm polyps detected at CTC screening, the exclusion of large polyps ($\geq$10 mm) already confers a very low CRC risk. For the concentrated cohort with a small polyp, the death rate was further reduced to 0.03% with the CTC surveillance strategy and 0.02% with immediate colonoscopy referral. However, for each additional cancer-related death prevented with immediate polypectomy versus CTC follow-up, 10,000 additional colonoscopy referrals would be needed, resulting in 10 perforations and an exorbitant incremental cost-effectiveness ratio of $372,853. These modeling simulations further support the practices of CTC surveillance for small polyps and for nonreporting of diminutive lesions.

The issue of "interval cancers" has received considerable attention in the recent GI literature and relates to a discussion on polyp natural history. An interval cancer may be defined as CRC diagnosed after a screening or surveillance examination in which no cancer was detected and before the date of the next recommended examination.[51] Possible explanations for interval CRCs following a negative OC (or CTC) examination would include missed lesions, incompletely resected lesions, and rapidly growing new lesions. It is generally accepted that most of the interval cancers following OC represent missed lesion at the index colonoscopy.[52] Most interval cancers are right-sided, some of which are likely related to the alternate serrated pathway. Although early on this has led some to hypothesize that SSP/As might therefore be fast growing,[53] it seems more likely that these lesions were repeatedly missed.[17] Issues relating to decreased protection from right-sided cancer at OC are well established.[54,55] In general, CTC has advantages over OC for evaluating the right colon (whereas the opposite may be true for the left colon), given its ability to distend the right colon and evaluate "behind" folds (see **Fig. 3**; **Fig. 9**).[25,56] Our experience with interval cancers following negative CTC suggest that the rates are lower relative to OC.[16,57]

In summary, the cumulative evidence on natural history shows that polyp growth assessment at CTC surveillance is a useful biomarker for determining the clinical importance of small polyps and that a 3-year interval is reasonable. Furthermore, diminutive lesions can safely be ignored for at least 5 years, and large lesions should generally be referred for polypectomy, even though their immediate risk is small unless masslike in appearance. This reinforces the initial recommendations made when the C-RADS classification system was first conceived.[37] Advanced adenomas, the primary target of CRC prevention, generally show more rapid growth than nonadvanced adenomas, whereas most other small polyps remain stable or regress. Flat lesions tend to be less aggressive but should eventually be removed when large in size. Collectively, these findings might allow for less invasive surveillance strategies, reserving polypectomy for lesions that show substantial or rapid growth. Further research is needed to regarding the ultimate fate of unresected small polyps without significant growth at initial follow-up. To that end, the authors now have another 5 to 6 years of additional polyp follow-up data, with CTC surveillance on over 750 total polyps, which they are currently in the process of further analyzing.

RADIOGENOMIC CORRELATION AND NOVEL TUMORIGENESIS THEORIES

The long-held classical view on CRC formation is that tumors arise via the gradual stepwise accumulation of mutations.[58,59] At each step, a new mutation was thought to generate a more advantageous subclone that would outcompete less-fit clones in a Darwinian fashion. Under such a stepwise or linear evolution model, all tumors should have the potential to progress from a benign to malignant state, typically over a decade or two, and the resulting cancers should be homogeneous, based on natural selection of fitness. However, emerging technologies and "big data" solutions that allow for rapid analysis of DNA, RNA, and proteins are revealing vast amounts of intratumoral heterogeneity.[60] In concert, more recent experience with CTC surveillance consisting of multiple follow-up examinations has allowed us to see that colorectal polyps demonstrate a variety of growth behaviors. Some polyps will grow and progress, others may grow for a period of time and then remain static in size, whereas some may grow for a while and then regress below our limits of detection. Mutational analysis of polyps with varying fates by CTC has revealed subclonal mutations that must have arisen early on before the polyp was of a detectable size (**Fig. 10**).[61] In addition, other investigators have uncovered epigenetic methylation alterations early on in

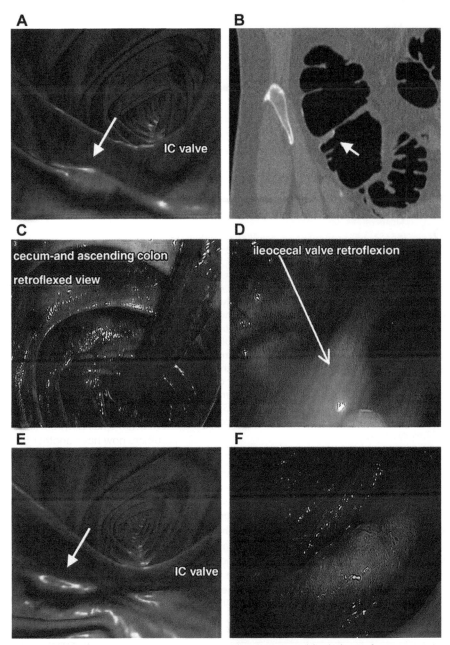

Fig. 9. Large advanced tubular adenoma missed at initial nonblinded OC after prospective detection at initial CTC screening. (*A*) Three-dimensional endoluminal CTC view shows a 2-cm sessile polyp (*arrow*) detected behind a cecal fold adjacent to the ileocecal valve. (*B*) Coronal 2D CTC image confirms a true mucosal-based polyp (*arrow*). A diminutive rectal lesion (not shown) was also detected and incidentally noted in the CTC report. (*C, D*) Retro-flexed images from same-day OC referral show the (*C*) cecum and ascending colon and (*D*) dedicated evaluation of the ileocecal valve fold (*arrow* in *D*). The polyp was not found despite previous knowledge of specific location and thorough inspection. The diminutive

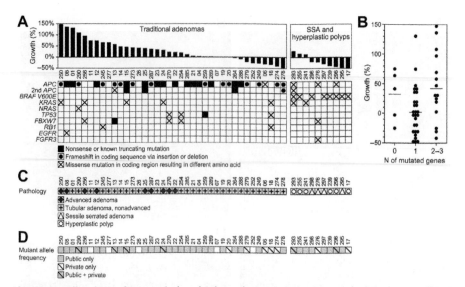

Fig. 10. Small polyps often carried multiple pathogenic mutations. (*A*) Mutation profile of polyps with known growth fates is shown. Only well-annotated, known pathogenic variants are included. (*B*) Small polyps had 0 to 3 pathogenic mutations. Horizontal lines represent the mean (*P* value = .044). The difference between polyps with 1 mutation and those with 2 or more was significant. (*C*) The pathology of polyps with known growth fates (*A*) compared with mutation frequency. (*D*) The mutations can be classified as public, that is, clonal with an adjusted allele frequency of greater than or equal to 30% or private, that is, subclonal with an adjusted allele frequency of 5% to 30%. Small polyps with only private mutation(s) tended to regress. Private only versus public only and public and private were significantly different. (*From* Sievers CK, Zou LS, Pickhardt PJ, et al. Subclonal diversity arises early even in small colorectal tumours and contributes to differential growth fates. Gut 2017;66:2132–40; with permission.)

benign and even nonneoplastic colonic tissue.[62] These findings indicate that some precursor lesions might be "born to be bad",[63] whereas early molecular events may dictate later tumor growth and progression. These new observations render the classic stepwise model of tumor evolution inadequate to explain the degree of molecular and phenotypic intra- and intertumoral heterogeneity observed in CRC tumorigenesis. In response, new evolutionary theories of tumorigenesis have been proposed, which may provide new insights into tumor formation and progression to invasive disease.

Two novel theories on colorectal tumorigenesis have been proposed in response to these newer observations, namely, the "big bang" and "punctuated equilibrium"

---

rectal lesion was confirmed and proved to be a hyperplastic polyp. The OC report recommended follow-up OC in 5 years. (*E*) Because of the standard expert discordant review process, repeat CTC with same-day OC, if needed, was recommended, and repeat CTC 9 months later shows the 2-cm polyp (*arrow*). (*F*) Repeat OC performed by a different gastroenterologist confirms the large polyp behind a fold, which was resected and proved to be a tubular adenoma, advanced according to size criteria (10 mm). (*From* Pooler BD, Kim DH, Weiss JM, et al. Colorectal polyps missed with optical colonoscopy despite previous detection and localization with CT colonography. Radiology 2016;278:422–9; with permission.)

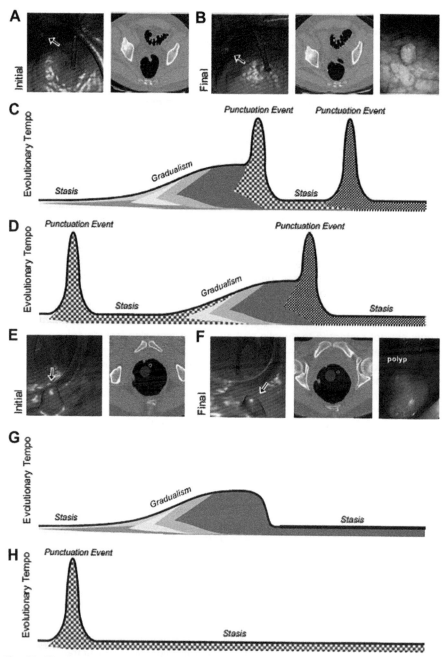

Fig. 11. The "cancer punctuated equilibrium" model of colon tumor evolution better explains the variability of colorectal polyp growth. CTC images from the initial (*A*) and final (*B*) scans from a patient with polyp that had an annual volumetric growth rate of 59% that was followed for more than 2.1 years before polypectomy. Black arrows point to the polyp that was followed longitudinally. (*C*) and (*D*) are possible evolutionary trajectories for a growing polyp. Shading under the line represents levels of intratumoral heterogeneity, with punctuation events creating the greatest amount of heterogeneity. Tumorigenesis may

models of tumor evolution.[60,64] The big bang theory asserts many mutations, and copy number alterations are generated within the first few neoplastic cell divisions leading to the development of an adenoma. Once all the necessary driver mutations are acquired, cancers grow from a single expansion of a diverse population of tumor cells, characterized by neutral evolution instead of Darwinian survival. This model helps to account for the presence of intratumoral heterogeneity not explained by the stepwise growth model, which arises as a function of time, and not as a function of increased fitness. As such, more recently acquired mutations will be at lower frequencies, often undetectable by bulk genomic methodologies. This possibility also might help explain why drug-resistant subclones are undetectable before treatment in the clinical setting. The big bang growth model also allows for variable tumor growth fates. More recently, the punctuated equilibrium theory was advanced as a more comprehensive model of tumor evolution. This model seeks to better explain how tumors evolve, including latent periods and gradual change, punctuated by rapid periods of transformation (**Fig. 11**). Three evolutionary phases are at work in this model: stasis, gradualism, and punctuation events. The stasis phase is characterized by the neutral accrual of passenger mutations, resulting in the stable phenotype. The gradualism phase is most similar to the classic stepwise growth model, in which molecular changes are acquired in a sequential manner, under natural selection, resulting in a quantifiable impact on the phenotype. Finally, punctuation events are derived from the big bang growth model, whereby periods of genomic instability result in many simultaneous molecular changes, often leading to dramatic phenotypic changes. These punctuation events are not restricted to genetic mutations, but may also include epigenetic and transcriptional alternations that result in a phenotypic change.

The inclusion of these 3 mechanisms of evolutionary change into this punctuated equilibrium model of CRC development seems to better explain the variability of polyp growth patterns at CTC and intratumoral heterogeneity. The clinical observation of different growth fates at CTC cannot be accounted for in the classical stepwise acquisition model, especially for static and regressing lesions. CTC also has the potential to assess intratumoral heterogeneity in vivo through texture analysis. Although typically applied to malignancy, either the primary cancer or metastatic foci,[65,66] CT texture analysis seems to be feasible even for benign colorectal polyps.[67,68] In summary, the punctuated equilibrium model of tumor evolution does seem to better fit what has been observed on both the molecular and gross tumor levels. However, the precise timing of these mechanisms during tumorigenesis and evolution, as well as the specific dynamics between multiple clones, remains unknown. By harnessing our unique CTC polyp surveillance experience, the authors hope to further investigate these questions. Specifically, they plan to further study our ongoing CTC-based cohort, correlating growth rates with whole exome sequencing, transcriptional profiling, and methylation profiling of the polyps when ultimately resected. With a

---

begin with a punctuation event or periods of stasis and gradualism, and a second punctuation event may provide enough molecular diversity allowing for malignant transformation. (*E*) and (*F*) are CTC images from the initial and final scans from a patient with polyp that had an annual volumetric growth rate of −33% that was followed for more than 0.9 years before polypectomy. (*G*) and (*H*) are possible evolutionary trajectories for a regressing polyp. Tumor regression may occur with the emergence of a negative or immunogenic phenotype acquired during a period of gradualism or via a punctuation event. (*From* Sievers CK, Grady WM, Halberg RB, et al. New insights into the earliest stages of colorectal tumorigenesis. Expert Rev Gastroenterol Hepatol 2017;11:723–9; with permission.)

greater understanding of polyp growth and progression behavior, screening intervals may increase or decrease for patients with certain low-risk or high-risk molecular characteristics. In addition, a deeper understanding of colorectal tumor evolution might allow for more precise and less-invasive screening strategies in the future.

SUMMARY

Substantial cross-sectional or static data exist on polyp features that correlate with increased cancer risk but are limited by the lack of longitudinal information. Cumulative natural history data from in vivo polyp surveillance have repeatedly shown the benign nature of sub-cm colorectal polyps, rendering diminutive lesions of little or no clinical relevance and demonstrating that in vivo surveillance of small (6–9 mm) polyps is a rational approach on both clinical and economic grounds. In terms of polyp management, this supports the CTC mantra of "ignore the tiny, watch the small, and remove the large." Emerging longitudinal polyp data from CTC surveillance and novel models of tumor evolution are challenging the classical theories of tumorigenesis. Further radiogenomic investigation should provide even further insights into cancer formation, which may one day alter clinical management strategies.

REFERENCES

1. Pickhardt PJ, Hain KS, Kim DH, et al. Low rates of cancer or high-grade dysplasia in colorectal polyps collected from computed tomography colonography screening. Clin Gastroenterol Hepatol 2010;8:610–5.
2. Pickhardt PJ, Kim DH. Colorectal cancer screening with CT colonography: key concepts regarding polyp prevalence, size, histology, morphology, and natural history. AJR Am J Roentgenology 2009;193:40–6.
3. Lieberman D, Moravec M, Holub J, et al. Polyp size and advanced histology in patients undergoing colonoscopy screening: implications for CT colonography. Gastroenterology 2008;135(4):1100–5.
4. Ponugoti PL, Cummings OW, Rex DK. Risk of cancer in small and diminutive colorectal polyps. Dig Liver Dis 2017;49:34–7.
5. Hassan C, Pickhardt PJ, Kim DH, et al. Systematic review: distribution of advanced neoplasia according to polyp size at screening colonoscopy. Aliment Pharmacol Ther 2010;31:210–7.
6. Pickhardt PJ, Lam VP, Weiss JM, et al. Carpet lesions detected at CT colonography: clinical, imaging, and pathologic features. Radiology 2014;270:435–43.
7. Burgess NG, Hourigan LF, Zanati SA, et al. Risk stratification for covert invasive cancer among patients referred for colonic endoscopic mucosal resection: a large multicenter cohort. Gastroenterology 2017;153:732–42.e1.
8. Soetikno RM, Kaltenbach T, Rouse RV, et al. Prevalence of nonpolypoid (flat and depressed) colorectal neoplasms in asymptomatic and symptomatic adults. JAMA 2008;299:1027–35.
9. Pickhardt PJ, Levin B, Bond JH. Screening for nonpolypoid colorectal neoplasms. JAMA 2008;299:2743 [author reply: 2743–4].
10. Pickhardt PJ, Kim DH, Robbins JB. Flat (Nonpolypoid) colorectal lesions identified at CT colonography in a US screening population. Acad Radiol 2010;17: 784–90.
11. Kim DH, Lubner MG, Cahoon AR, et al. Flat serrated polyps at CT colonography: relevance, appearance, and optimizing interpretation. Radiographics 2018;38(1): 60–74.

12. Kim DH, Matkowskyj KA, Lubner MG, et al. Serrated polyps at CT colonography: prevalence and characteristics of the serrated polyp spectrum. Radiology 2016; 280:455–63.

13. Snover DC, Jass JR, Fenoglio-Preiser C, et al. Serrated polyps of the large intestine - A morphologic and molecular review of an evolving concept. Am J Clin Pathol 2005;124:380–91.

14. Jass JR. Classification of colorectal cancer based on correlation of clinical, morphological and molecular features. Histopathology 2007;50:113–30.

15. Burgess NG, Pellise M, Nanda KS, et al. Clinical and endoscopic predictors of cytological dysplasia or cancer in a prospective multicentre study of large sessile serrated adenomas/polyps. Gut 2016;65:437–46.

16. Pickhardt PJ, Pooler BD, Mbah I, et al. Colorectal findings at repeat CT colonography screening after initial CT colonography screening negative for polyps larger than 5 mm. Radiology 2017;282:139–48.

17. Kahi CJ, Hewett DG, Norton DL, et al. Prevalence and variable detection of proximal colon serrated polyps during screening colonoscopy. Clin Gastroenterol Hepatol 2011;9:42–6.

18. Kim DH, Hinshaw JL, Lubner MG, et al. Contrast coating for the surface of flat polyps at CT colonography: a marker for detection. Eur Radiol 2014;24:940–6.

19. O'Connor SD, Summers RM, Choi JR, et al. Oral contrast adherence to polyps on CT colonography. J Comput Assist Tomogr 2006;30:51–7.

20. Ijspeert JEG, Bevan R, Senore C, et al. Detection rate of serrated polyps and serrated polyposis syndrome in colorectal cancer screening cohorts: a European overview. Gut 2017;66:1225–32.

21. Hassan C, Repici A. Recent advances in diagnostic colonoscopy for colorectal cancer screening: an update for radiologists. Am J Roentgenology 2017;209: 88–93.

22. Radaelli F, Paggi S, Hassan C, et al. Split-dose preparation for colonoscopy increases adenoma detection rate: a randomised controlled trial in an organised screening programme. Gut 2017;66:270–7.

23. Barclay RL, Vicari JJ, Doughty AS, et al. Colonoscopic withdrawal times and adenoma detection during screening colonoscopy. N Engl J Med 2006;355: 2533–41.

24. Pickhardt PJ, Taylor AJ, Gopal DV. Surface visualization at 3D endoluminal CT colonography: degree of coverage and implications for polyp detection. Gastroenterology 2006;130:1582–7.

25. Pickhardt PJ, Nugent PA, Mysliwiec PA, et al. Location of adenomas missed by optical colonoscopy. Ann Intern Med 2004;141:352–9.

26. Pooler BD, Kim DH, Weiss JM, et al. Colorectal polyps missed with optical colonoscopy despite previous detection and localization with CT Colonography. Radiology 2016;278(2):422–9.

27. Pooler BD, Kim DH, Hassan C, et al. Variation in diagnostic performance among radiologists at screening CT colonography. Radiology 2013;268:127–34.

28. Hassan C, Repici A. Defeating cancer by boosting the adenoma detection rate: the circle of life. Gastroenterology 2017;153:8–10.

29. Kaminski MF, Wieszczy P, Rupinski M, et al. Increased rate of adenoma detection associates with reduced risk of colorectal cancer and death. Gastroenterology 2017;153:98–105.

30. Hassan C, Pickhardt PJ, Rex DK. A resect and discard strategy would improve cost-effectiveness of colorectal cancer screening. Clin Gastroenterol Hepatol 2010;8:865–9.

31. Pickhardt PJ. Emerging stool-based and blood-based non-invasive DNA tests for colorectal cancer screening: the importance of cancer prevention in addition to cancer detection. Abdom Radiol (NY) 2016;41(8):1441–4.
32. Kim DH, Pickhardt PJ, Taylor AJ, et al. CT colonography versus colonoscopy for the detection of advanced neoplasia. N Engl J Med 2007;357:1403–12.
33. Pickhardt PJ, Choi JR, Hwang I, et al. Computed tomographic virtual colonoscopy to screen for colorectal neoplasia in asymptomatic adults. N Engl J Med 2003;349:2191–200.
34. Pickhardt PJ, Hassan C, Laghi A, et al. Small and diminutive polyps detected at screening CT colonography: a decision analysis for referral to colonoscopy. AJR Am J Roentgenol 2008;190:136–44.
35. Pickhardt PJ, Hassan C, Laghi A, et al. Cost-effectiveness of colorectal cancer screening with computed tomography colonography: the impact of not reporting diminutive lesions. Cancer 2007;109:2213–21.
36. Pickhardt PJ, Hassan C, Laghi A, et al. Clinical management of small (6- to 9-mm) polyps detected at screening CT colonography: a cost-effectiveness analysis. AJR Am J Roentgenol 2008;191:1509–16.
37. Zalis ME, Barish MA, Choi JR, et al. CT colonography reporting and data system: a consensus proposal. Radiology 2005;236:3–9.
38. Welin S, Youker J, Spratt JS Jr. The rates and patterns of growth of 375 tumors of the large intestine and rectum observed serially by double contrast enema study (Malmoe Technique). Am J Roentgenol Radium Ther Nucl Med 1963;90:673–87.
39. Hofstad B, Vatn M, Larsen S, et al. Growth of colorectal polyps - recovery and evaluation of unresected polyps of less-than 10 Mm, 1 year after detection. Scand J Gastroenterol 1994;29:640–5.
40. Hofstad B, Vatn MH, Andersen SN, et al. Growth of colorectal polyps: redetection and evaluation of unresected polyps for a period of three years. Gut 1996;39:449–56.
41. Knoernschild HE. Growth rate and malignant potential of colonic polyps: early results. Surg Forum 1963;14:137–8.
42. Hoff G, Foerster A, Vatn MH, et al. Epidemiology of polyps in the rectum and colon - recovery and evaluation of unresected polyps 2 years after detection. Scand J Gastroenterol 1986;21:853–62.
43. Bersentes K, Fennerty B, Sampliner RE, et al. Lack of spontaneous regression of tubular adenomas in two years of follow-up. Am J Gastroenterol 1997;92:1117–20.
44. Stryker SJ, Wolff BG, Culp CE, et al. Natural-history of untreated colonic polyps. Gastroenterology 1987;93:1009–13.
45. Loeve F, Boer R, Zauber AG, et al. National polyp study data: evidence for regression of adenomas. Int J Cancer 2004;111:633–9.
46. Togashi K, Shimura K, Konishi F, et al. Prospective observation of small adenomas in patients after colorectal cancer surgery through magnification chromocolonoscopy. Dis Colon Rectum 2008;51:196–201.
47. Pickhardt PJ, Lehman VT, Winter TC, et al. Polyp volume versus linear size measurements at CT colonography: Implications for noninvasive surveillance of unresected colorectal lesions. Am J Roentgenology 2006;186:1605–10.
48. Pickhardt PJ, Kim DH, Pooler BD, et al. Assessment of volumetric growth rates of small colorectal polyps with CT colonography: a longitudinal study of natural history. Lancet Oncol 2013;14:711–20.
49. Nolthenius CJT, Boellaard TN, de Haan MC, et al. Evolution of screen-detected small (6-9 mm) polyps after a 3-year surveillance interval: assessment of growth

with CT colonography compared with histopathology. Am J Gastroenterol 2015; 110:1682–90.

50. O'Brien MJ, Winawer SJ, Zauber AG, et al. Flat adenomas in the National Polyp Study: is there increased risk for high-grade dysplasia initially or during surveillance? Clin Gastroenterol Hepatol 2004;2:905–11.

51. Sanduleanu S, le Clercq CMC, Dekker E, et al. Definition and taxonomy of interval colorectal cancers: a proposal for standardising nomenclature. Gut 2015;64: 1257–67.

52. Adler J, Robertson DJ. Interval colorectal cancer after colonoscopy: exploring explanations and solutions. Am J Gastroenterol 2015;110:1657–64.

53. Jass JR. Serrated route to colorectal cancer: back street or super highway? J Pathol 2001;193:283–5.

54. Brenner H, Hoffmeister M, Arndt V, et al. Protection from right- and left-sided colorectal neoplasms after colonoscopy: population-based study. J Natl Cancer Inst 2010;102:89–95.

55. Bressler B, Paszat LF, Vinden C, et al. Colonoscopic miss rates for right-sided colon cancer: a population-based analysis. Gastroenterology 2004;127:452–6.

56. Pickhardt PJ, Hassan C, Halligan S, et al. Colorectal cancer: CT colonography and colonoscopy for detection–systematic review and meta-analysis. Radiology 2011;259:393–405.

57. Kim DH, Pooler BD, Weiss JM, et al. Five year colorectal cancer outcomes in a large negative CT colonography screening cohort. Eur Radiol 2012;22:1488–94.

58. Muto T, Bussey HJR, Morson BC. Evolution of cancer of colon and rectum. Cancer 1975;36:2251–70.

59. Vogelstein B, Fearon ER, Hamilton SR, et al. Genetic alterations during colorectal tumor development. N Engl J Med 1988;319:525–32.

60. Sievers CK, Grady WM, Halberg RB, et al. New insights into the earliest stages of colorectal tumorigenesis. Expert Rev Gastroenterol Hepatol 2017;11:723–9.

61. Sievers CK, Zou LS, Pickhardt PJ, et al. Subclonal diversity arises early even in small colorectal tumours and contributes to differential growth fates. Gut 2017; 66:2132–40.

62. Luo Y, Wong CJ, Kaz AM, et al. Differences in DNA methylation signatures reveal multiple pathways of progression from adenoma to colorectal cancer. Gastroenterology 2014;147:418–29.e8.

63. Sottoriva A, Kang H, Ma Z, et al. A Big Bang model of human colorectal tumor growth. Nat Genet 2015;47:209–16.

64. Cross WCH, Graham TA, Wright NA. New paradigms in clonal evolution: punctuated equilibrium in cancer. J Pathol 2016;240:126–36.

65. Lubner MG, Stabo N, Lubner SJ, et al. CT textural analysis of hepatic metastatic colorectal cancer: pre-treatment tumor heterogeneity correlates with pathology and clinical outcomes. Abdom Imaging 2015;40:2331–7.

66. Ng F, Ganeshan B, Kozarski R, et al. Assessment of primary colorectal cancer heterogeneity by using whole-tumor texture analysis: contrast-enhanced CT texture as a biomarker of 5-year survival. Radiology 2013;266:177–84.

67. Hu YF, Liang ZR, Song BW, et al. Texture feature extraction and analysis for polyp differentiation via computed tomography colonography. IEEE Trans Med Imaging 2016;35:1522–31.

68. Song BW, Zhang GP, Lu HB, et al. Volumetric texture features from higher-order images for diagnosis of colon lesions via CT colonography. Int J Comput Assist Radiol Surg 2014;9:1021–31.

Rectal MRI for Cancer Staging and Surveillance

Courtney C. Moreno, MD[a],*, Patrick S. Sullivan, MD[b,c], Pardeep K. Mittal, MD[a]

KEYWORDS

- Rectal adenocarcinoma • Staging MRI • Restaging MRI

KEY POINTS

- MRI is an integral part of the multidisciplinary treatment of rectal adenocarcinoma.
- Staging MRI establishes TMN stage and identifies prognostic factors (eg, circumferential resection margin status and presence of extramural vascular invasion) that determine which patients undergo preoperative neoadjuvant chemoradiation or systemic chemotherapy.
- Restaging MRI assesses for treatment response following neoadjuvant chemoradiation and may identify patients with no residual visible tumor who may be candidates for a "watch and wait" strategy in lieu of resection.

INTRODUCTION

There is a need for accurate clinical staging of rectal cancer to optimize individualized treatment. Although the incidence of rectal cancer is decreasing in the United States, approximately 40,000 new patients are diagnosed each year.[1] Surgical resection, chemoradiation, and systemic chemotherapy are the main treatment modalities for rectal cancer, and the combination of these treatments heavily depends on clinical staging. Innovations in surgical technique, including total mesorectal excision (TME), have resulted in lower rates of local recurrence.[2,3] Transanal endoscopic surgery techniques also offer the possibility of shorter recovery times and less morbidity in carefully selected patients.[4,5] With newer chemoradiation regimens, 10% to 30% of individuals experience a complete clinical response (no clinically detectable tumor) or a complete pathologic response (no detectable tumor in the resected specimen).[6–8]

Disclosure Statement: The authors have no relevant financial disclosures.
[a] Department of Radiology and Imaging Sciences, Emory University School of Medicine, 1365-A Clifton Road Northeast, Suite AT-627, Atlanta, GA 30322, USA; [b] Division of Surgical Oncology, Department of Surgery, Emory University School of Medicine, 1364 Clifton Road Northeast, Room B206, Atlanta, GA 30322, USA; [c] Division of Colorectal Surgery, Department of Surgery, Emory University School of Medicine, 1364 Clifton Road Northeast, Room B206, Atlanta, GA 30322, USA
* Corresponding author.
E-mail address: courtney.moreno@emoryhealthcare.org

Gastroenterol Clin N Am 47 (2018) 537–552
https://doi.org/10.1016/j.gtc.2018.04.005
0889-8553/18/© 2018 Elsevier Inc. All rights reserved.

gastro.theclinics.com

MRI is an important part of the multidisciplinary treatment of individuals with rectal cancer because it determines best treatment strategies for newly diagnosed patients. Characterization of the local extent of disease with imaging determines which patients would benefit from systemic chemotherapy or neoadjuvant chemoradiation before resection. MRI restaging after initial treatment informs the surgeon of threatened margins in preparation for resection. In addition, information obtained from restaging MRI helps determine which carefully selected patients may be candidates for an organ preserving "watch and wait" strategy than resection following neoadjuvant chemoradiation. This article describes technical considerations when performing rectal MRI, relevant anatomy, and TNM staging and concludes with an overview of treatment considerations.

TECHNICAL CONSIDERATIONS

High-resolution (slice thickness ≤3 mm) T2-weighted imaging is the primary sequence used to stage rectal cancer. Planning images should be acquired in the axial, coronal, and sagittal planes. These initial images are then used to select the plane of imaging to acquire axial images angled perpendicular to the tumor axis and coronal images angled parallel to the tumor axis.[9] Acquiring images angled based on the orientation of the tumor aids in assessment of depth of tumor invasion. For low rectal tumors, an additional coronal acquisition should be performed, angled parallel to the anal sphincter complex to assess the relationship of the tumor to the anal sphincter. In addition, a full field of view axial acquisition of the entire pelvis should be obtained to allow for the detection of pathologic lymph nodes located peripheral to the mesorectal fascia (eg, lateral pelvic sidewall lymph nodes). A diffusion-weighted sequence with a b-value greater than or equal to 800 should be obtained along with an apparent diffusion coefficient (ADC) map.[9] These diffusion-weighted images are especially helpful when comparing initial staging and restaging scans to assess for residual viable tumor following neoadjuvant chemoradiation.

Routine use of intravenous contrast material is not necessary because high-resolution noncontrast T2-weighted sequences are the primary images used to locally stage rectal cancer.[9] However, if the examination is also being performed to evaluate for distant metastatic disease (eg, liver metastases), intravenous contrast material should be administered. MRI staging of rectal cancer can be performed at either 1.5 T or 3 T.[10] Image acquisition should be performed with a surface coil and without an endorectal coil.[9]

Spasmolytics, endorectal distention with ultrasound gel, and a preprocedural enema are variably used. Spasmolytics (eg, glucagon or hyoscine butylbromide) can reduce bowel peristalsis and may be especially helpful for upper rectal tumors.[9] Both agents are administered intravenously or intramuscularly although duration of effectiveness is more predictable with intravenous administration.[11] Because of the short half-life of these medications, repeat administration may be necessary. Hyoscine butylbromide (Buscopan, Boehringer Ingelheim) is not available for use in the United States.

Endorectal distention with ultrasound gel improves visualization of rectal tumors, especially small tumors.[12,13] Endorectal distention may decrease the distance between normal rectal wall and the mesorectal fascia but does not significantly alter the distance between tumor and the mesorectal fascia.[13,14] Endorectal filling can be achieved via administration of 60 mLs of ultrasound gel using a small, pliable catheter inserted into the rectum. A preprocedural enema can reduce the amount of stool and air in the rectum although does not universally improve image quality.[15]

ANATOMIC CONSIDERATIONS

The rectum is approximately 15 cm long and is divided into the lower third (0–5 cm from the anal sphincter), middle third (5–10 cm), and upper third (10–15 cm). The anterior peritoneal reflection seems as a low signal intensity band that separates the intraperitoneal cavity from the extraperitoneal pelvis (**Fig. 1**).[16] Approximately one-third of the rectum is located above the anterior peritoneal reflection. Rectal masses that involve the anterior peritoneal reflection are staged as T4 tumors.

The 3 layers of the rectal wall are well-delineated with high-resolution T2-weighted imaging (**Fig. 2**). Moving from the lumen outward, the innermost mucosal layer seems as a low–signal-intensity band, and the submucosal layer seems as a high-signal-intensity band. The muscularis propria seems as a low-signal-intensity band that surrounds the rectum and serves as the boundary between the rectum and the perirectal fat. Moving further outward, the mesorectal fascia is a low-signal-intensity band that encircles the perirectal fat and is an important anatomic landmark because it serves as the dissection plane for a TME (**Fig. 3**).

The rectum ends at the anal sphincter complex, which is composed of internal and external sphincters. The internal anal sphincter is a continuation of the muscularis propria. The external sphincter is composed of the inferior portion of the levator ani muscles, puborectalis sling, and external sphincter musculature. The anal verge is defined as the inferior most level of the anal sphincter complex and is the level at which the skin meets the anal mucosa. The anal verge is an important anatomic landmark because masses palpable during a digital rectal examination or encountered at sigmoidoscopy or colonoscopy are generally reported with respect to their distance from the anal verge.

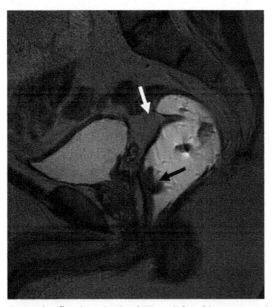

Fig. 1. Anterior peritoneal reflection. Sagittal T2-weighted image acquired after administration of ultrasound gel per rectum demonstrates the low-signal-intensity band of the anterior peritoneal reflection (*white arrow*). Low rectal mass partially imaged (*black arrow*).

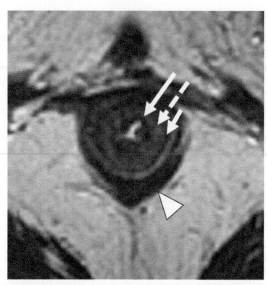

Fig. 2. Rectal wall layers. Axial high-resolution T2-weighted image obtained at the level of the anal sphincter demonstrates the low-signal-intensity mucosa (*solid long arrow*), intermediate to high-signal-intensity submucosa (*dashed arrow*), and the low-signal-intensity band of the muscularis propria (*short arrow*). The external anal sphincter musculature also seems as a low-signal-intensity band (*arrowhead*).

INITIAL STAGING

The role of staging MRI is to (1) establish TNM staging; (2) characterize the distance between the tumor and the anal sphincter; (3) assess prognostic factors including the circumferential resection margin; and (4) assess for sites of disease that could alter

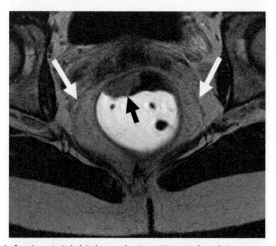

Fig. 3. Mesorectal fascia. Axial high-resolution T2-weighted image acquired following administration of ultrasound gel per rectum demonstrates the low-signal-intensity band of the mesorectal fascia (*white arrows*) surrounding the perirectal fat. The patient has a T2 rectal adenocarcinoma (*black arrow*) that did not violate the low-signal-intensity band of the muscularis propria.

the surgical approach (eg, lateral pelvic lymph nodes). A structured reporting template is useful because a detailed report precisely describing these tumor features is critical to the multidisciplinary management of patients with rectal adenocarcinoma.[17] Resources are available with sample structured reporting templates that can be modified based on the needs of a particular practice.[18]

TNM Stage

Rectal cancer is staged based on the TNM classification system where T stage refers to local tumor extent, N stage refers to regional lymph node status, and M stage refers to the presence or absence of distant metastatic disease (**Box 1**).

T stage

T1 tumors invade the submucosa, whereas T2 tumors extend into but not beyond the muscularis propria (**Figs. 4** and **5**). T3 tumors extend through the muscularis propria into the perirectal fat. Disruption of the low-signal-intensity band of the muscularis propria by tumor is diagnostic of T3 disease (see **Figs. 4** and **5**). By comparison, if the low-signal-intensity band of the muscularis propria is intact, the tumor is either a T1 or T2 lesion. Tumor involvement of adjacent organs or structures or tumor involvement of the anterior peritoneal reflection is diagnostic of T4 disease (see **Fig. 4**; **Fig. 6**).

Endorectal ultrasound is considered superior for differentiating T1 and T2 tumors, whereas MRI is superior for characterizing the distance of tumor extension beyond the rectal wall. In a meta-analysis, MRI demonstrated 87% sensitivity (95% confidence interval [CI]; 81%–92%) and 75% specificity (95% CI; 68%–80%) for T stage.[19] In an evaluation of 90 patients, endoscopic ultrasound was 76% accurate for staging

---

Box 1
TMN staging of rectal cancer

- Tx: Cannot assess primary tumor
- T0: No evidence of primary tumor
- Tis: Carcinoma in situ
- T1: Tumor invades submucosa
- T2: Tumor invades muscularis propria
- T3: Tumor extension beyond muscularis propria into mesorectal fat
- T4a: Tumor involves the anterior peritoneal resection
- T4b: Tumor invades other organs or structures
- Nx: Regional lymph nodes cannot be assessed
- N0: No regional lymph nodes involved
- N1: Tumor in 1 to 3 regional lymph nodes or tumor deposits in the perirectal tissues
- N2: Tumor in 4 or more regional lymph nodes
- Mx: Metastatic disease cannot be assessed
- M0: No distant metastasis
- M1: Distant metastatic disease

From American Joint Committee on Cancer (AJCC). Colon and Rectum Cancer Staging. 7th edition. 2009. Available at: https://cancerstaging.org/references-tools/quickreferences/Documents/ColonMedium.pdf. Accessed January 17, 2018; with permission.

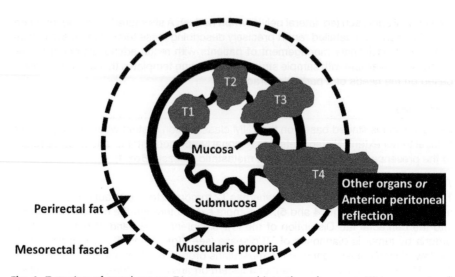

Fig. 4. T staging of rectal cancer. T1 tumors extend into the submucosa. T2 tumors extend into but not beyond the muscularis propria. T3 tumors extend beyond the muscularis propria. T4 tumors involve other organs or the anterior peritoneal reflection.

T2 and T3 disease, whereas MRI demonstrated 77% accuracy for T2 disease and 83% accuracy for T3 disease.[20] In the landmark Magnetic Resonance Imaging and Rectal Cancer European Equivalence (MERCURY) Study, MRI and histopathologic assessment of tumor spread in patients who underwent primary resection were considered equivalent to within 0.5 mm.[21] MRI and endorectal ultrasound should not be thought of as mutually exclusive in staging early rectal cancer, rather they should be thought of as being complementary.

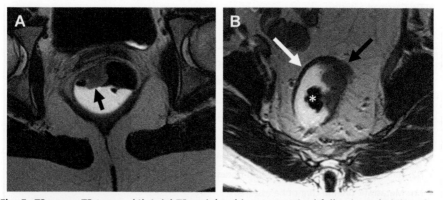

Fig. 5. T2 versus T3 tumor. (*A*) Axial T2-weighted image acquired following administration of ultrasound gel per rectum demonstrates an intermediate signal intensity tumor (*arrow*). The low-signal-intensity band of the muscularis propria is intact indicating that this is a T2 tumor. (*B*) Fecal debris (*asterisk*). Axial T2-weighted image also acquired after administration of ultrasound gel per rectum demonstrates intermediate signal intensity tumor (*black arrow*) extending into the perirectal fat compatible with a T3 tumor. Elsewhere, the low-signal-intensity band of the muscular propria is intact (*white arrow*).

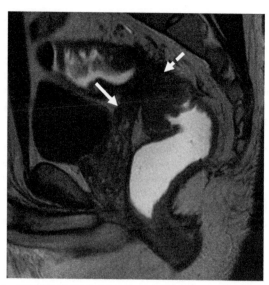

Fig. 6. T4 tumor. Sagittal T2-weighted image acquired after administration of ultrasound gel per rectum demonstrates a low-signal-intensity mass (*dashed arrow*) extending to involve the right seminal vesicle (*solid arrow*).

In the United States, the accurate differentiation of T1/T2 tumors from T3/T4 tumors is important because patients with T3 or T4 tumors or node-positive disease undergo neoadjuvant chemoradiation before resection. By comparison, patients with T1 or T2 tumors undergo resection without preoperative neoadjuvant chemoradiation.

N stage

N0 disease is defined as no pathologic regional lymph nodes. N1 disease is defined as 1 to 3 pathologic regional lymph nodes, whereas N2 disease is defined as 4 or more pathologic regional lymph nodes. For MRI staging purposes, differentiating between N0 and N1 disease is important because patients with pathologic lymph nodes typically undergo preoperative neoadjuvant chemoradiation before resection regardless of T stage. The precise number of pathologic lymph nodes (eg, N1 vs N2 disease) is determined by the pathologist following surgical resection.

MRI is less sensitive and specific in the assessment of N stage as compared with T stage, likely because of the variability in criteria used for lymph node assessment.[19,22] Lymph node size, by itself, is poorly predictive of nodal status as there is overlap in the size of normal and pathologic lymph nodes.[23] The old adage that "any visible perirectal lymph node is abnormal" is no longer believed to be true. Patients undergoing MRI for rectal cancer staging have usually recently undergone colonoscopy or sigmoidoscopy with tissue sampling and may have mildly prominent, reactive lymph nodes as a result of a recent invasive procedure.

Evaluation of lymph node size in combination with lymph node morphology is important to optimize interpretation accuracy. Morphologically abnormal lymph nodes that seem heterogeneous or demonstrate irregular margins are considered diseased.[23,24] Using criteria of irregular border or mixed signal intensity, MRI was found to have a sensitivity of 85% (95% CI; 74%–92%) and specificity of 97% (95% CI; 95%–99%) for pathologic lymph nodes.[23] According to the Society of Abdominal Radiology rectal cancer staging reporting template, a lymph node can be categorized as positive based on one of 3 criteria: (1) short axis greater than or equal to 9 mm; (2) short axis 5 to 9 mm and at least 2 abnormal morphologic features (heterogeneous signal intensity, irregular border, or round shape); or (3) short axis less than 5 mm and all 3 abnormal morphologic features (heterogeneous signal intensity, irregular border, and round shape).[18] Most of the pathologic lymph nodes within the mesorectum are at or proximal to the site of the primary tumor because it is less common to see pathologic lymph nodes with caudal descent inferior to the primary tumor. The reason for this has to do with the lymphatic drainage and venous drainage of the rectum going in a cranial direction.

Perirectal and internal iliac lymph nodes are considered regional lymph nodes in the setting of rectal cancer, whereas inguinal, external iliac, common iliac, and periaortic lymph nodes are considered nonregional lymph nodes.[25] It is also important to describe the presence and location of any pathologic lymph nodes located peripheral to the mesorectal fascia (eg, pelvic sidewall lymph nodes) in the staging MRI report because such nodes would not be within the resection of a TME and would warrant a more extensive resection so that all abnormal lymph nodes could be removed.

M stage

M stage refers to the presence of distant metastatic disease. M0 indicates no metastatic disease, whereas M1 indicates the presence of metastatic disease. The most common sites of metastatic disease for rectal cancer are liver and lung.[26] Computed tomography (CT) of the abdomen with intravenous contrast material, or in some centers contrast-enhanced abdominal MRI, is performed to assess for abdominal metastatic disease. Chest CT without intravenous contrast is generally performed to assess for pulmonary metastatic disease. Patients identified to have pathologic lymph nodes outside of the regional lymph node basin of the mesorectum and internal iliac (including common iliac, external iliac, inguinal, and periaortic) are considered for initial systemic therapy because these lymph node basins are considered metastatic systemic disease.

Circumferential Resection Margin

The status of the circumferential resection margin (CRM) is a prognostic factor for rectal cancer. Tumors extending close to or involving the CRM generally have a poorer prognosis as compared with tumors located more distant from the CRM.[27] MRI is accurate for the prediction of tumor involvement of the CRM (eg, the mesorectal fascia for a TME).[28,29] Tumor located within 1 mm of the mesorectal fascia (eg, direct extension of the primary tumor, an abnormal lymph node, or a tumor deposit) is defined as tumor involvement of the CRM (**Fig. 7**). A positive pathologic CRM is the worst prognostic factor for local recurrence and should be avoided. Drawing the surgeon's attention to the site of CRM tumor involvement is important because the surgeon will generally modify the dissection plane to ensure that the tumor is removed completely and is not violated by dissecting through tumor. A threatened circumferential resection margin is defined as tumor less than or equal to 2 mm of the mesorectal fascia.[30]

Extramural Vascular Invasion

Extramural vascular invasion is also a prognostic factor for rectal cancer. Tumors that demonstrate extramural vascular invasion (defined as tumor within endothelium-lined blood vessels extending beyond the muscularis propria of the rectum) are associated with higher rates of distant disease and poorer overall survival.[31,32] On high-resolution T2-weighted MRI, extramural vascular invasion seems as abnormally thickened and sometimes nodular vessels extending away from the rectal wall at the site of the tumor

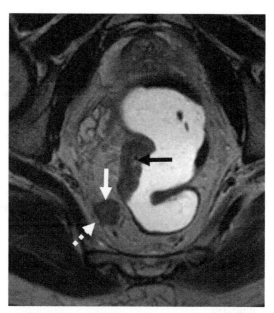

Fig. 7. Involved circumferential resection margin. Axial T2-weighted image acquired after administration of ultrasound gel per rectum demonstrates the primary rectal mass (*black arrow*) and a separate tumor implant (*white arrow*) involving the mesorectal fascia (*dashed arrow*).

(**Fig. 8**).[31] Intermediate tumor signal may be visible within the expanded vessel.[33] Using criteria of intermediate tumor signal intensity within expanded vessels or irregular or nodular vessel contour due to tumor, MRI was found to be 54% sensitive and 96% specific for the detection of extramural vascular invasion in veins greater than or equal

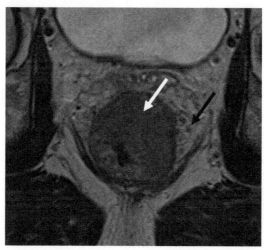

Fig. 8. Extramural vascular invasion. Axial high-resolution T2-weighted image demonstrates a large rectal mass (*white arrow*). Perirectal vascular structure (*black arrow*) demonstrates intermediate signal within it and irregular margins compatible with extramural vascular invasion. In contiguous images (not shown), this structure overall seemed tubular and therefore compatible with a vascular structure.

to 3 mm in diameter.[33] It is difficult to differentiate extramural vascular invasion from tumor-associated desmoplasia. Tumor-associated desmoplasia may seem fine and wispy, whereas extramural vascular invasion seems more cordlike.[31]

Mucinous Adenocarcinoma

Mucinous adenocarcinoma is a subtype of rectal adenocarcinoma and is defined as greater than 50% of tumor volume composed of mucinous material.[34] Approximately 5% to 10% of rectal adenocarcinomas are of the mucinous subtype.[34] Mucinous adenocarcinomas may be less responsive to neoadjuvant chemoradiation because most of the neoplasm is acellular mucin.[34] At T2-weighted imaging, mucinous tumors demonstrate high signal intensity similar to fluid (**Fig. 9**). An awareness of this appearance (in both the primary tumor and sites of metastatic disease) is important so as to avoid mistaking tumor for fluid. In addition, necrotic posttreatment changes demonstrating high T2 signal intensity should not be mistaken for a primary mucinous tumor.

RESTAGING MRI

Following neoadjuvant chemoradiation, patients generally undergo restaging MRI to assess for treatment response and for preoperative planning. Most patients will demonstrate a decrease in tumor size and 10% to 30% will demonstrate a pathologic complete response (**Fig. 10**).[35]

The same imaging protocol should be used for staging and restaging scans. A detailed reporting template also should be used for restaging scans and should include the same details provided in the staging report (eg, TNM stage, tumor size, tumor location, sphincter involvement, circumferential resection margin status, etc.). An additional consideration on restaging scans is the differentiation of residual tumor from posttreatment fibrosis. Utilization of diffusion-weighted imaging (DWI) has been

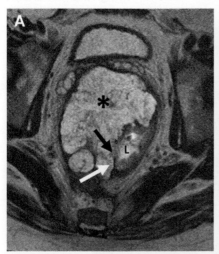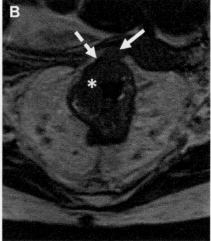

Fig. 9. Mucinous versus nonmucinous adenocarcinoma. Axial T2-weighted imaging. (*A*) Large high T2 signal intensity mucinous adenocarcinoma (*asterisk*). Tumor (*black arrow*) disrupts the low-signal-intensity band of the muscularis propria (*white arrow*) compatible with a T3 lesion. (*B*) Nonmucinous adenocarcinoma demonstrates low signal intensity (*asterisk*). Tumor (*solid arrow*) disrupts the low-signal band of the muscularis propria (*dashed arrow*) compatible with a T3 lesion. L, rectal lumen.

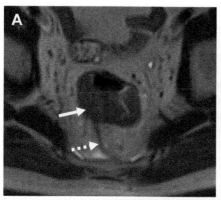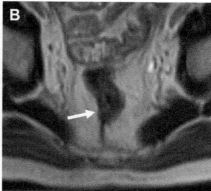

Fig. 10. Positive treatment response. (*A*) Axial T2-weighted image from staging examination demonstrates a large rectal mass (*solid arrow*) with extramural vascular invasion (*dashed arrow*). (*B*) Axial T2-weighted image from restaging scan following neoadjuvant chemoradiation demonstrates decreased size of the rectal mass (*arrow*).

shown to improve the diagnostic accuracy of the assessment of a complete response on restaging scans.[36] Areas of high signal intensity on DWI and corresponding low signal intensity on the ADC map indicate areas of residual tumor.[36] By comparison, areas of posttreatment fibrosis demonstrate low T2 signal intensity and no restricted diffusion. Restaging studies for mucinous adenocarcinomas can be challenging to interpret because it can be difficult to differentiate residual tumor from acellular mucin. Tumor response grading scales are being investigated as a way to improve the interpretation of restaging examinations for mucinous adenocarcinomas.[37] Endoscopic mucosal assessment is generally considered complementary to MRI for detection of posttreatment recurrence.

TREATMENT OVERVIEW

The 2 major treatment decisions that must be made for patients with newly diagnosed rectal adenocarcinoma are as follows: (1) what type of resection should be performed and (2) should neoadjuvant chemoradiation be administered before resection. The appearance of the tumor on staging and restaging MRI informs both of these decisions.

Total Mesorectal Excision

TME is the primary surgical approach used to remove rectal cancers. TME results in removal of the rectal tumor and perirectal fat with the mesorectal fascia serving as the dissection plane. TME reduces rates of local recurrence as compared with older surgical techniques that did not remove as much perirectal tissue.[2,3,38] MRI allows surgeons to visualize the TME plain and plan accordingly for areas that may be close or threatened. It has been demonstrated through pathologic assessment that the more intact the investing fascia of the rectum of the TME is, the lower the rate of local recurrence.[39] As part of the standardized pathologic reporting synoptic, the grade of TME is now becoming standard of care. The rectal specimen is graded as an incomplete TME (exposure of the muscularis propria is evident), near-complete (defects within the TME but not reaching the muscularis propria), or complete (a completely intact TME without divots). Accurate description of the relationship of the tumor to the mesorectal fascia is important so that the dissection plane is altered if necessary to encompass all tumor and obtain a negative resection margin during TME.

TME can be performed as part of low anterior resection (LAR) or abdominal perineal resection (APR). Performance of an LAR requires that the tumor is far enough away from the anal sphincter complex such that the tumor can be removed with enough rectum left above the sphincter to perform an end-to-end anastomosis. An LAR with complete TME excision includes resection of the rectum with associated lymph nodes in the mesorectal fat. This technique includes a high ligation of the superior rectal vascular pedicle and complete excision of the rectum by dissecting the loose areolar plane encompassing the circumference of the mesorectum as a complete unit. This ensures complete excision of the peritumoral lymph node packet. The distal rectum is divided below the cancer. The specimen is removed, and the proximal and distal bowel anastomosed to maintain continuity. For carefully selected low-lying rectal cancers, the intersphincteric plane, between the internal and external sphincters, is dissected to ensure a negative distal margin. A coloanal anastomosis between the proximal colon and the external sphincter is completed after the distal and circumferential radial margins are confirmed by frozen section to be clear of disease. A distal 1 cm margin and negative circumferential radial margin is acceptable to perform a coloanal reconstruction.

An APR is reserved for patients with low-lying rectal cancers that involve the anal sphincter in which a distal or circumferential radial margin would be threatened if a coloanal reconstruction were attempted. During an APR, dissection is performed along the mesorectal fascia to remove the rectum and continued distally to include the rectal mass and adjacent pelvic floor and anal sphincter. An APR results in definitive closure of the anus as well as a permanent end colostomy. The decision of whether to perform an APR or LAR is generally made based on an assessment of the distance between the tumor and the anal sphincter as determined by MRI, digital rectal examination, and/or endoscopy.

Tumors that invade surrounding structures (eg, prostate or uterus) may be removed with a pelvic exenteration including resection of the involved adjacent structures. In addition, pathologic lymph nodes located outside the mesorectal fascia (eg, pelvic sidewall lymph nodes) will be removed at the time of resection and a pelvic lymph node dissection performed along with TME. The single most important prognostic factor for local recurrence is a positive margin. The surgeon needs to study the imaging before resection to be informed about what adjacent organs need to be resected in order to ensure a negative margin.

Transanal Techniques

Other less invasive, transanal techniques also have been developed for removal of rectal cancers. These techniques require subspecialized training, are performed at a small number of centers, and are generally reserved for early, favorable T1N0 rectal cancers without high-risk pathologic features (including high-grade morphology, lymphovascular invasion, perineural invasion, signet cell features, and mucin). Other less favorable early rectal cancers (high-risk T1 or T2) may be treated with transanal excision; however, these patients should also receive neoadjuvant chemoradiation to decrease the risk of local recurrence, because a local recurrence rate can be as high as 40%.[40] Adjuvant chemoradiation can also be offered if after resection the pathologic assessment of the cancer identifies a T1 lesion with high-risk pathologic features or a T2 cancer. Another alternative is to offer the patient a transabdominal TME, excising the lesion and the entire lymph node packet. All T1 lesions with high-risk pathologic features and T2 lesions should be offered additional therapy, either chemoradiation or TME, given the increased risk of local recurrence with transanal resection alone. Because transanal excision only removes full-thickness rectal wall, a pathologic assessment of lymph nodes is not part of this operation. Therefore, it is important to determine on MRI that there are no pathologic lymph nodes.

Transanal endoscopic surgery is performed with transanal endoscopic microsurgery (TEM) or with transanal minimally invasive surgery (TAMIS). TEM, first developed in the 1980s, is performed by resecting the rectal cancer using a transanal approach with specialized instruments.[41] TAMIS is a more recent technique using an anal access port and conventional laparoscopic instruments to resect rectal pathology.[4,5] TAMIS is performed by insufflating the rectum with carbon dioxide. A camera and laparoscopic instruments are then inserted via the anus, and the tumor is resected full-thickness into the mesorectum.[5] Advantages of TAMIS are that it is minimally invasive surgery that does not require an abdominal wall incision. The complication rate is much less and recovery time shorter following TAMIS as compared with an LAR or APR.

Preoperative Neoadjuvant Chemoradiation

A final consideration is whether the patient should undergo preoperative neoadjuvant chemoradiation before surgical resection. Preoperative neoadjuvant chemoradiation has been shown to reduce rates of local recurrence and, in some studies, cancer-specific survival.[42–45] In the United States, preoperative neoadjuvant chemoradiation is generally administered to patients with T3 or T4 disease or node positive disease as determined by staging MRI.

Patients with no residual tumor observed on restaging MRI, endoscopy, and digital rectal examination and who are considered high risk for surgery may wish to undergo "watch and wait" strategy in lieu of resection.[46] Watchful waiting generally entails serial MRI examinations and endoscopy with tissue sampling to assess for recurrent tumor.

SUMMARY

In conclusion, rectal MRI is an integral part of the multidisciplinary treatment of rectal cancer. TNM stage as established by staging MRI determines which patients will undergo preoperative neoadjuvant chemoradiation. Local tumor extent and lymph node involvement as assessed with staging and restaging MRI informs surgical resection technique and may also identify patients who are candidates for watchful waiting in lieu of resection.

REFERENCES

1. Siegel RL, Miller KD, Jemal A. Cancer statistics, 2017. CA Cancer J Clin 2017;67: 7–30.
2. Heald RJ, Ryall RDH. Recurrence and survival after total mesorectal excision for rectal cancer. Lancet 1986;327:1479–82.
3. Heald RJ, Husband EM, Ryall RDH. The mesorectum in rectal cancer surgery–the clue to pelvic recurrence? Br J Surg 1982;69:613–6.
4. Atallah S, Albert M, Larach S. Transanal minimally invasive surgery: a giant leap forward. Surg Endosc 2010;24:2200–5.
5. Gill S, Stetler JL, Patel A, et al. Transanal minimally invasive surgery (TAMIS): standardizing a reproducible procedure. J Gastrointest Surg 2015;19:1528–36.
6. Maas M, Lambregts DM, Nelemans PJ, et al. Assessment of clinical complete response after chemoradiation for rectal cancer with digital rectal examination,

endoscopy, and MRI: selection for organ-saving treatment. Ann Surg Oncol 2015; 22:3873–80.

7. Habr-Gama A, Perez RO, Nadalin W, et al. Operative versus nonoperative treatment for stage 0 distal rectal cancer following chemoradiation therapy: long-term results. Ann Surg 2004;240:711–7.

8. Gerard JP, Chamorey E, Gourgou-Bourgade S, et al. Clinical complete response (cCR) after neoadjuvant chemoradiotherapy and conservative treatment in rectal cancer. Findings from the ACCORD 12/PRODIGE 2 randomized trial. Radiother Oncol 2015;115:246–52.

9. Beets-Tan RGH, Lambregts DMJ, Maas M, et al. Correction to: magnetic resonance imaging for clinical management of rectal cancer: updated recommendations from the 2016 European Society of Gastrointestinal and Abdominal Radiology (ESGAR) consensus meeting. Eur Radiol 2017. https://doi.org/10.1007/s00330-017-5026-2.

10. Maas M, Lambregts DM, Lahaye MJ, et al. T-staging of rectal cancer: accuracy of 3.0 Tesla MRI compared with 1.5 Tesla. Abdom Imaging 2012;37:475–81.

11. Gutzeit A, Binkert CA, Koh D-M, et al. Evaluation of the anti-peristaltic effect of glucagon and hyoscine on the small bowel: comparison of intravenous and intramuscular drug administration. Eur Radiol 2012;22:1186–94.

12. Kim SH, Lee JM, Lee MW, et al. Sonography transmission gel as endorectal contrast agent for tumor visualization in rectal cancer. Am J Roentgenol 2008; 191:186–9.

13. Ye F, Zhang H, Liang X, et al. Preoperative MRI evaluation of primary rectal cancer: intrasubject comparison with and without rectal distention. Am J Roentgenol 2016;207:32–9.

14. Slater A, Halligan S, Taylor SA, et al. Distance between the rectal wall and mesorectal fascia measured by MRI: effect of rectal distention and implications for preoperative prediction of a tumour-free circumferential resection margin. Clin Radiol 2006;61:65–70.

15. Lim C, Quon J, McInnes M, et al. Does a cleansing enema improve image quality of 3T surface coil multiparametric prostate MRI? J Magn Reson Imaging 2015;42: 689–97.

16. Gollub MJ, Maas M, Weiser M, et al. Recognition of the anterior peritoneal reflection at rectal MRI. AJR Am J Roentgenol 2013;200:97–101.

17. Sahni VA, Silveira PC, Sainani NI, et al. Impact of a structured report template on the quality of MRI reports for rectal cancer staging. AJR Am J Roentgenol 2015; 205:584–8.

18. Available at: http://c.ymcdn.com/sites/www.abdominalradiology.org/resource/resmgr/docs/UPDATEDmri_primary_rectal_ca.pdf. Accessed December 22, 2017.

19. Al-Sukhni E, Milot L, Fruitman M, et al. Diagnostic accuracy of MRI for assessment of T category, lymph node metastases, and circumferential resection margin involvement in patients with rectal cancer: a systematic review and meta-analysis. Ann Surg Oncol 2012;19:2212–23.

20. Fernandez-Esparrach G, Avuso-Colella JR, Sendino O, et al. EUS and magnetic resonance imaging in the staging of rectal cancer: a prospective and comparative study. Gastrointest Endosc 2011;74:347–54.

21. MERCURY Study Group. Extramural depth of tumor invasion at thin-section MR in patients with rectal cancer: results of the MERCURY study. Radiology 2007;243: 132–9.

22. Bipat S, Glas AS, Slors FJM, et al. Rectal cancer: local staging and assessment of lymph node involvement with endoluminal US, CT, and MR imaging-a meta-analysis. Radiology 2004;232:773–83.

23. Brown G, Richards CJ, Bourne MW, et al. Morphologic predictors of lymph node status in rectal cancer with use of high-spatial-resolution MR imaging with histopathologic comparison. Radiology 2003;227:371–7.

24. Kim JH, Beets GL, Kim MJ, et al. High-resolution MR imaging for nodal staging in rectal cancer: are there any criteria in addition to the size? Eur J Radiol 2004;52: 78–83.

25. McMahon CJ, Rofsky NM, Pedrosa I. Lymphatic metastases from pelvic tumors: anatomic classification, characterization, and staging. Radiology 2010;254: 31–46.

26. Riihimaki M, Hemminki A, Sundquist J, et al. Patterns of metastasis in colon and rectal cancer. Sci Rep 2016;6:29765.

27. Bernstein TE, Endreseth BH, Romundstad P, et al, Norwegian Colorectal Cancer Group. Circumferential resection margin as a prognostic factor in rectal cancer. Br J Surg 2009;96:1348–57.

28. Beets-Tan RGH, Beets GL, Vliegen RFA, et al. Accuracy of magnetic resonance imaging in prediction of tumor-free resection margin in rectal cancer surgery. Lancet 2001;357:497–504.

29. MERCURY Study Group. Diagnostic accuracy of preoperative magnetic resonance imaging in predicting curative resection of rectal cancer: a prospective observational study. BMJ 2006;333:779.

30. Dresen RC, Beet GL, Rutten HJT, et al. Locally advanced rectal cancer: MR imaging for restaging after neoadjuvant radiation therapy with concomitant chemotherapy part 1. Are we able to predict tumor confined to the rectal wall? Radiology 2009;252:71–80.

31. Smith NJ, Shihab O, Arnaout A, et al. MRI for detection of extramural vascular invasion in rectal cancer. Am J Roentgenol 2008;191:1517–22.

32. Talbot IC, Ritchie S, Leighton MH, et al. The clinical significance of invasion of veins by rectal cancer. Br J Surg 1980;67:439–42.

33. Jhaveri KS, Hosseini-Nik H, Thipphavong S, et al. MRI detection of extramural venous invasion in rectal cancer: correlation with histopathology using elastin stain. Am J Roentgenol 2016;206:747–55.

34. Simha V, Kapoor R, Gupta R, et al. Mucinous adenocarcinoma of the rectum: a poor candidate for neo-adjuvant chemoradiation? J Gastrointest Oncol 2014;5: 276–9.

35. Reerink O, Verschueren RC, Szabo BG, et al. A favourable pathological stage after neoadjuvant radiochemotherapy in patients with initially irresectable rectal cancer correlates with a favourable prognosis. Eur J Cancer 2003;39:192–5.

36. Kim SH, Lee JM, Hong SH, et al. Locally advanced rectal cancer: added value of diffusion-weighted MR imaging in the evaluation of tumor response to neoadjuvant chemo- and radiation therapy. Radiology 2009;253:116–25.

37. Park SH, Lim JS, Lee J, et al. Rectal mucinous adenocarcinoma: MR imaging assessment of response to concurrent chemotherapy and radiation therapy–A hypothesis-generating study. Radiology 2017;285:124–33.

38. Heald RJ, Moran BJ, Ryall RDH, et al. Rectal cancer: the Basingstoke experience of total mesorectal excision, 1978-1997. Arch Surg 1998;133:894–9.

39. Quirke P, Steele R, Monson J, et al. Effect of the plane of surgery achieved on local recurrence in patients with operable rectal cancer: a prospective study

using data from the MRC CR07 and NCIC-CTG CO16 randomised clinical trial. Lancet 2009;373:821–8.

40. Mellgren A, Sirivongs P, Rothenberger DA, et al. Is local excision adequate therapy for early rectal cancer? Dis Colon Rectum 2000;43:1064–71.
41. Buess G, Kipfmuller K, Hack D, et al. Technique of transanal endoscopic microsurgery. Surg Endosc 1988;2:71–5.
42. Sauer R, Becker H, Hohenberger W, et al. Preoperative versus postoperative chemoradiotherapy for rectal cancer. N Engl J Med 2004;351:1731–40.
43. Braendengen M, Tveit KM, Berglund A, et al. Randomized phase III study comparing preoperative radiotherapy with chemoradiotherapy in nonresectable rectal cancer. J Clin Oncol 2008;26:3687–94.
44. Roh MS, Colangelo LH, O'Connell MJ, et al. Preoperative multimodality therapy improves disease-free survival in patients with carcinoma of the rectum: NSABP R-03. J Clin Oncol 2009;27:5124–30.
45. Bosset JF, Collette L, Calais G, et al. Chemotherapy with preoperative radiotherapy in rectal cancer. N Engl J Med 2006;355:1114–23.
46. Habr-Gama A, Sao Juliao GP, Perez RO. Nonoperative management of rectal cancer: identifying the ideal patients. Hematol Oncol Clin North Am 2015;29: 135–51.

Defecography
An Overview of Technique, Interpretation, and Impact on Patient Care

Nathan Y. Kim, MD[a], David H. Kim, MD[a], Perry J. Pickhardt, MD[a],
Evie H. Carchman, MD[b], Arnold Wald, MD[c],
Jessica B. Robbins, MD[a],*

KEYWORDS

- Defecography • Fluoroscopy • Rectum • Pelvic floor

KEY POINTS

- Pelvic floor and defecatory dysfunction are exceedingly common in the female population.
- Barium defecography provides real-time, functional, and morphologic assessment of defecation and pelvic floor function.
- Barium defecography is a cost-effective, widely available, and well-established examination for assessing defecation and pelvic floor disorders.

INTRODUCTION

Defecatory and pelvic organ dysfunctions are common ailments, particularly in women. Advanced age, obesity, prior obstetric injuries, multiparity, chronic constipation, irritable bowel syndrome, nutritional deficiencies, and psychiatric disorders are the associated risk factors.[1–3] Nearly 24% of women of all ages report symptoms of at least one pelvic floor disorder and it increases to nearly 50% of women older than 80 years.[4] It is reported that defecatory dysfunction affects 20% to 81% of patients with chronic constipation.[5] Furthermore, of the women evaluated for chronic constipation, approximately 11% undergo at least one surgical procedure for pelvic floor dysfunction.[6] Accurate assessment of these abnormalities is vital in selecting

Disclosures: Dr P.J. Pickhardt is the co-founder of VirtuoCTC; advisor to Check-Cap and Bracco; and shareholder in SHINE, Elucent, and Cellectar Biosciences. Dr N.Y. D. Kim is the co-founder of VirtuoCTC and shareholder in Elucent and Cellectar Biosciences.
[a] Department of Radiology, University of Wisconsin School of Medicine & Public Health, 600 Highland Avenue, Madison, WI 53792, USA; [b] Department of Surgery, University of Wisconsin School of Medicine & Public Health, 600 Highland Avenue, Madison, WI 53792, USA; [c] Department of Medicine, University of Wisconsin School of Medicine & Public Health, 600 Highland Avenue, Madison, WI 53792, USA
* Corresponding author.
E-mail address: jrobbins@uwhealth.org

the appropriate surgical procedure because failure to detect a relevant abnormality may contribute to the relative high rate of repeat surgery in these patients. However, functional alterations may be difficult to identify on physical examination and static anatomic imaging and are better observed with dynamic imaging techniques.

Barium defecography, also known as evacuation proctography, is a fluoroscopy-based examination that allows for evaluation of the anatomic structure and function of the anorectum and pelvic floor. It assesses the relationship between the pelvic structures at rest, with increased intraabdominal and intrapelvic pressure, and during defecation. More importantly, it allows for real-time, functional assessment of the mechanics of defecation in a physiologic position while seated on a commode, which is not possible in most other radiologic settings such as a closed-bore MRI system. Given the close relationship between defecatory dysfunction and pelvic floor disorders, defecography serves as a useful tool to evaluate a spectrum of pathologies of the anorectum and pelvic floor.

Although barium defecography serves as a robust functional assessment of defecation, it can only infer the structural components of the complex pelvic floor anatomy. In contrast, MRI offers direct visualization of the pelvic organs and muscles. When combined with dynamic sequences, it can also be used to evaluate pelvic floor dysfunction.[7] A traditional MRI of the pelvis with dynamic sequences requires defecation in a nonphysiologic supine position, thus affecting the evaluation of defecatory function. Specialized systems allowing MRI to be performed with the patient in an upright position are uncommon. Therefore, the high cost, necessity of specialized equipment, and variability of measurements have limited MR defecography from being universally adopted. For the evaluation of defecatory dysfunction, the most recent American College of Radiology (ACR) appropriateness criteria consider MR defecography with rectal contrast to be equivalent to barium defecography as the most appropriate examination only if the MRI can be performed with the patient in an upright and seated position.[8]

Although it lacks the anatomic detail afforded by MRI, barium defecography continues to serve an important role in that it provides specialized information in the evaluation of both defecatory and pelvic floor disorders. In this article, the authors describe the normal anatomy and physiology of the pelvic floor and the techniques they use when performing barium defecography, review the pathology that can be detected with this examination, and discuss its clinical implications. Because the patients who present with these disorders will be predominately women, the techniques, findings, and diagnoses discussed herein are focused on the female patient; however, they are all applicable to the male population as well.

ANATOMY AND PHYSIOLOGY

The pelvis is divided into 3 compartments: anterior, middle, and posterior. The anterior compartment contains the bladder and urethra, the middle compartment is composed of the uterus, cervix, and vagina, and the anorectum comprises the posterior compartment.

The pelvic floor is a complex structure composed of fascia and ligaments, which provide passive support, and muscles, which provide active support.[9] The levator ani is the main muscle complex of the pelvic floor, consisting of the pubococcygeus, iliococcygeus, and puborectalis muscles, which surround the rectum, bladder, and uterus (**Fig. 1**). The pubococcygeus and iliococcygeus comprise the major structural component of the pelvic floor. The pubococcygeus fans out from the superior pubic ramus to the coccyx and the iliococcygeus extends from the ischial spine to the

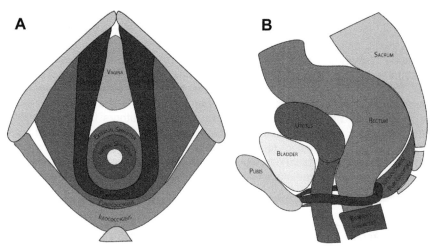

Fig. 1. Schematic axial (*A*) and sagittal (*B*) anatomy of the female pelvis and pelvic floor musculature.

anococcygeal body. The puborectalis attaches to the pubic symphysis and forms a sling around the anal canal, pulling it anteriorly to form the anorectal angle (see **Fig. 1**B). Along with the internal sphincter contraction at rest, the angulation of the anorectal junction provides the mechanical barrier for the flow of stool and maintains normal fecal continence.[10] Voluntary external sphincter and pelvic floor contraction can help increase resistance against defecation.

The rectum measures approximately 12 to 15 cm in length and extends from the rectosigmoid junction to the level of the levator ani, which anchors the rectum in the pelvis. The anal canal measures approximately 4 cm and extends from the levator ani to the anal verge.[11] The internal and external anal sphincters (see **Fig. 1**) comprise the bulk of the anal canal, and the internal sphincter is a continuation of the inner muscular layer of the rectum.

Normal defecation requires coordination between the rectum, pelvic floor, sphincter muscles, and nervous system. Distension from the fecal bolus in the rectum relaxes the internal anal sphincter. Evacuation is then initiated via voluntary activity including abdominal straining and pelvic floor relaxation, which allows the anorectal junction to descend. When the puborectalis relaxes, the anorectal angle straightens. Once the anal canal opens, stool empties from the rectum. After evacuation is complete, tone is restored to the sphincters and levator ani, the pelvic floor is restored to its resting position, and the anorectal angle returns to its acute angulation. Incoordination or weakness during this process or damage to these structures may result in defecation disorders.

EXAMINATION COMPONENTS AND TECHNIQUE
History

Common indications for defecography include a myriad of defecation disorders, such as chronic constipation, sense of incomplete or obstructive defecation, fecal incontinence, mucous or bloody discharge, perineal pain, or discomfort. In addition, defecography may be useful in surgical planning for patients undergoing pelvic floor surgery or as a follow-up of patients who have previously undergone surgery in the pelvic region.[12,13]

It is important to obtain a focused history before the examination, because it helps to understand the patient's perspective of their difficulty in defecation as well as the chronicity of their symptoms. It is important to inquire if the patient undertakes any maneuvers to help in fecal evacuation so that the maneuver can be investigated during the examination. Knowledge of prior interventions, such as pelvic physical therapy, and/or surgeries, is helpful. In addition, this personal interaction establishes rapport to help the patient feel more at ease with an examination that may be perceived as embarrassing. The authors found it helpful to stress that this is a routine examination that many patients undergo and that it provides important information for the surgeon or treating physician. They also emphasize that they explain everything that is happening, and the patient should feel free to notify the radiologist if they are uncomfortable or confused by the instructions.

Patient Preparation

In order to prepare the bowel for barium defecography, the patient is asked to undergo a bowel-cleansing regimen. They are instructed to follow a clear liquid diet beginning the morning before the examination, to ingest a cathartic agent (10 ounces magnesium citrate) and a laxative (20 mg bisacodyl) in the evening, and to cease all oral intakes after midnight. One hour before the examination, 350 mL of thin barium is administered orally to opacify the small bowel. At the time of the examination, female patients are placed on an examination table in a supine lithotomy position. A lubricated enema tip is inserted into the vagina and 40 to 60 mL of thick barium paste is instilled. All patients are then placed in a lateral decubitus position and a rectal examination is performed to assess rectal tone and evaluate for distal rectal mass. A lubricated enema tip is inserted into the rectum and 60 mL of thin barium is instilled, followed by approximately 180 mL of thick barium paste or until the patient can no longer tolerate further administration of contrast.

Examination

The patient is placed on a radiolucent fluoroscopy commode and the X-ray tube is centered on the pelvis from a lateral projection. Care must be taken to ensure that the skin of the perineum, the coccyx, and pubic bones are included in the field of view (**Fig. 2**). A scout image is obtained once the patient is optimally positioned to allow for assessment of the pelvic anatomy at rest (see **Fig. 2**A). Subsequently, multiple cine clips are obtained during full cycles of (1) squeeze, where the patient maximally contracts the anal sphincters and pelvic floor; (2) strain, where the patient strains but does not evacuate, in other words, performs a Valsalva maneuver; and (3) defecation, where the patient is instructed to evacuate completely and without interruption. In addition, if the patient senses they are unable to completely evacuate and identifies any maneuvers that assist with defecation, a cine clip should be repeated with the patient performing these maneuvers.

Because the radiologist asks the patient to perform specific maneuvers during the examination, verbal prompts in layman's terminology can be helpful to successfully communicate with the patient. For example, during the "squeeze" maneuver, the patient should maximally contract the anal sphincters and pelvic floor. An appropriate verbal prompt could be as follows: "squeeze your bottom as if you have a sense of urgency to have a bowel movement, but you cannot immediately get to a restroom." With straining, the objective is to increase intraabdominal and intrapelvic pressures to determine if this will elicit pathology. Therefore, the radiologist may ask the patient to perform a Valsalva maneuver with a verbal prompt such as "flex your abdominal

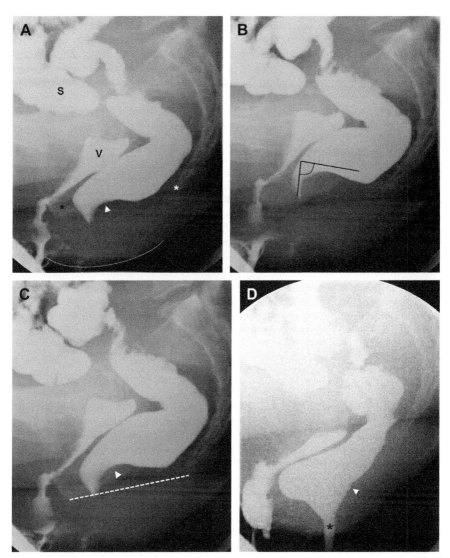

Fig. 2. Sagittal images from defecography. (*A*) Rest. The skin of the perineum (*dashed line*), the coccyx (*white asterisk*), and the pubis (*black asterisk*) are included in the field of view. The impression from the puborectalis (*arrowhead*) forms the anorectal angle. Contrast fills the vagina (V) and orally ingested contrast fills the small bowel (S). (*B*) Squeeze. Contraction of puborectalis increases the angulation of the anorectal angle. (*C*) Strain. The anorectal angle (*arrowhead*) returns to its resting state, and the pelvic organs do not descend below the pelvic floor denoted by pubococcygeal line (*dashed line*). (*D*) Evacuation. With evacuation, the anorectal angle (*arrowhead*) opens, descends, and the anal canal opens (*black asterisk*).

muscles like you are trying to have a bowel movement while at the same time trying to keep everything in." Finally, the defecation phase is intended to replicate physiologic defecation. As such, the patient may be asked to fully evacuate their rectum with as little interruption as possible.

Normal Defecogram Findings

At rest, the anus should be completely closed with the impression of the puborectalis on the posterior wall of the rectum forming the anorectal angle (see **Fig. 2**A). The anorectal angle ranges from approximately 90° to 140° at rest[14,15] when approximated along the central axis of the lumen. Given the degree of variability in the anorectal angle at rest, it is often not measured in practice.

During the squeeze phase, the pelvic floor contracts. Contraction of the puborectalis lifts the anorectal angle anteriorly and cranially and causes it to become more acute[14] (see **Fig. 2**B). This increase in angulation aids in maintenance of fecal continence.

During the strain phase, the anorectal angle should assume its resting configuration (see **Fig. 2**C). Straining, in effect, tests the integrity of the pelvic floor. Because the pelvic floor musculature is inconspicuous at fluoroscopy, the pubococcygeal line is used as the surrogate reference for the pelvic floor. The plane extending from the last coccygeal joint to the inferior margin of the pubis defines the pubococcygeal line[16] (see **Fig. 2**C). This line is a static representation of the expected location of the approximate margins of the pelvic floor, and thus the pelvic organs should remain superior to the pubococcygeal line at rest, during squeeze and throughout a Valsalva maneuver.[16] If, on the other hand, the pelvic structures descend below the pubococcygeal line at rest or there is excessive descent, greater than 3 cm, during evacuation, pathology should be suspected.[14,16] The strain sequence also allows for evaluation of integrity of the middle compartment of the pelvis. When the middle compartment is intact, the vagina remains in close apposition to the rectum throughout the examination, especially during strain (see **Fig. 2**C).

During evacuation, the puborectalis relaxes and the anorectal angle becomes more obtuse, the puborectalis impression becomes less conspicuous, and the rectum descends[14] (see **Fig. 2**C). In conjunction with the relaxation of both anal sphincters, the anus opens, through which the entirety of the rectal contents should pass. At the conclusion of the evacuation effort, the anal sphincters contract, closing the anus, and the puborectalis pulls the anorectum cranially and anteriorly back to its resting position.[14]

Abnormal Findings/Pathology

Rectocele

A rectocele is a protrusion of the anterior rectal wall due to weakness in the rectovaginal septum (**Fig. 3**). It is found almost exclusively in multiparous women, often as a result of obstetric trauma, with an incidence of 78% to 99% in parous women.[17–19] Rectoceles less than 2 cm in size are considered clinically insignificant and within normal limits, whereas rectoceles larger than 2 cm are often associated with evacuation disorders. Most patients with rectoceles have coexisting pathology, including rectal intussusception and dyssynergic defecation. As a result, the mere presence of a rectocele on defecography may not necessarily account for a patient's evacuation symptoms,[20] but the pattern of rectal deformation and the degree of rectal emptying observed during defecography may be helpful in determining if the rectocele is likely to account for the patient's symptoms. Finally, the size of a rectocele does not directly correlate with symptoms.[18]

Patients with rectoceles may be asymptomatic or present with nonspecific symptoms, such as pelvic pain, constant pelvic pressure, backache, and constipation. Some patients will describe requiring digital pressure on/in the vagina, the perineum, or rectum to complete evacuation.[20] If the patient requires manual pressure, the impact of such maneuvers can be observed during defecography.

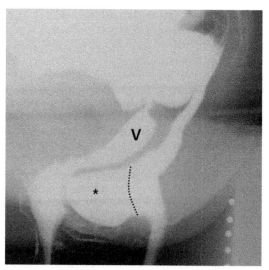

Fig. 3. Rectocele. The rectocele (*asterisk*) protrudes anteriorly beyond the expected contour of the anterior rectal wall (*dashed line*). The rectocele exerts significant mass effect on the vagina (V). Note that the vagina remains in close apposition to the rectum during the evacuation phase, excluding a coexisting middle compartment defect.

Surgical repair of a rectocele is generally performed transvaginally or transanally. The defect of the rectovaginal septal fascia is repaired, with or without mesh, and the rectal redundancy plicated.[21]

Enterocele

Enteroceles represent herniation of the peritoneal sac into the rectovaginal space or posterior cul-de-sac (**Fig. 4**). When filled with sigmoid colon, they are referred to as sigmoidoceles. Women who have undergone previous gynecologic procedures,

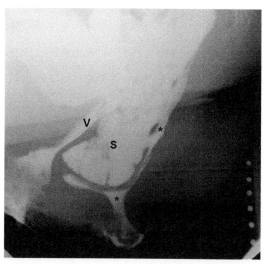

Fig. 4. Enterocele. At the end of evacuation, small bowel (S) herniates into the Pouch of Douglas displacing the vagina (V) anteriorly and exerting mass effect on the rectum (*asterisks*).

such as hysterectomy or urethropexy are at increased risk for development of enterocele because both procedures involve opening of the posterior cul-de-sac.[13,22,23] One study demonstrated enterocele in 64% of patients with prior hysterectomy and 27% of patients with prior cystopexy.[24]

Unlike rectoceles, enteroceles are difficult to detect on physical examination. Enteroceles are often more evident at the end of evacuation, when the rectum is nearly empty yielding space into which the peritoneal contents can herniate.[16,25] As a result, some enteroceles may only become evident fluoroscopically on postevacuation images with maximal straining. The mass effect of the small bowel on the rectal or vaginal wall can result in an associated rectal or vaginal vault prolapse.

Typical symptoms associated with enteroceles include pelvic pain, heaviness on standing, pelvic pressure during straining, incomplete evacuation, and postevacuation discomfort.[20] It is unclear if these symptoms can be entirely, or even partially, attributed to the presence of an enterocele. Some studies have suggested that enteroceles do not impair evacuation[26–28] and are not related to symptoms of bowel dysfunction.[29] Nevertheless, other studies have reported symptomatic improvement with surgical repair although in a limited series of patients.[13]

Treatment options for these patients include avoidance of heavy lifting and straining, a pessary, or surgical intervention. The goal of surgical intervention is to obliterate the Pouch of Douglas, sometimes with the assistance of mesh; the surgical approach is either transabdominal or transvaginal.[28]

Intussusception

Intussusception occurs when there is an invagination of the rectal wall during defecation or straining. The location of the intussusception can vary, remaining within the rectum (rectorectal intussusception) (**Fig. 5**), extending into the anus (anorectal intussusception) or extending past the anal canal (rectal prolapse) (**Figs. 6** and **7**). Because of the internal nature of the first 2 types of intussusception, defecography is often the only means of making this diagnosis. However, intussusception can occasionally be difficult to distinguish from normal rectal mucosal folds, especially when the rectum

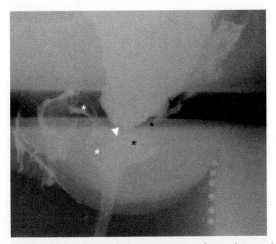

Fig. 5. Rectorectal intussusception. Late in the evacuation phase, the proximal rectum (*black asterisks*) telescopes into the distal rectum (*white asterisks*) with invagination of the anterior aspect of the distal rectal wall (*arrowhead*) toward the anal canal.

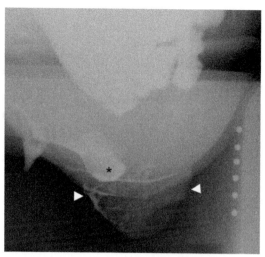

Fig. 6. Rectal prolapse. The distal rectum has prolapsed through the anal canal (*arrowheads*). Residual contrast coats the prolapsed rectal mucosa. The vaginal apex (*asterisk*) is also prolapsed.

seems to in-fold, because this may represent collapse of the rectum on itself.[16] Like an enterocele, an intussusception may only become apparent during the late phases of defecation.

Rectal intussusception is frequently associated with solitary rectal ulcer syndrome, occurring in 45% to 80% of patients.[20] Chronic straining results in ischemia and

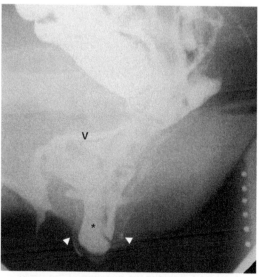

Fig. 7. Rectal prolapse, rectal intussusception, and enterocele. In the final phase of defecation, multiple loops of small bowel descend between the vagina (V) and rectum forming an enterocele. Along with the proximal rectum, a portion of the enterocele (*asterisk*) telescopes into the distal rectum (rectal intussusception) and the entire complex prolapses through the anal canal (*arrowheads*).

mucosal injury to the anterior wall of the rectum, in the region where it is repeatedly exposed to pressure and trauma. The chronic insult of the anterior rectal wall is thought to cause erosions and eventually ulceration. Solitary ulcer syndrome is a misnomer, because only 35% of cases have the characteristic solitary ulceration, 22% to 30% of patients have several ulcerations, 25% may have a polypoid lesion, and nearly 20% may merely have hyperemic mucosa.[30,31]

Patients with rectal intussusception may report symptoms of obstructed defecation, incomplete evacuation, rectal pain, and/or hematochezia. Rectal intussusception is itself not pathologic as it has been demonstrated in up to 50% to 60% of healthy volunteers.[15] As a result, care must be taken before attributing symptoms to an intussusception. Conservative treatment with behavioral therapy and biofeedback are commonplace.[31] A fiber-rich diet may be helpful but, in isolation, is generally not effective.[31] The role of surgery is more controversial with numerous procedures, including rectopexy, transrectal excision, and laparoscopic resection rectopexy, showing poor improvement in symptoms despite resolution of the intussusception.[20]

Rectal prolapse

Rectal prolapse is defined as protrusion of all layers of the rectal wall through the anal canal[20] (see **Fig. 6**). The pathophysiology of rectal prolapse is still not well delineated because progression of an internal rectal intussusception, an abnormally deep anterior cul-de-sac, redundant sigmoid colon, weakened pelvic floor, and insufficient rectal-sacral attachments have all been implicated.[20,22,32,33] Rectal prolapse can occur either in isolation or in association with prolapse of other pelvic organs such as the vagina/uterus and/or bladder or small bowel (see **Fig. 7**). Defecography is able to delineate the extent of pelvic prolapse.

Rectal prolapse is rare, occurring in approximately 0.5% of the population, with the highest incidence in elderly women.[33] Although prolapse is often attributed to obstetric injury, approximately one-third of female patients with prolapse are nulliparous.[33] The peak age in men is less than 40 years of age with a predilection in patients with autism and developmental delay.[33]

Patients will often report protrusion of the rectum through the anus with passage of blood and mucus, which can result in debilitating discomfort due to internal and external symptoms. Digital manipulation may be necessary to reduce the prolapsed segment of rectum. Fecal incontinence and constipation are common, affecting approximately 50% to 75% and 25% to 50% of patients with prolapse, respectively.[33,34]

The primary surgical approaches to rectal prolapse are transabdominal and transanal and are the only curative treatment of rectal prolapse. A transabdominal approach is associated with lower rates of recurrence, but a transanal approach is preferred in a patient with significant comorbidities.[33] For a transabdominal procedure the options include rectopexy (open or minimally invasive approach) or resection with rectopexy.[33] For the rectopexy portion of the procedure, it is up to surgeon preference to determine if mesh (Anterior Sling Rectopexy (Ripstein Procedure), Posterior Mesh Rectopexy or Ventral Rectopexy) or sutures should be used.[33] Transperineal procedures include the Delorme procedure and the Perineal Rectosigmoidectomy (Altemeier Procedure).[33] The Delorme procedure is a mucosal sleeve resection and is preferred for short segment or hem circumference rectal prolapses in high-risk patients.[33] The Altemeier procedure involves full thickness excision of the prolapsing rectum, resulting in a coloanal anastomosis.[33] This procedure is combined with levatorplasty to tighten the pelvic floor muscles and decrease fecal incontinence.[33] The specific procedure is generally dictated by the surgeon's preference and experience as well as the patient's comorbidities and age.[33]

Descending perineum syndrome

Descending perineum syndrome results from excessive descent of the perineum at rest and during defecation as a result of pelvic floor hypotonia[12] (**Fig. 8**). Perineal descent has been linked to chronic straining, followed by a sense of obstruction, resulting in a cycle of straining and constipation.[13] In older patients, the pelvic floor is lower at rest and there is lesser descent at evacuation, which can make the findings subtle during defecation.[35] Descending perineum syndrome is usually defined as more than 3 to 4 cm of descent during evacuation or when the anorectal junction sits 3 cm below its normal position at rest.[16,36]

Patients may present with painful or impaired defecation, excessive straining, incomplete evacuation, or fecal incontinence, which are accompanied by mucoid discharge and bleeding. Hysterectomy is a likely predisposing factor in its development.[37] Because of the pelvic floor hypotonia, perineal descent is often associated with other anorectal disorders, such as rectocele, solitary rectal ulcer syndrome, enterocele, and rectal prolapse.[38]

The treatment of descending perineum syndrome mainly consists of conservative measures aimed at correcting chronic straining, namely biofeedback.[38] Another option is a specialized commode that consists of 2 separate holes for passing urine and stool with a built-in hump to support the perineum that has been shown to improve symptoms in approximately 50% of patients.[31] There is currently no surgical intervention for perineal descent syndrome.[36]

Pelvic floor dyssynergia

In pelvic floor dyssynergia, also known as nonrelaxing puborectalis syndrome, spastic pelvic floor syndrome, puborectalis dyskinesia, or anismus, there is a poor coordination of abdominal and pelvic floor muscles to evacuate stool. Various underlying abnormalities may include inadequate propulsive forces, paradoxic anal sphincter contraction, and/or inadequate anal sphincter relaxation[39] (**Fig. 9**). The most common symptoms include excessive straining, incomplete evacuation, and abdominal bloating.[39]

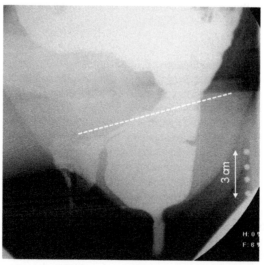

Fig. 8. Descending perineum. There is approximately 6 cm of descent of the vagina and anorectum below the anticipated position of the pelvic floor as denoted by the pubococcygeal line (*dashed line*).

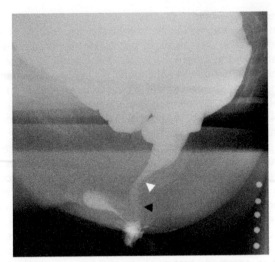

Fig. 9. Pelvic floor dyssynergia. Continued impression of the puborectalis (*white arrowhead*) at the anorectal junction and contraction of the anal sphincters (*black arrowhead*) precluding evacuation of contrast despite maximal strain during attempted evacuation.

Defecography is often used in conjunction with physiologic testing, such as anal manometry, electromyography, and balloon expulsion to diagnose pelvic floor dyssynergia. During defecography, the indentation of the puborectalis tends to remain during evacuation because of paradoxic persistent muscular contraction and there is prolonged retention or incomplete evacuation of barium.[40,41]

Similar to descending perineum syndrome, management is focused on conservative therapy, namely biofeedback therapy, with the goal of improving rectal and pelvic floor coordination.[42] Use of laxatives and stool softeners are inferior to biofeedback because they do not address the underlying abnormality.[42,43] There are currently no surgical options for the treatment of pelvic floor dyssynergia.

CLINICAL APPLICATIONS

Pelvic floor dysfunction is estimated to affect 24% to 37% of community-dwelling women with approximately 60% of these women experiencing defecatory dysfunction.[4,44,45] Approximately 11% of patients whom have been evaluated for their defecatory disorder have undergone at least one surgery, most commonly enterocele or rectocele repair, and nearly 30% of these patients ultimately undergo repeat surgery for recurrence.[6] Although the exact cause for the high rate of recurrence is not well understood, it may reflect a failure to recognize the full extent of pathology before surgical intervention. Pelvic floor disorders are often multicompartmental and, therefore, often benefit from a multidisciplinary team approach consisting of a gastroenterologist and colorectal, urologic, and gynecologic surgeons to evaluate and treat the patient.

The role of barium defecography in surgical planning remains unclear. One report found defecography to be of major benefit in 40% of patients, enabling surgical management to be substituted by medical management in 14% of cases.[46] Furthermore, the report found defecography to improve diagnostic confidence and clarify the initial clinical assessment in a significant percentage of patients referred for the examination.

Although one study has shown that coexisting asymptomatic defects can become symptomatic if a comprehensive repair is not performed,[47] this must be balanced with the myriad of findings that can be seen in asymptomatic patients, including small intra-rectal intussusceptions, small rectoceles, and small enteroceles. Therefore, treatment should be targeted to the patient's symptoms instead of solely imaging results, especially when small or isolated abnormalities are noted.[48,49]

Barium defecography is recommended by the American College of Gastroenterology (ACG) when the clinical features suggest a defecatory disorder but the results of anorectal manometry and balloon expulsion test are equivocal.[50] A recent study has shown significant disagreement between anorectal manometry and balloon expulsion[50,51] and other studies have demonstrated that defecography can identify defecatory dysfunction in symptomatic patients with normal manometry.[52,53] As such, no single test is sufficient for diagnosing all forms of defecatory dysfunction. For example, in the setting of fecal incontinence, barium defecography serves a limited role in the diagnostic evaluation except to identify structural alterations of the pelvic floor.[5] On the other hand, in the assessment of rectal prolapse, defecography may identify internal pelvic organ prolapse, not readily identifiable on physical examination, which may prompt a multidisciplinary surgical team evaluation.[54]

LIMITATIONS

There are several limitations of barium defecography that have precluded more routine utilization of this examination. First, the artificial setting required for defecography can potentially embarrass and inhibit the patient from their normal defecatory process, reducing its physiologic representation. Second, defecography suffers from a lack of accepted standards of reference with which to make definitive diagnoses. As a result, there have been attempts to establish a range of normal parameters using healthy volunteers,[14,15,19] although a small study found poor interobserver reliability.[55] Although defecography lacks the soft tissue characterization and multiplanar capabilities of more advanced imaging, such as ultrasound and MRI, when performed properly, it can yield many of the same diagnoses. In addition, the consistency of the barium paste may not represent the consistency of normal stool for all patients, which is why the balloon expulsion test is complementary.

SUMMARY

Barium defecography is a cost-effective, widely available, and well-established examination for assessing defecation and pelvic floor disorders. Despite its limitations, it provides real-time, functional, and morphologic assessment of defecation. It continues to play a significant role in the workup of these disorders, complementing physical examination and other examinations, such as manometry, balloon expulsion, and electromyography.

REFERENCES

1. Nygaard I, Bradley C, Brandt D, Women's Health Initiative. Pelvic organ prolapse in older women: prevalence and risk factors. Obstet Gynecol 2004;104(3):489–97.
2. Swift S, Woodman P, O'Boyle A, et al. Pelvic Organ Support Study (POSST): the distribution, clinical definition, and epidemiologic condition of pelvic organ support defects. Am J Obstet Gynecol 2005;192(3):795–806.
3. Silva AC, Maglinte DD. Pelvic floor disorders: what's the best test? Abdom Imaging 2013;38(6):1391–408.
4. Nygaard I, Barber MD, Burgio KL, et al. Prevalence of symptomatic pelvic floor disorders in US women. JAMA 2008;300(11):1311–6.

5. Rao SS, Bharucha AE, Chiarioni G, et al. Functional anorectal disorders. Gastroenterology 2006;130(5):1510–8.

6. Olsen AL, Smith VJ, Bergstrom JO, et al. Epidemiology of surgically managed pelvic organ prolapse and urinary incontinence. Obstet Gynecol 1997;89(4): 501–6.

7. Khatri G, de Leon AD, Lockhart ME. MR imaging of the pelvic floor. Magn Reson Imaging Clin N Am 2017;25(3):457–80.

8. Pannu HK, Javitt MC, Glanc P, et al. ACR appropriateness criteria pelvic floor dysfunction. J Am Coll Radiol 2015;12(2):134–42.

9. Stoker J, Halligan S, Bartram CI. Pelvic floor imaging. Radiology 2001;218(3): 621–41.

10. Patcharatrakul T, Rao SSC. Update on the pathophysiology and management of anorectal disorders. Gut Liver 2017. [Epub ahead of print].

11. Solan P, Davis B. Anorectal anatomy and imaging techniques. Gastroenterol Clin North Am 2013;42(4):701–12.

12. Faccioli N, Comai A, Mainardi P, et al. Defecography: a practical approach. Diagn Interv Radiol 2010;16(3):209–16.

13. Jorge JM, Habr-Gama A, Wexner SD. Clinical applications and techniques of cinedefecography. Am J Surg 2001;182(1):93–101.

14. Bartram CI, Turnbull GK, Lennard-Jones JE. Evacuation proctography: an investigation of rectal expulsion in 20 subjects without defecatory disturbance. Gastrointest Radiol 1988;13(1):72–80.

15. Shorvon PJ, McHugh S, Diamant NE, et al. Defecography in normal volunteers: results and implications. Gut 1989;30(12):1737–49.

16. Maglinte DD, Hale DS, Sandrasegaran K. Comparison between dynamic cystocolpoproctography and dynamic pelvic floor MRI: pros and cons: which is the "functional" examination for anorectal and pelvic floor dysfunction? Abdom Imaging 2013;38(5):952–73.

17. Kelvin FM, Maglinte DD, Hornback JA, et al. Pelvic prolapse: assessment with evacuation proctography (defecography). Radiology 1992;184(2):547–51.

18. Kenton K, Shott S, Brubaker L. The anatomic and functional variability of rectoceles in women. Int Urogynecol J Pelvic Floor Dysfunct 1999;10(2):96–9.

19. Palit S, Bhan C, Lunniss PJ, et al. Evacuation proctography: a reappraisal of normal variability. Colorectal Dis 2014;16(7):538–46.

20. Felt-Bersma RJ, Tiersma ES, Cuesta MA. Rectal prolapse, rectal intussusception, rectocele, solitary rectal ulcer syndrome, and enterocele. Gastroenterol Clin North Am 2008;37(3):645–68, ix.

21. Grossi U, Horrocks EJ, Mason J, et al. Surgery for constipation: systematic review and practice recommendations: results IV: recto-vaginal reinforcement procedures. Colorectal Dis 2017;19(Suppl 3):73–91.

22. Yang XM, Partanen K, Farin P, et al. Defecography. Acta Radiol 1995;36(5):460–8.

23. Karasick S, Karasick D, Karasick SR. Functional disorders of the anus and rectum: findings on defecography. AJR Am J Roentgenol 1993;160(4):777–82.

24. Hock D, Lombard R, Jehaes C, et al. Colpocystodefecography. Dis Colon Rectum 1993;36(11):1015–21.

25. Takahashi T, Yamana T, Sahara R, et al. Enterocele: what is the clinical implication? Dis Colon Rectum 2006;49(10 Suppl):S75–81.

26. Halligan S, Bartram C, Hall C, et al. Enterocele revealed by simultaneous evacuation proctography and peritoneography: does "defecation block" exist? AJR Am J Roentgenol 1996;167(2):461–6.

27. Gosselink MJ, van Dam JH, Huisman WM, et al. Treatment of enterocele by obliteration of the pelvic inlet. Dis Colon Rectum 1999;42(7):940–4.
28. Oom DM, van Dijl VR, Gosselink MP, et al. Enterocele repair by abdominal obliteration of the pelvic inlet: long-term outcome on obstructed defaecation and symptoms of pelvic discomfort. Colorectal Dis 2007;9(9):845–50.
29. Chou Q, Weber AM, Piedmonte MR. Clinical presentation of enterocele. Obstet Gynecol 2000;96(4):599–603.
30. Goei R, Baeten C, Janevski B, et al. The solitary rectal ulcer syndrome: diagnosis with defecography. AJR Am J Roentgenol 1987;149(5):933–6.
31. Schey R, Cromwell J, Rao SS. Medical and surgical management of pelvic floor disorders affecting defecation. Am J Gastroenterol 2012;107(11):1624–33 [quiz p: 1634].
32. Neill ME, Parks AG, Swash M. Physiological studies of the anal sphincter musculature in faecal incontinence and rectal prolapse. Br J Surg 1981;68(8):531–6.
33. Bordeianou L, Paquette I, Johnson E, et al. Clinical practice guidelines for the treatment of rectal prolapse. Dis Colon Rectum 2017;60(11):1121–31.
34. Madoff RD, Mellgren A. One hundred years of rectal prolapse surgery. Dis Colon Rectum 1999;42(4):441–50.
35. Pinho M, Yoshioka K, Ortiz J, et al. The effect of age on pelvic floor dynamics. Int J Colorectal Dis 1990;5(4):207–8.
36. Chaudhry Z, Tarnay C. Descending perineum syndrome: a review of the presentation, diagnosis, and management. Int Urogynecol J 2016;27(8):1149–56.
37. Pucciani F, Boni D, Perna F, et al. Descending perineum syndrome: are abdominal hysterectomy and bowel habits linked? Dis Colon Rectum 2005;48(11):2094–9.
38. Rao SS, Go JT. Treating pelvic floor disorders of defecation: management or cure? Curr Gastroenterol Rep 2009;11(4):278–87.
39. Rao SS, Tuteja AK, Vellema T, et al. Dyssynergic defecation: demographics, symptoms, stool patterns, and quality of life. J Clin Gastroenterol 2004;38(8):680–5.
40. Halligan S, Malouf A, Bartram CI, et al. Predictive value of impaired evacuation at proctography in diagnosing anismus. AJR Am J Roentgenol 2001;177(3):633–6.
41. Jorge JM, Wexner SD, Ger GC, et al. Cinedefecography and electromyography in the diagnosis of nonrelaxing puborectalis syndrome. Dis Colon Rectum 1993;36(7):668–76.
42. Rao SS, Seaton K, Miller M, et al. Randomized controlled trial of biofeedback, sham feedback, and standard therapy for dyssynergic defecation. Clin Gastroenterol Hepatol 2007;5(3):331–8.
43. Chiarioni G, Whitehead WE, Pezza V, et al. Biofeedback is superior to laxatives for normal transit constipation due to pelvic floor dyssynergia. Gastroenterology 2006;130(3):657–64.
44. Lawrence JM, Lukacz ES, Nager CW, et al. Prevalence and co-occurrence of pelvic floor disorders in community-dwelling women. Obstet Gynecol 2008;111(3):678–85.
45. Kepenekci I, Keskinkilic B, Akinsu F, et al. Prevalence of pelvic floor disorders in the female population and the impact of age, mode of delivery, and parity. Dis Colon Rectum 2011;54(1):85–94.
46. Harvey CJ, Halligan S, Bartram CI, et al. Evacuation proctography: a prospective study of diagnostic and therapeutic effects. Radiology 1999;211(1):223–7.
47. Gill EJ, Hurt WG. Pathophysiology of pelvic organ prolapse. Obstet Gynecol Clin North Am 1998;25(4):757–69.

48. Agachan F, Pfeifer J, Wexner SD. Defecography and proctography. Results of 744 patients. Dis Colon Rectum 1996;39(8):899–905.

49. Renzi A, Izzo D, Di Sarno G, et al. Cinedefecographic findings in patients with obstructed defecation syndrome. A study in 420 cases. Minerva Chir 2006;61(6): 493–9.

50. Wald A, Bharucha AE, Cosman BC, et al. ACG clinical guideline: management of benign anorectal disorders. Am J Gastroenterol 2014;109(8):1141–57 [quiz: 1058].

51. Palit S, Thin N, Knowles CH, et al. Diagnostic disagreement between tests of evacuatory function: a prospective study of 100 constipated patients. Neurogastroenterol Motil 2016;28(10):1589–98.

52. Bordeianou L, Savitt L, Dursun A. Measurements of pelvic floor dyssynergia: which test result matters? Dis Colon Rectum 2011;54(1):60–5.

53. Chiarioni G, Kim SM, Vantini I, et al. Validation of the balloon evacuation test: reproducibility and agreement with findings from anorectal manometry and electromyography. Clin Gastroenterol Hepatol 2014;12(12):2049–54.

54. Vogler SA. Rectal prolapse. Dis Colon Rectum 2017;60(11):1132–5.

55. Muller-Lissner SA, Bartolo DC, Christiansen J, et al. Interobserver agreement in defecography–an international study. Z Gastroenterol 1998;36(4):273–9.

Multidetector Computed Tomography for Retrospective, Noninvasive Staging of Liver Fibrosis

Meghan G. Lubner, MD*, Perry J. Pickhardt, MD

KEYWORDS

- MDCT • Liver fibrosis • Liver segmental volume ratio (LSVR)
- Liver surface nodularity • CT texture analysis • Elastography

KEY POINTS

- Noninvasive assessment of hepatic fibrosis currently includes laboratory tests, clinical data, and cross-sectional imaging, particularly magnetic resonance or ultrasound elastography techniques.
- Computed tomography (CT) is fast, accessible, robust, and commonly used for a variety of abdominal indications. CT metrics are captured retrospectively without special equipment.
- Subjective assessment of morphologic changes of liver disease is relatively insensitive, particularly for early or intermediate stages of fibrosis; however, new CT tools or metrics allowing quantitative assessment of these features may improve detection.
- Liver segmental volume ratio (Volume of segments I–III/Segments IV–VIII) quantifies regional hepatic volume changes and allows detection of significant fibrosis (≥METAVIR fibrosis stage 2).
- Quantification of liver surface nodularity on CT can accurately identify intermediate stages of fibrosis and was the best performing metric in a multiparametric model.

INTRODUCTION

Liver disease resulting in hepatic fibrosis is a common problem that is important to identify early to halt progression and, with continued improvements in therapy, potentially reverse the process. Assessing the degree of hepatic fibrosis is useful in

Disclosures: M.G. Lubner receives grant funding from Philips, Ethicon. P.J. Pickhardt is the cofounder of VirtuoCTC and advisor to Check-Cap and Bracco, as well a shareholder in SHINE, Elucent, and Cellectar Biosciences.
Department of Radiology, University of Wisconsin School of Medicine and Public Health, E3/311 Clinical Sciences Center, 600 Highland Avenue, Madison, WI 53792, USA
* Corresponding author. Department of Radiology, University of Wisconsin School of Medicine and Public Health, E3/311 Clinical Sciences Center, 600 Highland Avenue, Madison, WI 53792.
E-mail address: mlubner@uwhealth.org

Gastroenterol Clin N Am 47 (2018) 569–584
https://doi.org/10.1016/j.gtc.2018.04.012
0889-8553/18/© 2018 Elsevier Inc. All rights reserved.

determining treatment and prognosis.[1,2] Liver biopsy remains the gold standard in diagnosing and staging hepatic fibrosis; however, this method is invasive, expensive, and may be subject to sampling error.[3,4] Pathologic scoring of fibrosis is commonly reported as fibrosis stage (F)-0 through F4, corresponding to absent (F0), early or mild (F1), significant (≥F2), advanced (≥F3), and cirrhotic (F4) levels. However, there has been a growing interest in noninvasive staging of liver disease, with great strides made in the last decade, particularly with respect to medical imaging. A variety of noninvasive strategies exists, ranging from serum laboratory tests to techniques assessing liver stiffness such as magnetic resonance (MR) and ultrasound (US) elastography.[2] Although not traditionally used in the assessment of hepatic fibrosis, computed tomography (CT) can also be a valuable tool in the assessment of liver disease.

NONINVASIVE ASSESSMENT OF LIVER DISEASE
Laboratory Tests or Biochemical Markers

The first and easiest step in assessing liver disease is often the use of routine serologic biochemical tests.[1] Several different models or scoring systems combining blood-based laboratory values exist and rely on evaluation of common functional alterations of liver to identify significant fibrosis or cirrhosis.[5–8] Two of the most frequently used scoring systems, extensively studied in viral hepatitis, include AST to platelet ratio index (APRI) (platelets, aspartate aminotransferase (AST)) or Fibrosis 4 (FIB-4) (age, platelets, AST, alanine aminotransferase (ALT)) scores.[9,10] These scores may suggest significant fibrosis (≥F2, area under the curve [AUC] 0.63–0.86) but cannot stage individual fibrosis levels and typically cannot detect mild or early stages of fibrosis that are at risk for progression.[9,10] Serum markers measuring products of extracellular matrix synthesis, or degradation products and enzymes that regulate production have been found to be increased in patients with advanced fibrosis, which has led to the development of new and potentially improved serum assays.[5,6,8,11] Again, the main limitation of these tests is the inability to identify early stages of fibrosis. In addition, these more advanced assays may not be available in all clinical laboratories.[1]

Imaging Techniques: Magnetic Resonance and Ultrasound Elastography

Use of elastography techniques for measuring liver stiffness has increased for assessment of hepatic fibrosis. Transient US elastography (eg, Fibroscan, Echosens, Paris France) is widely used in Europe.[12] Mechanical vibrations are transmitted to tissues, which induces a shear wave that propagates in the liver. The measured velocity of wave propagation is directly related to liver tissue stiffness (shear waves travel faster in stiffer tissues).[1] This technique has shown moderate performance in detecting significant fibrosis (≥F2) with an AUC of approximately 0.72 to 0.91 in patients with Hepatitis C virus (HCV).[12–16] Another US-based elastography technique generates shear waves by focusing an acoustic radiation force inside the tissue of interest.[17] This technique allows real-time conventional hepatic US for window placement of elastography and shows similar or improved performance compared with transient elastography, with AUCs for significant fibrosis (≥F2) of 0.85 to 0.87 in meta-analyses.[16,18,19] The downside to US assessment is that it can be limited by the acoustic window (often performed from an intercostal approach) or by patient body habitus.

MR elastography uses a similar technique to transient US elastography, in which shear waves are generated by applying a mechanical vibration to the surface of the body. However, with MR elastography, these shear waves are generated continuously and are tracked by acquiring images with motion sensitive phase-contrast sequences used to create wave images and subsequent elastograms.[17] MR elastography performs as well or better than US elastography in identifying significant fibrosis (≥F2), with AUCs of 0.88 to 0.98 in meta-analyses.[16,20,21] MRI does not require a specific acoustic window and is more operator-independent than US.[1] However, MR elastography is associated with higher cost, longer examination time, and lower accessibility than US. Wagner and colleagues[22] reported that, even in expert hands, a 3.5% (1.5 T) and 15.3% (3.0 T) technical failure rate for MR elastography is seen with associated factors, including body mass index, liver iron deposition, massive ascites, and the presence of cirrhosis. In addition, both US and MR elastography techniques require special equipment and must be prospectively planned and applied. Elastography techniques use stiffness as a surrogate for fibrosis; however, other entities such as inflammation and congestion can also lead to increased liver stiffness.[2]

MULTIDETECTOR COMPUTED TOMOGRAPHY FOR ASSESSMENT OF HEPATIC FIBROSIS

Multidetector CT (MDCT) is widely available, robust, repeatable, time-efficient, and has high temporal and spatial resolution with multiple postprocessing capabilities.[23] This is currently the workhorse modality for myriad indications in abdominal imaging, in which liver disease may or may not be present, suspected, or the primary focus of imaging.[24] A variety of CT parameters, many of which can be measured retrospectively and without specific equipment or technique, can therefore be harnessed in the assessment of liver disease, and these features are the emphasis of the remainder of this review article. CT uses ionizing radiation and, in many cases, intravenous (IV) iodine-based contrast media, which must be taken into consideration when choosing CT as an evaluation modality in this setting.

Morphologic Features of Liver Disease on Computed Tomography

A variety of morphologic features of advanced fibrosis and cirrhosis can be subjectively identified on cross-sectional imaging. These include relative atrophy of the right lobe and medial left lobe (Couinaud segments IV–VIII) with associated hypertrophy of the left lateral section and caudate (segments I–III); liver surface nodularity (LSN); hepatic fissural widening, including expansion of the gallbladder fossa and the hilar periportal space; narrowing of the hepatic veins; and development of a right hepatic posterior notch[2,25–30] (**Fig. 1**). Although many of these assessments are subjective, some can be objectively quantified. For example, when assessing the periportal space, a unidimensional measurement is taken from the anterior wall of the right portal vein to the posterior margin of the medial segment of the left hepatic lobe. The line of the measurement is made perpendicular to the midpoint of the anterior wall of the right portal vein on transverse images (**Fig. 2**). A measurement greater than 10 mm is considered a widened distance and demonstrates a sensitivity of 93%, specificity of 92%, accuracy of 92%, and a positive predictive value of 91% for a diagnosis of early cirrhosis.[31] In later stages of fibrosis, findings of portal hypertension can also be identified, including splenomegaly and development of portosystemic collaterals. However, many of these findings, particularly those that are subjective, may lack interobserver reproducibility, leading to variability in accuracy. In addition, these tend to be features of cirrhosis and may not be present or easily identifiable in earlier stages of fibrosis.[2] Even in the setting of cirrhosis, studies have shown that these features may or may not be present, with 15% to 20% of subjects showing advanced fibrosis or cirrhosis on biopsy, elevated liver stiffness on elastography, but no morphologic features of cirrhosis on cross-sectional imaging.[32,33]

Because development of hepatic fibrosis and cirrhosis is a continuous process, one could hypothesize that these changes are occurring very gradually and are present but

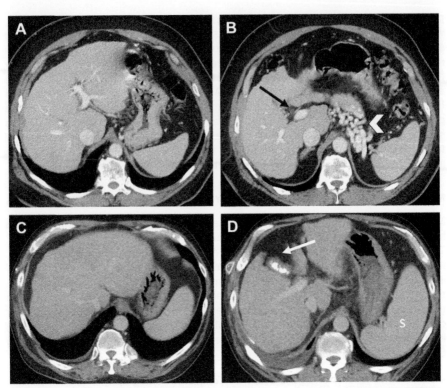

Fig. 1. Two different patients with cirrhosis demonstrating multiple morphologic features on CECT. (*A, B*) Hypertrophy of the left lateral section and caudate with comparable atrophy of the right and medial left lobe. Surface nodularity, hepatic fissural prominence, and expansion of the periportal space (*arrow, B*), with multiple portosystemic collaterals seen (*arrowhead, B*) are apparent. (*C, D*) A different patient with hypertrophy of the left lateral liver (segments II and III) and surface nodularity (*C*) but also expansion of the gallbladder fossa (*arrow, D*) and splenomegaly (*S*).

challenging to visually identify in early stages. Objective CT-based tools and metrics for quantification of these morphologic changes have emerged that have shown more promise in identifying earlier stages of liver disease. Conceivably, some of these measurements could also be performed on MRI but have been evaluated more extensively on CT.

Volumetric Assessment of the Liver and Spleen on Computed Tomography

Because of the known relative changes of atrophy of the right lobe and medial left lobe with compensatory hypertrophy of the left lateral section and caudate, a measurement termed the caudate–right-lobe (CRL) ratio was devised to capture this.[34,35] The method for obtaining the CRL ratio, as detailed by Harbin and colleagues,[34] is to draw a line through the right lateral wall of the main portal vein, with a second line through the most medial margin of the caudate lobe. A third line is drawn perpendicular to lines 1 and 2, midway between the portal vein and the inferior vena cava. The distances along line 3 between lines 1 and 2 (width of caudate) and along line 3 between the right lateral margin of the liver and line 1 (width of right lobe) are measured and expressed as a ratio, termed the CRL ratio (**Fig. 3**). In that original study, the mean

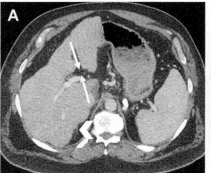 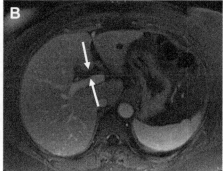

Fig. 2. Measurement of the hilar periportal space in 2 different patients. CECT image (*A*) of a 64-year-old man with HCV and alcohol-related cirrhosis demonstrates a widened hilar peri-portal space (*arrows*) measuring 17 mm. Note some of the other stigmata of cirrhosis, including surface nodularity and a prominent right posterior notch (*arrowhead*). T1-weighted postcontrast MRI image (*B*) in a 54-year-old woman with hepatitis B virus dem-onstrates some hepatic fissural prominence; however, the hilar periportal space (*arrows*) measures 8 mm and liver biopsy demonstrated stage 2 fibrosis. Other stigmata of cirrhosis are largely absent.

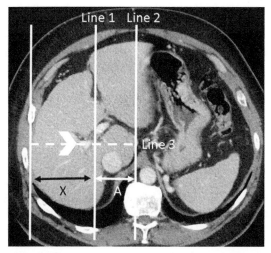

Fig. 3. CRL and modified CRL ratio. CECT image in a patient with cirrhosis demonstrates measurement of the CRL ratio. Line 1 is drawn through the right lateral wall of the main portal vein, parallel to the midsagittal plane of the body, with line 2 drawn through the most medial margin of the caudate lobe and parallel to line 1. Line 3 (*dashed*) is drawn perpendicular to lines 1 and 2, midway between the portal vein and the inferior vena cava. The distances along line 3 between lines 1 and 2 (A) and along line 3 between the right lateral margin of the liver and line 1 (X) are measured and expressed as the ratio A/X, termed the CRL ratio. In this patient, the CRL ratio measured 0.8, similar to the cirrhotic patients in Harbin and colleagues[2], Horowitz and colleagues.[34] For the modified CRL ratio, it was proposed to move line 1 to the lateral margin of the right portal vein (*arrowhead*); however, this modification did not improve performance.[36]

CRL ratio in normal livers was 0.3, compared with 0.8 in cirrhotic livers. In a subsequent study, a threshold of 0.9 for identifying cirrhosis showed a sensitivity of 71%, a specificity of 77%, and an accuracy of 74%.[35] A modified CRL ratio was subsequently proposed, in which the right portal vein was used as the boundary rather than the main portal vein (see **Fig. 3**); however, this did not perform as well in diagnosing cirrhosis or predicting clinical severity as the original CRL ratio.[36]

Torres and colleagues[28] took this concept a step further to perform a volumetric assessment of cirrhotic livers compared with normal livers. They found that the mean percentage of the total liver occupied by the right lobe decreased by 15% and by the medial left lobe decreased by 11% in cirrhotics. The mean percentage of total liver occupied by the caudate and lateral left lobe increased by 192% and 56%, respectively. These changes were statistically significantly different from normal controls. However, these approaches fail to capture the full effect of volumetric changes in segments IV to VIII relative to I to III.

Furusato Hunt and colleagues[37] also looked at a cohort of cirrhotic versus normal livers but with a new metric designed to better capture segmental changes in the liver. Segmental volumes were measured in a semiautomated fashion and a liver segmental volume ratio (LSVR) was calculated. The LSVR, a natural extension of the work of Torres and colleagues,[28] is defined as a volume ratio of Couinaud segments I to III (lateral left lobe and caudate) to segments IV to VIII (medial left and right lobe) (**Fig. 4**). Differences between cirrhotics and normal controls were again highly statistically significantly different (LSVR 0.55 vs 0.27, respectively), with an AUC of 0.916 for identifying cirrhosis. Using an LSVR threshold of 0.35 or greater had a sensitivity of 81.5% and specificity of 88.7% for cirrhosis. This performed significantly better than CRL ratio and total liver volume, which were not statistically significantly different between the 2 groups.[37] This proof-of-concept study established that regional volumetric assessment was better than standard linear measures or total liver volume. In addition, an assessment of interobserver reproducibility was performed in a subset of subjects with 3 readers of varying levels of experience with high interclass correlation seen for total liver volume, LSVR, and splenic volume.[37]

This was followed by a study looking at LSVR in intermediate stages of pathologic fibrosis (F1–F3), in which both LSVR and total splenic volumes were measured in 624 subjects with varying stages of fibrosis.[38] The LSVR steadily increased with increasing stage of fibrosis, as did total splenic volume (**Fig. 5**). For discriminating advanced fibrosis ($\geq$F3), LSVR, splenic volume, and LSVR-splenic volume combined demonstrated receiver operating characteristic (ROC) AUC values of 0.86, 0.89, and 0.95, respectively. For discriminating significant fibrosis ($\geq$F2), LSVR, splenic volume, and combined LSVR-splenic volume showed ROC AUC values of 0.85, 0.85, and 0.91, respectively, performing much better than total liver volume (**Table 1**). Thresholds for LSVR and splenic volume of 0.34 and 311.5 mL showed sensitivity and specificity of 68.3% and 87.9%, and 71.6 % and 85.9%, respectively, for detecting significant fibrosis. In both of these studies, volumes were retrospectively obtained using a fairly rapid, semiautomated technique.[37,38]

Quantification of Liver Surface Nodularity on Computed Tomography

As previously described, it has long been recognized that the development of LSN is seen in cirrhotic patients; however, previously this had primarily been a subjective assessment and was challenging to identify in earlier stages of fibrosis. However, more recently, Smith and colleagues[39] devised and tested a tool that can objectively measure surface nodularity of the liver on MDCT. In this study, a customized semiautomated postprocessing software tool was developed and tested wherein the user

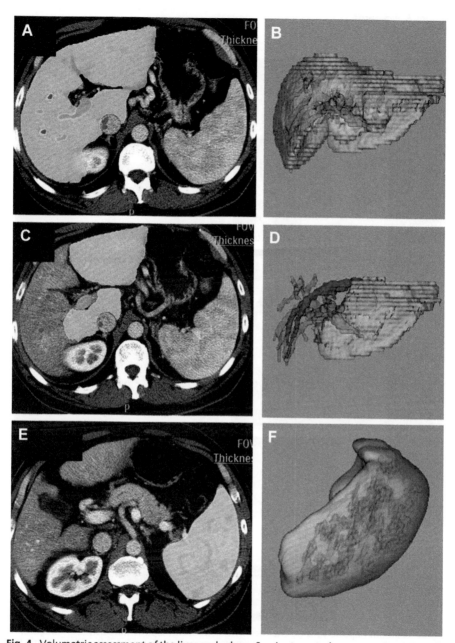

Fig. 4. Volumetric assessment of the liver and spleen. Semiautomated segmentation is initially performed on the whole liver (axial CECT, *A*; volume rendering, *B*). The medial left lobe and right lobe, segments IV to VIII, are then removed to give a volume for the caudate and left lateral section or segments I to III (axial CECT, *C*; volume rendering, *D*). The volume of segments I to III is subtracted from the total to give the volume of segments IV to VIII, and the LSVR is calculated by taking the volume of segments I to III divided by the volume of segments IV to VIII. The spleen can then be segmented for a total splenic volume (axial CECT, *E*; volume rendering, *F*). In this 57-year-old man with nonalcoholic fatty liver disease (NAFLD)-based nonalcoholic steatohepatitis and cirrhosis, the total liver volume was measured at 1683 mL, segments I to III at 624 mL, segments IV to VIII at 1060 mL. LSVR was calculated at 0.589. Splenic volume was measured at 1158 mL. This LSVR is compatible with a diagnosis of cirrhosis, well above the reported threshold of 0.35.[37] This splenic volume supports a diagnosis of cirrhosis as well, above the mean reported value of 790.7 mL for the F4 group.[38]

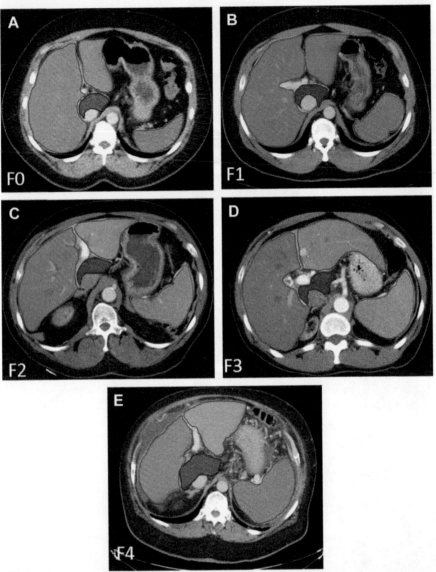

Fig. 5. Regional hepatic volume changes with increasing hepatic fibrosis. CECT images in 5 different patients with increasing stages of fibrosis, F0 (*A*), F1 (*B*), F2 (*C*), F3 (*D*), and F4 (*E*). Note the gradual hypertrophy of the left lateral section (*blue*) and caudate (*red*) with increasing stages of fibrosis, with the concurrent atrophy of segments IV to VIII (*green*). Because of these inverse changes, the LSVR increases while the overall liver volume stays relatively constant. The splenic volume (*orange*) also increases with increasing fibrosis. These visual findings were borne out numerically in the pooled cohort that included intermediate fibrosis stages, in which the mean LSVR and splenic volume for the F0 group was 0.26 and 149 mL, for F1 0.29 and 212 mL, for F2 0.33 and 261 mL, for F3 0.39 and 412 mL, and for F4 0.60 and 978 mL. (*From* Pickhardt PJ, Malecki K, Hunt OF, et al. Hepatosplenic volumetric assessment at MDCT for staging liver fibrosis. European Radiol 2017;27(7):3062; with permission.)

Table 1
Performance of quantitative computed tomography features in assessing hepatic fibrosis

Fibrosis Stage Measurement	F0 vs F1–F4	F0–1 vs F2–F4	F0–2 vs F3–4	F0-3 vs F4
		ROC AUC Values		
CRL ratio	—	—	—	0.567[37]
Total liver volume	0.533[38]	0.512[38]	0.506[38]	0.598,[37] 0.617[38]
LSVR	0.782[38]	0.854[38]	0.880[38]	0.916,[37] 0.904[38]
Splenic 1D measure	—	—	—	0.909[37]
SV	0.825[38]	0.848[38]	0.901[38]	0.938,[37] 0.920,[38] 0.835[39]
LSVR plus SV	0.865[38]	0.908[38]	0.947[38]	0.986,[37] 0.965[38]
LSN score	0.903[41]	0.902[41]	0.932[41]	0.959,[41] 0.929[39]
CTTA[44]	0.78 (mean), 0.74 (entropy)	0.73 (mean)	0.73 (mean)	0.84 (mean), 0.87 (skewness), 0.86 (kurtosis)
CT perfusion	—	—	0.79[47]	0.78,[47] 0.78–0.89,[48] 0.732[51]
fECS	—	0.832[52]	0.757[54]	0.953,[51] 0.775[54]
MP 3 (LSN, SV, PPS)[57]	—	0.856	0.897	0.938
MP 4 (LSN, SV, PPS, CTTA)[57]	—	0.873	0.911	0.957
MP 11[57]	—	0.905	0.936	0.972

Abbreviations: CTTA, CT texture analysis; fECS, fractional extracellular space; MP, multiparametric; PPS, periportal space; SV, splenic volume.

paints along the liver surface for a distance of approximately 8 to 10 cm. The liver edge is detected by the software and the distance between the detected edge and a generated smooth polynomial line is measured on a pixel-by-pixel basis. The mean distance for each section is measured and constitutes the basis for the LSN score. Approximately 10 measurements are performed and the final LSN score is the arithmetical mean of the measurements in each section (**Fig. 6**).[39] LSN scores were measured in a cohort of normal and largely cirrhotic subjects. Mean LSN scores were significantly higher in cirrhotics than normal, with an ROC AUC value of 0.93 for identifying cirrhosis. In addition, this study measured LSN on varying slice thickness and on CT images with and without IV contrast. LSN scores from all protocol types were highly correlated. Images were also evaluated repeatedly by a single reader and by 2 separate readers, with high interobserver and intraobserver intraclass correlation coefficients.[39]

Smith and colleagues[40] performed a follow-up study in subjects with compensated cirrhosis. In their cohort, 40% developed decompensation during a median follow-up period of 4.2 years, and 61% died in a median follow-up of 2.3 years. LSN score was an independent predictor of hepatic decompensation and death in this cohort. Subjects at low, intermediate, and high risk of decompensation and death showed significantly different LSN scores.[40]

In addition to identifying and predicting clinical outcomes in cirrhosis, LSN has demonstrated utility in differentiating intermediate stages of fibrosis (F1–F3).[41] In a cohort of pooled causes of liver disease with varying stages of pathologic fibrosis, LSN scores increased with increasing stages of fibrosis. For discriminating significant fibrosis (≥F2), advanced fibrosis (≥F3), and cirrhosis, the scores demonstrated ROC AUC values of 0.90, 0.93, and 0.96, respectively. Using a threshold LSN score of 2.38,

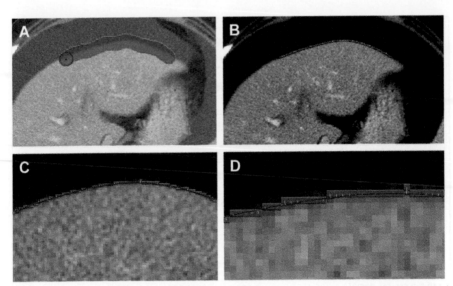

Fig. 6. Assessment of LSN score. Using a simple region of interest tool, a green line is painted along the surface of the liver (*A*) on an axial CT image. The software then autodetects the liver edge and draws a line following the true surface, as well as an associated smooth polynomial line (*B–D*; progressively zoomed). The distance between the detected edge and the smooth polynomial line is measured on a pixel-by-pixel basis, and the mean distance for each section is measured. Approximately 10 measurements are performed and the final LSN score is the arithmetical mean of the measurements in each section.

a sensitivity and specificity of 80% and 80%, respectively, was seen for identifying significant fibrosis (≥F2) (**Fig. 7**).[41] Similar results were seen in a cause-specific cohort of subjects with HCV and intermediate stages of fibrosis (see **Table 1**).

Computed Tomography Texture Analysis for Assessment of Hepatic Fibrosis

CT texture analysis (CTTA) is a technique that quantifies heterogeneity in a given region of interest. It does this by analyzing the distribution and relationship of pixel or voxel-gray levels in the image based on histogram analysis.[42] First-order descriptors of the pixel histogram include mean gray level intensity, standard deviation, skewness (symmetry), and kurtosis (peakedness). Entropy is also a descriptor of the irregularity of the pixel histogram. Second and higher level CTTA features take pixel location and relationship into account and include things such as run length matrix and gray level co-occurrence matrix. These quantitative descriptors have been evaluated for numerous oncologic and a growing number of nononcologic applications.[42] Several groups have looked at applying CTTA to assessment of hepatic fibrosis on CT.

In a group of subjects with chronic liver disease and varying degrees of hepatic fibrosis, 19 different texture features demonstrated statistically significant differences for discriminating between hepatic fibrosis groupings, with the highest AUC values in the range of fair performance.[43] In a separate cohort of 289 adults with pooled causes of liver disease and varying stages of hepatic fibrosis, several texture features, including mean gray level intensity, entropy, kurtosis, and skewness, showed some promise in identifying and discriminating the stage of fibrosis, particularly at advanced levels.[44] For detecting significant fibrosis (≥F2), mean gray level intensity showed ROC AUC values ranging from 0.71 to 0.73. Kurtosis and skewness showed AUC

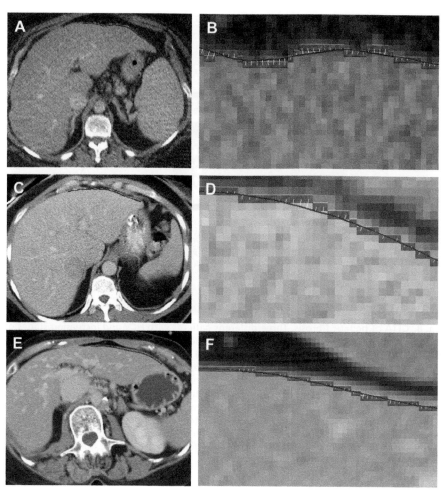

Fig. 7. LSN measurements in varying stages of fibrosis. Three different patients with NAFLD and associated fibrosis with LSN quantification demonstrate decreasing LSN scores with decreasing degrees of fibrosis. A 43-year-old woman with F4 fibrosis and an LSN score of 5.34 (*A, B*), a 49-year-old woman with F3 fibrosis and LSN score of 3.70 (*C, D*), and a 72-year-old woman with F2 fibrosis and LSN score of 2.86 (*E, F*) are shown. This is similar to what was seen in a pooled cause cohort of patients with F0–F4 stage fibrosis, in which the mean LSN score for F0 was 2.0 ± 0.28, F1 2.34 ± 0.39, F2 2.37 ± 0.39, F3 2.88 ± 0.68, and F4 4.11 ± 0.95. (*Data from* Pickhardt PJ, Malecki K, Kloke J, et al. Accuracy of liver surface nodularity quantification on MDCT as a noninvasive biomarker for staging hepatic fibrosis. AJR Am J Roentgenol 2016;207(6):1194–9.)

values of 0.86 and 0.87 for cirrhosis.[44] In this study, because of the known changes in hepatic morphology and the demonstrated efficacy of LSVR, CTTA features were measured in the total liver, segments IV to VIII and segments I to III (**Fig. 8**; see **Table 1**). The most predictive measurement seemed to be the measurement of segments IV to VIII on portal venous phase.[44] Similar results were demonstrated in an HCV-specific cohort of more than 500 subjects. Like LSVR and LSN, CTTA can be performed retrospectively. However, there are many different CTTA software platforms

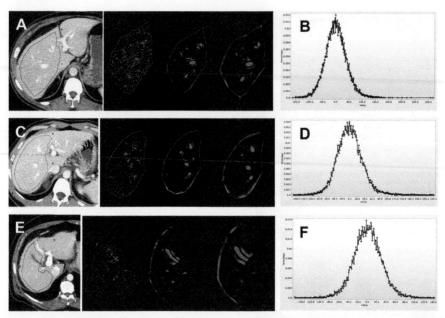

Fig. 8. CTTA of hepatic fibrosis. Three different patients with HCV and increasing stages of histologic fibrosis with associated texture maps and pixel histograms measured from segments IV to VIII during portal venous phase. (*A, B*) A patient with stage F2 fibrosis, (*C, D*) stage F3 fibrosis, and (*E, F*) stage F4 fibrosis. The texture maps demonstrate fine, medium-sized, and coarse-sized features (*left* to *right panels*) in which blue and purple represent negative pixels and pink and red represent positive pixels. These livers show gradually increasing mean gray level intensity and entropy with increasing fibrosis, and decreasing skewness and kurtosis, particularly in advanced fibrosis. This similar to the results seen a pooled cohort containing intermediate fibrosis stages. (*Data from* Lubner MG, Malecki K, Kloke J, et al. Texture analysis of the liver at MDCT for assessing hepatic fibrosis. Abdom Radiol (NY) 2017;42(8):2069–78.)

and metrics. Therefore, further study and standardization of CTTA methodology is needed.[42]

Computed Tomography Perfusion

With increasing fibrosis, there is increasing intrahepatic resistance, which can in turn alter or decrease portal venous flow and increase hepatic arterial flow.[2,45,46] CT perfusion involves repeated imaging of the liver after injection of IV contrast, which allows for measurements of increased arterial flow, arterial fractional flow, and mean transit time, which have shown association with liver fibrosis and portal hypertension.[47,48] In a study of subjects with chronic HCV, mean transit time showed some promise in differentiating minimal from intermediate fibrosis, with a sensitivity of 71% and specificity of 65% at a threshold of 13.4 seconds (see **Table 1**).[49] However, there was considerable overlap between fibrosis groups. Unlike the CT parameters previously discussed, CT perfusion must be prospectively obtained and requires increased radiation and significant postprocessing.[2] These issues temper enthusiasm for this approach relative to the retrospective measures previously described (ie, volumetrics, surface nodularity, and texture analysis).

Fractional Extracellular Space or Volume

With increasing hepatic fibrosis, there is increased deposition of collagen and expansion of the extracellular space.[2] Assessment of the fractional extracellular space can be performed with or without dual-energy CT (DECT), and requires a noncontrast CT scan followed by a delayed or equilibrium phase scan (performed at least 5 minutes post-IV contrast). Fractional extracellular space is calculated as the enhancement of (liver or aorta)*(1-Hct) during the equilibrium phase.[50] In the setting of fibrosis, there is increased enhancement or abnormally high attenuation of the liver during the equilibrium phase. Quantification of the fractional extracellular space or volume has been shown to be associated with the Model for End Stage Liver Disease (MELD) score and has demonstrated an AUC of 0.953 for predicting cirrhosis.[51] This has also shown some association with intermediate stages of fibrosis (see **Table 1**).[52–54] Using a fractional extracellular volume threshold of 28.8%, sensitivity of 88% and specificity of 71% for significant fibrosis was demonstrated (ROC AUC = 0.832).[52]

In theory, use of DECT may allow for imaging of the single equilibrium phase and replacement of true noncontrast phase with virtual unenhanced images.[2] DECT also allows for iodine quantification, with higher quantities of iodine associated with higher stages of fibrosis.[55,56] As with CT perfusion techniques, this type of protocol requires prospective planning and acquisition.

Multiparametric Assessment

Ideally, an assessment of hepatic fibrosis on CT would be multiparametric and include a combination of the most promising CT features, particularly those that are available retrospectively. In a cohort of 469 subjects with HCV, 11 CT features were assessed, including hepatosplenic volumetrics, CT texture features, LSN score, and linear CT measurements (eg, periportal space). In a model combining all 11 parameters, the ROC AUC values for significant fibrosis ($\geq$F2), advanced fibrosis ($\geq$F3), and cirrhosis (F4) were 0.905, 0.936, and 0.972, respectively. A simple model combining 3 basic parameters that are readily available retrospectively (ie, LSN score, splenic volume, and periportal space) demonstrated corresponding AUC values of 0.856, 0.897, and 0.938, respectively (see **Table 1**). Of all the parameters, LSN score showed the best individual performance.[57]

SUMMARY

In summary, although several methods exist for noninvasive assessment of liver disease, a variety of CT parameters show great promise in identifying and stratifying stages of fibrosis. These are attractive not only for their association with hepatic fibrosis but also because CT is readily accessible and commonly performed at many institutions. Furthermore, the most promising of these CT features, including hepatosplenic volumetric assessment, and LSN assessment, can be retrospectively obtained.

REFERENCES

1. Martinez SM, Crespo G, Navasa M, et al. Noninvasive assessment of liver fibrosis. Hepatology 2011;53(1):325–35.
2. Horowitz JM, Venkatesh SK, Ehman RL, et al. Evaluation of hepatic fibrosis: a review from the society of abdominal radiology disease focus panel. Abdom Radiol (NY) 2017;42(8):2037–53.
3. Bedossa P, Dargere D, Paradis V. Sampling variability of liver fibrosis in chronic hepatitis C. Hepatology 2003;38(6):1449–57.

4. Cadranel JF, Rufat P, Degos F. Practices of liver biopsy in France: results of a prospective nationwide survey. For the Group of Epidemiology of the French Association for the Study of the Liver (AFEF). Hepatology 2000;32(3):477–81.

5. Adams LA, Bulsara M, Rossi E, et al. Hepascore: an accurate validated predictor of liver fibrosis in chronic hepatitis C infection. Clin Chem 2005;51(10):1867–73.

6. Cales P, Oberti F, Michalak S, et al. A novel panel of blood markers to assess the degree of liver fibrosis. Hepatology 2005;42(6):1373–81.

7. Forns X, Ampurdanes S, Llovet JM, et al. Identification of chronic hepatitis C patients without hepatic fibrosis by a simple predictive model. Hepatology 2002; 36(4 Pt 1):986–92.

8. Imbert-Bismut F, Ratziu V, Pieroni L, et al. Biochemical markers of liver fibrosis in patients with hepatitis C virus infection: a prospective study. Lancet 2001; 357(9262):1069–75.

9. Sterling RK, Lissen E, Clumeck N, et al. Development of a simple noninvasive index to predict significant fibrosis in patients with HIV/HCV coinfection. Hepatology 2006;43(6):1317–25.

10. Wai CT, Greenson JK, Fontana RJ, et al. A simple noninvasive index can predict both significant fibrosis and cirrhosis in patients with chronic hepatitis C. Hepatology 2003;38(2):518–26.

11. Rosenberg WM, Voelker M, Thiel R, et al. Serum markers detect the presence of liver fibrosis: a cohort study. Gastroenterology 2004;127(6):1704–13.

12. Sandrin L, Fourquet B, Hasquenoph JM, et al. Transient elastography: a new noninvasive method for assessment of hepatic fibrosis. Ultrasound Med Biol 2003;29(12):1705–13.

13. Talwalkar JA, Kurtz DM, Schoenleber SJ, et al. Ultrasound-based transient elastography for the detection of hepatic fibrosis: systematic review and meta-analysis. Clin Gastroenterol Hepatol 2007;5(10):1214–20.

14. Friedrich-Rust M, Ong M-F, Martens S, et al. Performance of transient elastography for the staging of liver fibrosis: a meta-analysis. Gastroenterology 2008; 134(4):960–74.

15. Tsochatzis EA, Gurusamy KS, Ntaoula S, et al. Elastography for the diagnosis of severity of fibrosis in chronic liver disease: a meta-analysis of diagnostic accuracy. J Hepatol 2011;54(4):650–9.

16. Tang A, Cloutier G, Szeverenyi NM, et al. Ultrasound elastography and MR elastography for assessing liver fibrosis: part 2, diagnostic performance, confounders, and future directions. Am J Roentgenol 2015;205(1):33–40.

17. Tang A, Cloutier G, Szeverenyi NM, et al. Ultrasound elastography and MR elastography for assessing liver fibrosis: part 1, principles and techniques. AJR Am J Roentgenol 2015;205(1):22–32.

18. Friedrich-Rust M, Nierhoff J, Lupsor M, et al. Performance of acoustic radiation force impulse imaging for the staging of liver fibrosis: a pooled meta-analysis. J Viral Hepat 2012;19(2):E212–9.

19. Bota S, Herkner H, Sporea I, et al. Meta-analysis: ARFI elastography versus transient elastography for the evaluation of liver fibrosis. Liver Int 2013;33(8): 1138–47.

20. Wang Q-B, Zhu H, Liu H-L, et al. Performance of magnetic resonance elastography and diffusion-weighted imaging for the staging of hepatic fibrosis: a meta-analysis. Hepatology 2012;56(1):239–47.

21. Singh S, Venkatesh SK, Wang Z, et al. Diagnostic performance of magnetic resonance elastography in staging liver fibrosis: a systematic review and

meta-analysis of individual participant data. Clin Gastroenterol Hepatol 2015; 13(3):440–51.

22. Wagner M, Corcuera-Solano I, Lo G, et al. Technical failure of MR elastography examinations of the liver: experience from a large single-center study. Radiology 2017;284(2):401–12.

23. Kartalis N, Brehmer K, Loizou L. Multi-detector CT: liver protocol and recent developments. Eur J Radiol 2017;97:101–9.

24. Moreno CC, Hemingway J, Johnson AC, et al. Changing abdominal imaging utilization patterns: perspectives from medicare beneficiaries over two decades. J Am Coll Radiol 2016;13(8):894–903.

25. Ito K, Mitchell DG, Kim MJ, et al. Right posterior hepatic notch sign: a simple diagnostic MR finding of cirrhosis. JMRI 2003;18(5):561–6.

26. Ito K, Mitchell DG, Gabata T, et al. Expanded gallbladder fossa: simple MR imaging sign of cirrhosis. Radiology 1999;211(3):723–6.

27. Tan KC. The right posterior hepatic notch sign. Radiology 2008;248(1):317–8.

28. Torres WE, Whitmire LF, Gedgaudas-McClees K, et al. Computed tomography of hepatic morphologic changes in cirrhosis of the liver. J Comput Assist Tomogr 1986;10(1):47–50.

29. Dodd GD 3rd, Baron RL, Oliver JH 3rd, et al. Spectrum of imaging findings of the liver in end-stage cirrhosis: part I, gross morphology and diffuse abnormalities. AJR Am J Roentgenol 1999;173(4):1031–6.

30. Yu JS, Shim JH, Chung JJ, et al. Double contrast-enhanced MRI of viral hepatitis-induced cirrhosis: correlation of gross morphological signs with hepatic fibrosis. Br J Radiol 2010;83(987):212–7.

31. Tan KC. Enlargement of the hilar periportal space. Radiology 2008;248(2): 699–700.

32. Rustogi R, Horowitz J, Harmath C, et al. Accuracy of MR elastography and anatomic MR imaging features in the diagnosis of severe hepatic fibrosis and cirrhosis. Journal of magnetic resonance imaging. J Magn Reson Imaging 2012;35(6):1356–64.

33. Venkatesh SK, Yin M, Takahashi N, et al. Non-invasive detection of liver fibrosis: MR imaging features vs. MR elastography. Abdom Imaging 2015;40(4):766–75.

34. Harbin WP, Robert NJ, Ferrucci JT Jr. Diagnosis of cirrhosis based on regional changes in hepatic morphology: a radiological and pathological analysis. Radiology 1980;135(2):273–83.

35. Giorgio A, Amoroso P, Lettieri G, et al. Cirrhosis: value of caudate to right lobe ratio in diagnosis with US. Radiology 1986;161(2):443–5.

36. Awaya H, Mitchell DG, Kamishima T, et al. Cirrhosis: modified caudate-right lobe ratio. Radiology 2002;224(3):769–74.

37. Furusato Hunt OM, Lubner MG, Ziemlewicz TJ, et al. The liver segmental volume ratio for noninvasive detection of cirrhosis: comparison with established linear and volumetric measures. J Comput Assist Tomogr 2016;40(3):478–84.

38. Pickhardt PJ, Malecki K, Hunt OF, et al. Hepatosplenic volumetric assessment at MDCT for staging liver fibrosis. Eur Radiol 2017;27(7):3060–8.

39. Smith AD, Branch CR, Zand K, et al. Liver surface nodularity quantification from routine CT images as a biomarker for detection and evaluation of cirrhosis. Radiology 2016;280(3):771–81.

40. Smith AD, Zand KA, Florez E, et al. Liver surface nodularity score allows prediction of cirrhosis decompensation and death. Radiology 2017;283(3):711–22.

41. Pickhardt PJ, Malecki K, Kloke J, et al. Accuracy of liver surface nodularity quantification on MDCT as a noninvasive biomarker for staging hepatic fibrosis. AJR Am J Roentgenol 2016;207(6):1194–9.

42. Lubner MG, Smith AD, Sandrasegaran K, et al. CT texture analysis: definitions, applications, biologic correlates, and challenges. Radiographics 2017;37(5): 1483–503.

43. Daginawala N, Li B, Buch K, et al. Using texture analyses of contrast enhanced CT to assess hepatic fibrosis. Eur J Radiol 2016;85(3):511–7.

44. Lubner MG, Malecki K, Kloke J, et al. Texture analysis of the liver at MDCT for assessing hepatic fibrosis. Abdom Radiol (NY) 2017;42(8):2069–78.

45. Richter S, Mucke I, Menger MD, et al. Impact of intrinsic blood flow regulation in cirrhosis: maintenance of hepatic arterial buffer response. Am J Physiol Gastrointest Liver Physiol 2000;279(2):G454–62.

46. Gulberg V, Haag K, Rossle M, et al. Hepatic arterial buffer response in patients with advanced cirrhosis. Hepatology 2002;35(3):630–4.

47. Bonekamp D, Bonekamp S, Geiger B, et al. An elevated arterial enhancement fraction is associated with clinical and imaging indices of liver fibrosis and cirrhosis. J Comput Assist Tomogr 2012;36(6):681–9.

48. Van Beers BE, Leconte I, Materne R, et al. Hepatic perfusion parameters in chronic liver disease: dynamic CT measurements correlated with disease severity. AJR Am J Roentgenol 2001;176(3):667–73.

49. Ronot M, Asselah T, Paradis V, et al. Liver fibrosis in chronic hepatitis C virus infection: differentiating minimal from intermediate fibrosis with perfusion CT. Radiology 2010;256(1):135–42.

50. Varenika V, Fu Y, Maher JJ, et al. Hepatic fibrosis: evaluation with semiquantitative contrast-enhanced CT. Radiology 2013;266(1):151–8.

51. Zissen MH, Wang ZJ, Yee J, et al. Contrast-enhanced CT quantification of the hepatic fractional extracellular space: correlation with diffuse liver disease severity. AJR Am J Roentgenol 2013;201(6):1204–10.

52. Yoon JH, Lee JM, Klotz E, et al. Estimation of hepatic extracellular volume fraction using multiphasic liver computed tomography for hepatic fibrosis grading. Invest Radiol 2015;50(4):290–6.

53. Bandula S, Punwani S, Rosenberg WM, et al. Equilibrium contrast-enhanced CT imaging to evaluate hepatic fibrosis: initial validation by comparison with histopathologic sampling. Radiology 2015;275(1):136–43.

54. Guo SL, Su LN, Zhai YN, et al. The clinical value of hepatic extracellular volume fraction using routine multiphasic contrast-enhanced liver CT for staging liver fibrosis. Clin Radiol 2017;72(3):242–6.

55. Lamb P, Sahani DV, Fuentes-Orrego JM, et al. Stratification of patients with liver fibrosis using dual-energy CT. IEEE Trans Med Imaging 2015;34(3):807–15.

56. Lv P, Lin X, Gao J, et al. Preliminary studies in the liver cirrhosis. Korean J Radiol 2012;13(4):434–42.

57. Pickhardt PJ, Graffy PM, Said A, et al. Multi-parametric CT for noninvasive staging of liver fibrosis from HCV: correlation with the Histopathologic METAVIR score society of abdominal radiology; 2018; Scottsdale, AZ.

Role of Imaging in Surveillance and Diagnosis of Hepatocellular Carcinoma

Mohit Gupta, MD[a], Helena Gabriel, MD[a], Frank H. Miller, MD[b],*

KEYWORDS

- Hepatocellular carcinoma • Screening • Liver • MR • Ultrasound • LI-RADS

KEY POINTS

- Prognosis for hepatocellular carcinoma (HCC) is dependent on tumor stage at diagnosis, with small, localized, early-stage tumors more amenable to curative treatment options.
- Screening guidelines have been made by various organizations to improve early detection in at-risk populations.
- Ultrasound is the most commonly used screening tool with increased interest in use of MRI in specific populations.
- Imaging-based diagnosis of HCC has been incorporated into all recent clinical guidelines and is used to determine the extent of tumor burden, guide treatment options, and prioritize patients for organ transplantation.
- The Liver Imaging Reporting and Data System (LI-RADS) was created by the radiology community as a tool for standardized reporting and consistent lexicon; its expanded use necessitates further evaluation and validation of its categories.

INTRODUCTION

Hepatocellular carcinoma (HCC) is the second leading cause of cancer mortality worldwide with more than 700,000 deaths each year.[1] The global distribution closely follows the distribution of hepatitis B (HBV) and hepatitis C (HCV) infections, with the greatest burden in developing countries where these infections are endemic. Interestingly, recent trends have shown a decline in viral hepatitis in East Asian countries, such as China and Korea, owing to the increased vaccination against HBV, whereas rates

Disclosures: The authors have nothing to disclose.
[a] Department of Radiology, Northwestern Memorial Hospital, Northwestern University Feinberg School of Medicine, 676 North Saint Clair Street, Suite 800, Chicago, IL 60611, USA;
[b] Body Imaging Section and Fellowship Program, MRI, Department of Radiology, Northwestern Memorial Hospital, Northwestern University Feinberg School of Medicine, 676 North Saint Clair Street, Suite 800, Chicago, IL 60611, USA
* Corresponding author.
E-mail address: frank.miller@nm.org

Gastroenterol Clin N Am 47 (2018) 585–602
https://doi.org/10.1016/j.gtc.2018.04.013
0889-8553/18/© 2018 Elsevier Inc. All rights reserved.

have rapidly increased in developed countries, such as the United States and Japan, where a large aging adult population acquired HCV infection through intravenous drug use and blood transfusions between the 1960s and 1980s. Recent advances in the treatment of HCV may alter this trend; however, antiviral treatment is projected to decrease the number of cases of cirrhosis by only 5%, as most patients are unaware of their infection status and do not receive treatment.[2] Additionally, the epidemic of metabolic syndrome and subsequent development of nonalcoholic fatty liver disease (NAFLD) increasingly contributes to the rise in HCC in developed countries.[3–5] Regardless of etiology, underlying liver cirrhosis is the single most important risk factor for development of HCC, identified in approximately 80% to 90% of all cases.[6]

The prognosis for patients with HCC is dependent on tumor stage at diagnosis. Early-detected HCCs are amenable to curative resection and transplantation, with a 5-year survival rate of nearly 70%, compared with a median survival of less than 1 year with advanced HCC.[7] Early detection, however, can be difficult, as many HCCs remain subclinical until more advanced stages or are only seen incidentally on imaging.[6,8–15] Thus, it is important to have close active surveillance in high-risk patients to diagnose cirrhosis and HCC when the disease burden is small.

HEPATOCELLULAR CARCINOMA SCREENING AND SURVEILLANCE

The World Health Organization established tenets of cancer screening approximately 50 years ago, emphasizing that the success of a screening program is dependent on identification of a disease that has high associated morbidity and mortality; effective and available treatment; and an acceptable, safe, and relatively inexpensive surveillance tool.[16] Cancer screening and surveillance programs, such as for breast, colon, and prostate cancer, have traditionally focused on a cost-effective method to reduce mortality, and have often been implemented with high degrees of success.[17] However, there are limitations that include poor availability and utilization rate, suboptimal sensitivity of screening tests, and limited access to treatment options. For example, the fecal occult blood test and the prostate-specific antigen, although widely available and relatively inexpensive, have received substantial criticism due to downstream physical, psychological, and financial harm. Further analysis of screening programs has resulted in ongoing revised clinical practice.[18]

In contrast to prospective trials that have proven screening efficacy with other malignancies, such as breast cancer, studies evaluating screening for HCC are more limited. One large-scale randomized controlled trial performed in China by Zhang and colleagues[19] demonstrated survival benefit in patients with chronic hepatitis B in a study population of approximately 19,000 patients undergoing screening and surveillance with ultrasound and alpha-fetoprotein (AFP) every 6 months. Despite poor patient compliance, there was a significant 37% reduction in mortality in the screened group. Despite these promising results, this patient population was that of HBV and not cirrhosis. To date, there are no similar large-scale trials evaluating screening in cirrhosis.

Many worldwide professional organizations have produced HCC screening guidelines in at-risk groups in which the incidence of HCC is sufficiently high enough for a surveillance program to be deemed cost-effective.[20–23] These guidelines provide both an evidence-based and consensus approach to HCC screening, and have been supported by a number of studies that have concluded a survival benefit due to earlier diagnosis.[19,24–26] Although there is substantial overlap among the different guidelines, variation does exist in HCC surveillance recommendations, specifically the targeted population and means of screening (**Table 1**). The 2017 guideline update

Table 1
Population and screening

Strategy	AASLD 2017[22]	APASL 2017[21]	JHS 2014[20]	EASL 2012[23]
Target population	Cirrhosis, chronic HBV	Cirrhosis	Super high-risk: HBV or HCV cirrhosis High-risk: Cirrhosis (other etiology) Chronic HBV or HCV	Cirrhosis, chronic HBV, chronic HCV with advanced liver fibrosis F3
Screening modality	Abdominal US ± AFP	Abdominal US + AFP	Super high-risk: US + tumor markers[a] and Gd-EOB-DTPA-MRI High-risk: US + tumor markers	Abdominal US
Serum tumor markers	Yes	Yes	Yes[a]	No
Screening intervals, mo	6	6	Super high-risk: US + tumor markers-3 to 4 Gd-EOB-DTPA-MRI - 6 to 12 High-risk: 6	6

Abbreviations: AASLD, American Association for the Study of Liver Disease; AFP, alpha-fetoprotein; APASL, Asian Pacific Association for the Study of the Liver; EASL, European Association for the Study of the Liver; Gd-EOB-DTPA, gadolinium ethoxybenzyl diethylenetriamine pentaacetic acid; HBV, hepatitis B virus; HCV, hepatitis C virus; JSH, Japan Society of Hepatology; US, ultrasound.
[a] Tumor markers = AFP, des-gamma carboxyprothrombin (DCP, also known as PIVKA-II).

from the American Association for the Study of Liver Disease (AASLD) includes surveillance of cirrhotic patients and noncirrhotic patients with chronic HBV using ultrasound, with or without AFP, every 6 months.[19,22,27,28] Surveillance is currently not recommended by the AASLD for noncirrhotic patients with HCV or NAFLD. Similar guidelines are proposed by the European Association for the Study of the Liver (EASL) and the Asian Pacific Association for the Study of the Liver (APASL), with the following variations: the EASL recommends surveillance with ultrasound alone and includes noncirrhotic patients with HCV with bridging fibrosis (Metavir F3),[23] and the APASL recommends surveillance with ultrasound in combination with serum AFP.[21] The role of serum biomarkers in HCC surveillance is not well determined. Of the serum biomarkers, AFP has been the most extensively studied.[29,30] A meta-analysis demonstrated that a combination of ultrasound imaging and AFP versus ultrasound alone did not statistically increase the sensitivity or ability to detect subclinical HCC, was less specific with an increased false-positive rate, and was less cost-effective.[31] Limited data exist for the added value of other serum biomarkers, including des-gamma carboxy prothrombin and AFP L3.[32–36]

Nearly all current practice guidelines recommend ultrasonography as the screening modality of choice for HCC.[19–21] Ultrasound is widely available, cost-effective,[28–31] and does not expose patients to excess radiation. These characteristics are important benchmarks in cancer screening and are vital for worldwide recommendations of HCC surveillance. HCC does not have a characteristic appearance on ultrasound. Most lesions are larger than 1 cm and typically hypoechoic relative to background parenchyma.[37] However, HCCs may be isoechoic, hyperechoic with or without a hypoechoic rim, or heterogeneous (**Fig. 1**). Lesions larger than 1 cm and not definitely benign require further investigation.[38]

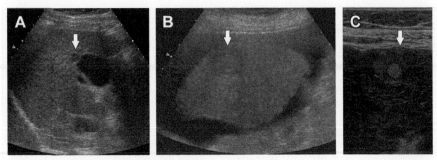

Fig. 1. Varying appearances of hepatocellular carcinoma on ultrasound. (*A*) A 67-year-old man with an approximately 1-cm hypoechoic lesion (*arrow*) adjacent to the gallbladder. (*B*) A 41-year-old woman with an isoechoic lesion with halo appearance (*arrow*). (*C*) A 62-year-old man with a heterogeneous lesion (*arrow*) on ultrasound. All 3 lesions were confirmed to be HCC on diagnostic MRI.

Although ultrasound has been shown to reduce mortality from HCC when used as a screening tool,[39] it is not a perfect test and its sensitivity for individual lesion detection is variable. A meta-analysis reported a pooled sensitivity of 94% for detection of HCC at any stage; however, only 63% in detection of early HCC in patients with cirrhosis.[31] A more recent meta-analysis in 2014 reiterated the prior findings with ultrasound alone and ultrasound plus AFP demonstrating similar rates of early detection of HCC.[25] The reduced sensitivity for detection of early HCC is multifactorial, both inherent to the imaging modality and to the patient population. Ultrasound imaging is operator-dependent and requires expert technique, which is difficult to standardize across facilities ranging from local community centers to tertiary-care hospitals. Studies also have shown that ultrasound has decreased sensitivity in the setting of advanced liver disease and obesity.[28,40–43] Cirrhotic patients have coarsened and nodular liver possibly obscuring subtle focal nodules or infiltrative tumors suspicious for HCC. There are also areas of the liver that can be relative blind spots limiting detection of lesions.[38,43] The advent of the new Ultrasound–Liver Imaging Reporting and Data System (US-LIRADS) guidelines has addressed the technical issues and sought a means of providing guidelines for consistent imaging and reporting.[44] US-LIRADS also has addressed the fact that not all patients scan consistently and that some patients have sonographic limitations. US-LIRADS, therefore, classifies each ultrasound screen examination done in 1 of 3 categories: no limitations, moderate limitation, and severe limitation. In this way, the referring clinician has a sense of the success of screening in that individual patient. US-LIRADS does not, however, offer alternative means of screening if the ultrasound examination is limited, namely the use of computed tomography (CT) or MRI.

There has been more recent interest in using MR for screening. The most recent consensus guideline provided by the Liver Cancer Study Group of Japan includes MRI as a first-line surveillance and diagnostic tool for HCC in select super high-risk patients.[20] Unlike other guidelines, the Japan Society of Hepatology guidelines subcategorize the at-risk population into 2 groups: super high-risk for HCC (HBV or HCV cirrhosis) and high-risk for HCC (chronic HBV or HCV and cirrhosis of other etiology). In addition to screening with ultrasound and serum biomarkers, it is suggested that the super high-risk group undergo surveillance with gadoxetic acid–enhanced MRI (dynamic contrast-enhanced CT is an alternative if MRI is not available or inadequate) every 6 to 12 months to pick up small HCCs that may be missed by ultrasound due to the poor sensitivity with cirrhotic liver morphology (**Fig. 2**). Gadoxetic acid–enhanced MR, however, can have limitations related to the small amount of gadolinium contrast administered and respiratory-associated artifacts in the arterial phase.[45]

The increased sensitivity of MR and CT has prompted some academic treatment centers in the United States to increasingly use CT and MRI for detection and characterization of HCC, especially in very high-risk patients. The sensitivity of MR imaging has substantially improved over the past decade. Advanced MR techniques (fat suppression, improved gradients, 3-dimensional gradient-recall echo sequences, diffusion-weighted imaging) and more reproducible dynamic contrast-enhanced imaging using fluoroscopic-preparatory timing with thinner slices have improved significantly the quality of MR examinations. The detection of smaller lesions and subsequent close follow-up with MRI also minimizes the role of biopsy in small lesions; biopsy has limitations in accuracy and is technically challenging, and introduces risks of bleeding, hepatic decompensation, and tumor peritoneal seeding.[46,47]

Although most models suggest that ultrasound remains the most cost-effective tool for surveillance around the world, a one-size-fits-all approach to HCC surveillance is unlikely to succeed in improving the quality of care and survival in all targeted populations. In the United States, sometimes limited ultrasound screening examinations (due to high prevalence of morbid obesity, NAFLD, and advanced cirrhosis), and the subsequent cost of treatment options with advanced-stage HCC highlights the need for consideration of all potential screening methods, particularly when the

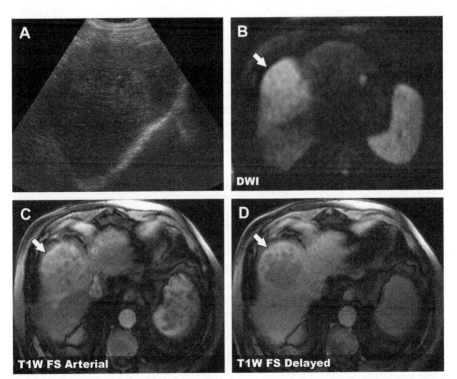

Fig. 2. Missed HCC on screening ultrasound. A 68-year-old man with cirrhosis. No lesion is identified on screening ultrasound (*A*). Follow-up MRI demonstrates a large area with increased signal (*arrow*) on diffusion-weighted imaging (*B*), heterogeneous arterial enhancement (*C*) and "washout" (*D*) (*arrows*), consistent with HCC.

ultrasound examination has limitations. Although initial work suggested that the cost per quality-adjusted life year (cost/QALY) approached $100,000 to $300,000 for CT and MRI,[27] well above the $50,000 threshold level for AASLD guidelines, more recent risk-stratified cost models have suggested that the cost/QALY in targeted populations has reached AASLD threshold level and is similar to ultrasound at the current utilization rate.[48] Recent advances in technology, decreased cost, and wider availability of MRI have largely contributed to the increased cost-effectiveness of MRI and substantiates the need for further investigation into MRI as a surveillance tool for HCC. The ability to detect small HCCs by MRI is especially imperative in transplant centers and institutions that may provide curable resection, hepatic transplantation, or therapies such as transarterial chemoembolization, radiofrequency ablation, and yttrium-90 radioembolization, all of which depend on accurate identification and characterization of the number and size of lesions.

HEPATOCELLULAR CARCINOMA DIAGNOSIS

Unlike many other malignancies, diagnostic imaging detects HCC with specificity levels similar to biopsy analysis without the physical complications associated with invasive procedures or possible tumor seeding.[49,50] Therefore, HCC may be diagnosed by imaging features alone, with histologic sampling reserved for indeterminate lesions. Diagnostic imaging also helps to determine the extent of tumor burden that guides treatment options and prioritizes patients for organ transplantation.[51,52]

Imaging-based diagnosis of HCC has been incorporated by nearly all clinical guidelines since 2001.[23,27,28,52–56] Most criteria stratify findings as positive, negative, or indeterminate for HCC based on the presence of "arterial-phase hyperenhancement" and "washout" after intravenous contrast administration on multiphasic CT or MRI, which is specific for the diagnosis of HCC. This simplified system does not account for the inherent variability in appearance and management of indeterminate lesions from HCC in clinical practice. For example, management of an indeterminate lesion suspicious for HCC, but not meeting definite criteria, will differ from an indeterminate lesion suspected to represent a benign lesion. In addition, the diagnosis of cholangiocarcinoma and distinction from HCC in cirrhotic patients is important.

Recognizing the challenges presented by multiple guidelines and lack of precise definitions, the radiology community, endorsed by the American College of Radiology (ACR), launched the Liver Imaging Reporting and Data System (LI-RADS) in March 2011.[57] The objective of LI-RADS is to provide a consistent lexicon and standardized reporting that may more effectively communicate imaging findings to the multidisciplinary team involved in the management of HCC. With input from radiologists, hepatologists, surgeons, and pathologists, LI-RADS has been increasingly accepted with expanded use and compatibility with the Organ Procurement and Transplantation Network (OPTN)[54] and AASLD clinical management guidelines. However, the lack of large prospective data and validation, as well as competing algorithms, has hindered adoption both within and across involved disciplines. A more detailed discussion of LI-RADS and its relationship to AASLD and OPTN clinical guidelines is described in subsequent sections.

LIVER IMAGING REPORTING AND DATA SYSTEM OVERVIEW

Unlike clinical management guidelines, LI-RADS is a tool for standardizing the performance, interpretation, and reporting of CT, MRI, and most recently contrast-enhanced ultrasound (CEUS) imaging findings. It is applied only to high-risk patients, defined by the ACR as "patients in whom the incidence of HCC is sufficient to justify screening or surveillance according to the AASLD guidelines."[58] LI-RADS uses a 5-point scale to assign a relative probability of HCC to an observation in the liver. The observation is ascribed to the scale based on a lexicon of precisely defined terms and imaging features supplemented by an imaging atlas. LI-RADS includes 5 major categories: LR-5 indicates a definite HCC; LR-1 indicates a definite benign lesion; and LR-4, LR-3, and LR-2 indicate decreasing likelihood of HCC. LR-1 and LR-2 observations include lesions such as cysts, hemangiomas, vascular anomalies, perfusion alteration, focal fat sparing or deposition, hypertrophic pseudomass, confluent fibrosis, or focal scarring. These are rarely reported using LI-RADS lexicon in radiology reports. LR-M indicates a probable malignancy not specific for HCC. An example of the LI-RADS M category is intrahepatic cholangiocarcinoma (**Fig. 3**), which has a higher incidence in patients with cirrhosis and is potentially treated differently than HCC, especially in relationship to transplantation. Observations that have undergone liver-directed

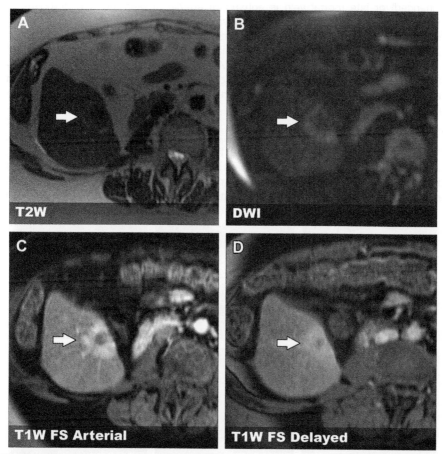

Fig. 3. LR-M category, intrahepatic cholangiocarcinoma. A 68-year-old woman with nonalcoholic steatohepatitis (NASH) cirrhosis. In segment VI of the liver, there is a 4.1 × 2.6-cm mass (*arrow*) demonstrating a "targetoid" appearance with mild hyperintense signal on T2-weighted imaging (*A*), a peripheral rim of increased signal (*arrow*) on diffusion-weighted imaging (*B*, B = 800), a rim of APHE (*arrow*) (*C*), and progressive delayed centripetal enhancement (*arrow*) (*D*) on postcontrast sequences.

therapy are evaluated using the treatment response algorithm, which was implemented into LI-RADS in the most recent 2017 update. Observations may be categorized as LR-TR nonevaluable, LR-TR nonviable, LR-TR equivocal, and LR-TR viable.[58,59]

LIVER IMAGING REPORTING AND DATA SYSTEM IMAGING FEATURES: MAJOR CRITERIA

Five major imaging features are ascribed to the LI-RADS algorithm: arterial phase enhancement, observation size (diameter), washout appearance, capsule, and threshold growth.

Arterial Phase Enhancement (Not Rim)

Arterial phase enhancement is one of the most important imaging features of HCC. Arterial phase enhancement is subdivided into early (the portal vein is not yet enhanced) or late (portal vein is enhanced) arterial phases. For the purposes of HCC diagnosis, late arterial phase enhancement is preferred. The degree of enhancement by an observation is relative to the surrounding background liver parenchyma. Observations are categorized as (1) arterial hypoenhancement or isoenhancement and (2) arterial phase hyperenhancement (APHE). Only observations with APHE may be categorized as LR-5 (**Fig. 4**). Subtraction images with appropriate coregistration may be helpful in observations that are hyperintense on precontrast T1-weighted imaging (**Fig. 5**).

Observation Size

When an observation demonstrates APHE, the key threshold diameter size is ≥10 mm. Observations smaller than 10 mm cannot be classified as LR-5. Observations that demonstrate arterial phase hypoenhancement or isoenhancement are classified as either smaller than 20 or larger than 20 mm in diameter, with additional major and

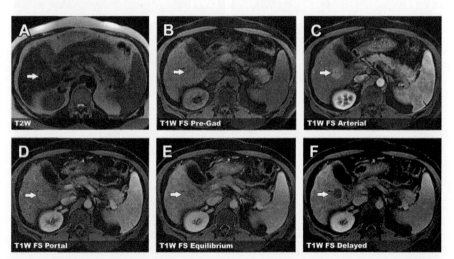

Fig. 4. LI-RADS major imaging features, APHE, and "washout." A 66-year-old man with alcoholic cirrhosis. In the posterior right hepatic lobe, there is a 3.3-cm mass (*arrow*) that demonstrates mild hyperintense signal on T2-weighted imaging (*A*). Precontrast (*B*) and postcontrast sequences demonstrate arterial enhancement (*C*) with progressive "washout" on delayed sequences (*D–F*). The lesion was biopsy-proven HCC.

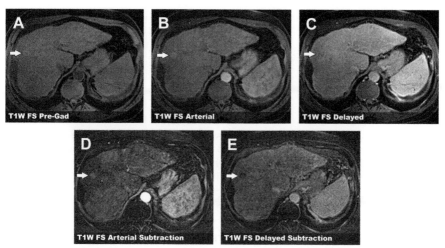

Fig. 5. Value of subtraction images for detection of APHE and "washout." Precontrast T1-weighted image demonstrates a lesion (*arrow*) in the anterior right hepatic lobe with a rim of hyperintense signal (*A*). Postcontrast images demonstrate mild increased signal in the arterial phase (*B*) and subtle hypointense signal relative to background liver parenchyma on delayed phase (*C*). However, these images alone would not qualify for definite APHE or "washout." By subtracting image (*A*) from images (*B*) and (*C*), we derive subtraction images (*D, E*) that demonstrates true APHE and "washout," consistent with HCC.

ancillary features determining whether they are categorized as LR-3 or LR-4 observations.

"Washout" (Not Peripheral)

Washout appearance is defined by the ACR as "nonperipheral visually assessed temporal reduction in enhancement relative to liver from an earlier to a later phase resulting in hypoenhancement in the extracellular phase" (see **Fig. 4**).[58] When using extracellular agents, evaluating for washout in the delayed phase may be helpful, as some observations may not demonstrate definite hypoenhancement on the portal venous phase.[60–62] If the radiologist is uncertain, observations should not be characterized as having washout appearance. Additional sequences, such as subtraction images, may be used to supplement visual evaluation (see **Fig. 5**).[63]

Enhancing "Capsule"

An enhancing "capsule" is defined by the ACR as a "smooth, uniform, sharp border around most or all of the observation, unequivocally thicker or more conspicuous than fibrotic tissue around background nodules, and visible as an enhancing rim on portal venous phase, delayed phase, or transitional phase" (**Fig. 6**).[58] An enhancing "capsule" has a high positive predictive value for HCC in high-risk patients.[64–66]

Threshold Growth

An observation with a diameter increase of a minimum of 5 mm and either ≥50% growth in ≤6 months or ≥100% growth after 6 months is considered threshold growth. Additionally, a new observation ≥10 mm is considered to have threshold growth. The OPTN guidelines, which use the same 5 major criteria, have stricter guidelines on threshold growth, only including lesions with ≥50% growth in ≤6 months.

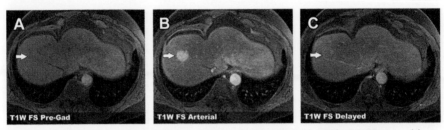

Fig. 6. LI-RADS major imaging features, APHE with enhancing "capsule." A 58-year-old man with cirrhosis secondary to hepatitis C virus. In segment VIII of the liver, there is a 2.8 × 2.3-cm well-circumscribed lesion (*arrow*) that demonstrates hyperintense signal on precontrast T1-weighted images (*A*). Postcontrast images demonstrate APHE (*B*) and washout with a smooth, uniform rim of enhancement on delayed phase (*C*), consistent with APHE and an enhancing "capsule."

LIVER IMAGING REPORTING AND DATA SYSTEM IMAGING FEATURES: MINOR CRITERIA

Ancillary features that may favor malignancy in general or HCC in particular may be applied to upgrade an observation by 1 or more categories (up to but not beyond LR-4). These features include hypointensity on hepatobiliary and transitional phase, mild-moderate hyperintense signal on T2-weighted imaging, restricted diffusion, intralesional fat (**Fig. 7**), lesional fat or iron sparing, hemorrhage, diameter increase less than threshold growth, and other features that specifically favor malignancy over benign causes in general. These imaging features are important considerations in atypical presentations of HCC. HCC lesions with atypical features, such as hypovascularity, are not uncommon, and ancillary features may be essential in differentiating HCC from mimics. Similarly, marked T2 hyperintensity, as well as diameter

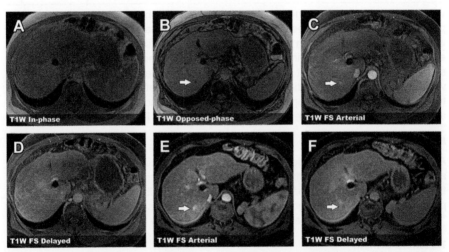

Fig. 7. LI-RADS ancillary features favoring malignancy. A 63-year-old man with cirrhosis. In segment VII of the liver, a 1.1-cm lesion (*arrow*) demonstrates signal loss on opposed-phase imaging (*A, B*), consistent with intralesional fat. Despite the lack of "washout" on delayed imaging (*C, D*), the presence of fat raised concern for HCC and close follow-up was recommended. An examination performed 3 months later demonstrates true APHE with "washout," (*E, F*) diagnostic of HCC.

stability ≥2 years are all considered ancillary features that favor benignity and may be applied to downgrade an observation by 1 or more categories.

LIVER IMAGING REPORTING AND DATA SYSTEM LIMITATIONS

LI-RADS has been successful in providing a standardized method of reporting and data collection for evaluation of HCC. The LR-5 category in the 2017 LI-RADS version maintains nearly 100% specificity and is equivalent to OPTN class 5 and AASLD-definite HCC.[67–72] The high specificity of the LR-5 category ensures that patients who obtain liver transplants do indeed have HCC malignancy at explantation. However, concerns remain by both radiologists and clinicians regarding the LR-3 and LR-4 categories, as they do not have well-defined clinical management implications. Many lesions that may have been simply reported by radiologists as highly suspicious for HCC are now reported as LR-3 or LR-4 observations. These observations do not provide exception points for transplantation and have a wide spectrum of management options, including routine surveillance, alternative imaging, or accelerated follow-up. Based on LI-RADS, biopsy or locoregional treatment may be considered only after multidisciplinary discussion. Additionally, not all HCCs have classic presentations and therefore do not appropriately fit into the LI-RADS criteria. A small but not insignificant percentage of HCCs are hypovascular,[73] which makes characterization more difficult, as all guidelines use dynamic arterial perfusion pattern in lesion evaluation. Some of the most advanced infiltrative HCCs lack arterial enhancement and washout and can have variant imaging features (**Fig. 8**).

More research is required to assess the LR-3 and LR-4 categories to address the concerns of radiologists and clinicians. Although LR-3 and LR-4 observations are not definitive for HCC, it is reasonable to suggest that other available guidelines, such as OPTN and AASLD, have similar or potentially more inherent limitations. For

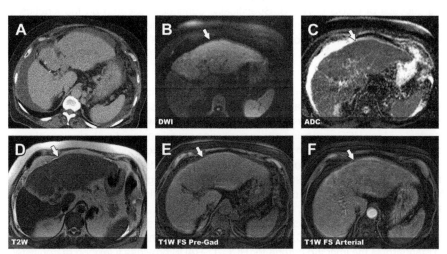

Fig. 8. Infiltrative HCC. A 69-year-old man with NASH cirrhosis. A CT performed at an outside hospital demonstrates cirrhotic liver morphology without definite evidence of a discrete lesion (*A*). Subsequent MRI performed approximately 1 month later shows restricted diffusion (B = 800) throughout the left hepatic lobe (*arrow*) (*B, C*) with associated mild hyperintense signal on T2-weighted imaging (*arrow*) (*D*) and mild heterogeneous arterial enhancement (*arrow*) (*E, F*), consistent with infiltrative HCC. Additional findings on this study included enhancing left and main portal venous thrombus.

example, some of the current AASLD guidelines encourage biopsies for lesions that do not meet the AASLD criteria for HCC. Based on LI-RADS criteria, these same lesions may be treated or have accelerated follow-up, which limits the associated complications and risks of biopsy. Future validation of these 2 categories will be important in the success of LI-RADS reporting.[74–77]

CONTRAST-ENHANCED ULTRASOUND LIVER IMAGING REPORTING AND DATA SYSTEM

Recently, a diagnostic algorithm was approved by the ACR for use of CEUS in patients at high risk for developing HCC.[78,79] The use of CEUS in diagnosis of HCC was initially removed by AASLD guidelines in 2010 because of concerns of misdiagnosing intrahepatic cholangiocarcinoma (ICC). However, since then, multiple studies have concluded that CEUS can be used for lesion characterization and diagnosis of HCC with high specificity, 93% to 100%.[38,78,80–85] As with CT and MRI, diagnostic accuracy may be lower for HCC lesions smaller than 2 cm.[85–87]

CEUS LI-RADS has many similar properties as LI-RADS v2017; however, one important distinction is that washout kinetics may be used to distinguish non-HCC malignant lesions (LR-M) from HCC (LR-5).[84,88–91] ICC has marked rapid washout, typically less than 60 seconds after contrast administration, whereas HCC lesions tend to have mild and delayed (greater than 60 seconds) washout. As a result, the AASLD acknowledged that although not widely used in North America, CEUS also may be used to diagnose HCC noninvasively, although further investigation is needed.[22]

CEUS provides many advantages, including real-time imaging (high temporal resolution); high spatial resolution, which increases lesion detection and characterization; repeated contrast injections due to the small volume of contrast agent; and use in patients with contraindications to CT or MRI. It is important to understand that CEUS LI-RADS may be applied only when the lesion in consideration is identified on conventional gray-scale ultrasound. Similar to LI-RADS v2017, further validation is needed for the success of CEUS LI-RADS. Specifically, continued research on the kinetics of arterial enhancement pattern in HCC and non-HCC malignancies is needed for it to be an effective tool in the workup of patients at high risk for HCC.

SUMMARY

HCC is a major cause of morbidity and mortality worldwide with more effective treatment options available for early-detected lesions. HCC surveillance using ultrasound for high-risk groups is widely accepted and has been shown to improve morbidity and mortality. Many HCC screening and surveillance guidelines exist with significant overlap in screening population, surveillance tools, and screening interval. However, further research is needed to evaluate screening methods for very high at-risk populations and cost-effectiveness of more advanced imaging modalities such as CT and MRI, especially in advanced centers where treatment options, such as transplantation and interventional oncology, are available.

As imaging-based diagnosis of HCC has been universally incorporated into management guidelines for HCC, the radiology community has made a concerted effort to standardize the imaging criteria for HCC. LI-RADS provides a lexicon of consistent terminology and a categorized algorithm that may reduce imaging interpretation variability and error, enhance communication with clinicians, and facilitate quality assurance and research. LI-RADS has been increasingly accepted with expanded use and compatibility with OPTN and AASLD clinical management guidelines; however, further work is needed to provide large prospective data and validation of LI-RADS categories.

REFERENCES

1. Ferlay J, Soerjomataram I, Dikshit R, et al. Cancer incidence and mortality worldwide: sources, methods and major patterns in GLOBOCAN 2012. Int J Cancer. 2015 Mar 1;136(5):E359-86.

2. El-Serag HB, Kanwal F. Epidemiology of hepatocellular carcinoma in the United States: where are we? where do we go? Hepatology 2014;60(5):1767–75.

3. Petrick JL, Braunlin M, Laversanne M, et al. International trends in liver cancer incidence, overall and by histologic subtype, 1978-2007. Int J Cancer 2016; 139(7):1534–45.

4. Siegel RL, Miller KD, Jemal A. Cancer statistics, 2017. CA Cancer J Clin 2017; 67(1):7–30.

5. Makarova-Rusher OV, Altekruse SF, McNeel TS, et al. Population attributable fractions of risk factors for hepatocellular carcinoma in the United States. Cancer 2016;122(11):1757–65.

6. El-Serag HB. Hepatocellular carcinoma. New Engl J Med 2011;365:1118–27.

7. Forner A, Llovet JM, Bruix J. Hepatocellular carcinoma. Lancet 2012;379(9822): 1245–55.

8. Meissner HI, Smith RA, Rimer BK, et al. Promoting cancer screening: learning from experience. Cancer 2004;101(5 Suppl):1107–17.

9. El-Serag HB, Davila JA. Surveillance for hepatocellular carcinoma: in whom and how? Therap Adv Gastroenterol 2011;4(1):5–10.

10. Ioannou GN, Perkins JD, Carithers RL Jr. Liver transplantation for hepatocellular carcinoma: impact of the MELD allocation system and predictors of survival. Gastroenterology 2008;134(5):1342–51.

11. Llovet JM, Bruix J. Early diagnosis and treatment of hepatocellular carcinoma. Baillieres Best Pract Res Clin Gastroenterol 2000;14(6):991–1008.

12. Llovet JM, Burroughs A, Bruix J. Hepatocellular carcinoma. Lancet 2003; 362(9399):1907–17.

13. Marrero JA, Fontana RJ, Barrat A, et al. Prognosis of hepatocellular carcinoma: comparison of 7 staging systems in an American cohort. Hepatology 2005; 41(4):707–16.

14. Marrero JA, Kudo M, Bronowicki JP. The challenge of prognosis and staging for hepatocellular carcinoma. Oncologist 2010;15(Suppl 4):23–33.

15. Mazzaferro V, Regalia E, Doci R, et al. Liver transplantation for the treatment of small hepatocellular carcinomas in patients with cirrhosis. N Engl J Med 1996; 334(11):693–9.

16. Wilson JM, Jungner YG. Principles and practice of mass screening for disease. Bol Oficina Sanit Panam 1968;65(4):281–393 [in Spanish].

17. Nelson HD, Fu R, Cantor A, et al. Effectiveness of breast cancer screening: systematic review and meta-analysis to update the 2009 U.S. Preventive Services Task Force recommendation. Ann Intern Med 2016;164(4):244–55.

18. Heleno B, Thomsen MF, Rodrigues DS, et al. Quantification of harms in cancer screening trials: literature review. BMJ 2013;347:f5334.

19. Zhang BH, Yang BH, Tang ZY. Randomized controlled trial of screening for hepatocellular carcinoma. J Cancer Res Clin Oncol 2004;130(7):417–22.

20. Kudo M, Matsui O, Izumi N, et al. JSH consensus-based clinical practice guidelines for the management of hepatocellular carcinoma: 2014 update by the Liver Cancer Study Group of Japan. Liver Cancer 2014;3(3–4):458–68.

21. Omata M, Cheng AL, Kokudo N, et al. Asia-Pacific clinical practice guidelines on the management of hepatocellular carcinoma: a 2017 update. Hepatol Int 2017; 11(4):317–70.

22. Heimbach JK, Kulik LM, Finn R, et al. AASLD guidelines for the treatment of hepatocellular carcinoma. Hepatology 2018;67(1):358–80.

23. European Association for the Study of the Liver, European Organisation for Research and Treatment of Cancer. EASL-EORTC clinical practice guidelines: management of hepatocellular carcinoma. J Hepatol 2012;56(4):908–43.

24. Mittal S, Kanwal F, Ying J, et al. Effectiveness of surveillance for hepatocellular carcinoma in clinical practice: a United States cohort. J Hepatol 2016;65(6): 1148–54.

25. Singal AG, Pillai A, Tiro J. Early detection, curative treatment, and survival rates for hepatocellular carcinoma surveillance in patients with cirrhosis: a meta-analysis. PloS Med 2014;11(4):e1001624.

26. van Meer S, de Man RA, Coenraad MJ, et al. Surveillance for hepatocellular carcinoma is associated with increased survival: results from a large cohort in the Netherlands. J Hepatol 2015;63(5):1156–63.

27. Bruix J, Sherman M, American Association for the Study of Liver Disease. Management of hepatocellular carcinoma: an update. Hepatology 2011;53(3):1020–2.

28. Bruix J, Sherman M. Practice Guidelines Committee American Association for the Study of Liver Diseases. Management of hepatocellular carcinoma. Hepatology 2005;42(5):1208–36.

29. Marrero JA. Screening tests for hepatocellular carcinoma. Clin Liver Dis 2005; 9(2):235–51, vi.

30. Trevisani F, D'Intino PE, Morselli-Labate AM, et al. Serum alpha-fetoprotein for diagnosis of hepatocellular carcinoma in patients with chronic liver disease: influence of HBsAg and anti-HCV status. J Hepatol 2001;34(4):570–5.

31. Singal A, Volk ML, Waljee A, et al. Meta-analysis: surveillance with ultrasound for early-stage hepatocellular carcinoma in patients with cirrhosis. Aliment Pharmacol Ther 2009;30(1):37–47.

32. Chaiteerakij R, Addissie BD, Roberts LR. Update on biomarkers of hepatocellular carcinoma. Clin Gastroenterol Hepatol 2015;13(2):237–45.

33. Chon YE, Choi GH, Lee MH, et al. Combined measurement of preoperative alpha-fetoprotein and des-gamma-carboxy prothrombin predicts recurrence after curative resection in patients with hepatitis-B-related hepatocellular carcinoma. Int J Cancer 2012;131(10):2332–41.

34. Sterling RK, Jeffers L, Gordon F, et al. Utility of Lens culinaris agglutinin-reactive fraction of alpha-fetoprotein and des-gamma-carboxy prothrombin, alone or in combination, as biomarkers for hepatocellular carcinoma. Clin Gastroenterol Hepatol 2009;7(1):104–13.

35. Oka H, Saito A, Ito K, et al. Multicenter prospective analysis of newly diagnosed hepatocellular carcinoma with respect to the percentage of Lens culinaris agglutinin-reactive alpha-fetoprotein. J Gastroenterol Hepatol 2001;16(12):1378–83.

36. Volk ML, Hernandez JC, Su GL, et al. Risk factors for hepatocellular carcinoma may impair the performance of biomarkers: a comparison of AFP, DCP, and AFP-L3. Cancer Biomark 2007;3(2):79–87.

37. McEvoy SH, McCarthy CJ, Lavelle LP, et al. Hepatocellular carcinoma: illustrated guide to systematic radiologic diagnosis and staging according to guidelines of the American Association for the Study of Liver Diseases. Radiographics 2013; 33(6):1653–68.

38. Fetzer DT, Rodgers SK, Harris AC, et al. Screening and surveillance of hepatocellular carcinoma: an introduction to ultrasound liver imaging reporting and data system. Radiol Clin North Am 2017;55(6):1197–209.

39. Cucchetti A, Trevisani F, Cescon M, et al. Cost-effectiveness of semi-annual surveillance for hepatocellular carcinoma in cirrhotic patients of the Italian liver cancer population. J Hepatol 2012;56(5):1089–96.

40. Del Poggio P, Olmi S, Ciccarese F, et al. Factors that affect efficacy of ultrasound surveillance for early stage hepatocellular carcinoma in patients with cirrhosis. Clin Gastroenterol Hepatol 2014;12(11):1927–33.e2.

41. Tong MJ, Blatt LM, Kao VW. Surveillance for hepatocellular carcinoma in patients with chronic viral hepatitis in the United States of America. J Gastroenterol Hepatol 2001;16(5):553–9.

42. Simmons O, Fetzer DT, Yokoo T, et al. Predictors of adequate ultrasound quality for hepatocellular carcinoma surveillance in patients with cirrhosis. Aliment Pharmacol Ther 2017;45(1):169–77.

43. Yu NC, Chaudhari V, Raman SS, et al. CT and MRI improve detection of hepatocellular carcinoma, compared with ultrasound alone, in patients with cirrhosis. Clin Gastroenterol Hepatol 2011;9(2):161–7.

44. Morgan TA, Maturen KE, Dahiya N, et al. US LI-RADS: ultrasound liver imaging reporting and data system for screening and surveillance of hepatocellular carcinoma. Abdom Radiol (NY) 2018;43(1):41–55.

45. Davenport MS, Khalatbari S, Liu PS, et al. Repeatability of diagnostic features and scoring systems for hepatocellular carcinoma by using MR imaging. Radiology 2014;272(1):132–42.

46. Stigliano R, Burroughs AK. Should we biopsy each liver mass suspicious for HCC before liver transplantation?–no, please don't. J Hepatol 2005;43(4):563–8.

47. Thampanitchawong P, Piratvisuth T. Liver biopsy: complications and risk factors. World J Gastroenterol 1999;5(4):301–4.

48. Goossens N, Singal AG, King LY, et al. Cost-effectiveness of risk score-stratified hepatocellular carcinoma screening in patients with cirrhosis. Clin Transl Gastroenterol 2017;8(6):e101.

49. Levy I, Greig PD, Gallinger S, et al. Resection of hepatocellular carcinoma without preoperative tumor biopsy. Ann Surg 2001;234(2):206–9.

50. Silva MA, Hegab B, Hyde C, et al. Needle track seeding following biopsy of liver lesions in the diagnosis of hepatocellular cancer: a systematic review and meta-analysis. Gut 2008;57(11):1592–6.

51. Kim WR, Lake JR, Smith JM, et al. OPTN/SRTR 2015 annual data report: liver. Am J Transplant 2017;17(Suppl 1):174–251.

52. Wald C, Russo MW, Heimbach JK, et al. New OPTN/UNOS policy for liver transplant allocation: standardization of liver imaging, diagnosis, classification, and reporting of hepatocellular carcinoma. Radiology 2013;266(2):376–82.

53. Song P, Tobe RG, Inagaki Y, et al. The management of hepatocellular carcinoma around the world: a comparison of guidelines from 2001 to 2011. Liver Int 2012; 32(7):1053–63.

54. Pomfret EA, Washburn K, Wald C, et al. Report of a national conference on liver allocation in patients with hepatocellular carcinoma in the United States. Liver Transpl 2010;16(3):262–78.

55. Kudo M, Izumi N, Kokudo N, et al. Management of hepatocellular carcinoma in Japan: consensus-based clinical practice guidelines proposed by the Japan Society of Hepatology (JSH) 2010 updated version. Dig Dis 2011;29(3):339–64.

56. Arslanoglu A, Seyal AR, Sodagari F, et al. Current guidelines for the diagnosis and management of hepatocellular carcinoma: a comparative review. AJR Am J Roentgenol 2016;207(5):W88–98.

57. Mitchell DG, Bruix J, Sherman M, et al. LI-RADS (Liver Imaging Reporting and Data System): summary, discussion, and consensus of the LI-RADS Management Working Group and future directions. Hepatology 2015;61(3):1056–65.

58. American College of Radiology. Liver imaging reporting and data system version 2017. Available at: http://www.acr.org/Quality-Safety/Resources/LIRADS. Accessed October 12, 2017.

59. Kielar A, Fowler KJ, Lewis S, et al. Locoregional therapies for hepatocellular carcinoma and the new LI-RADS treatment response algorithm. Abdom Radiol (NY) 2018;43(1):218–30.

60. Cereser L, Furlan A, Bagatto D, et al. Comparison of portal venous and delayed phases of gadolinium-enhanced magnetic resonance imaging study of cirrhotic liver for the detection of contrast washout of hypervascular hepatocellular carcinoma. J Comput Assist Tomogr 2010;34(5):706–11.

61. Monzawa S, Ichikawa T, Nakajima H, et al. Dynamic CT for detecting small hepatocellular carcinoma: usefulness of delayed phase imaging. AJR Am J Roentgenol 2007;188(1):147–53.

62. Furlan A, Marin D, Vanzulli A, et al. Hepatocellular carcinoma in cirrhotic patients at multidetector CT: hepatic venous phase versus delayed phase for the detection of tumour washout. Br J Radiol 2011;84(1001):403–12.

63. Elsayes KM, Hooker JC, Agrons MM, et al. 2017 Version of LI-RADS for CT and MR imaging: an update. Radiographics 2017;37(7):1994–2017.

64. Ishigami K, Yoshimitsu K, Nishihara Y, et al. Hepatocellular carcinoma with a pseudocapsule on gadolinium-enhanced MR images: correlation with histopathologic findings. Radiology 2009;250(2):435–43.

65. Khan AS, Hussain HK, Johnson TD, et al. Value of delayed hypointensity and delayed enhancing rim in magnetic resonance imaging diagnosis of small hepatocellular carcinoma in the cirrhotic liver. J Magn Reson Imaging 2010;32(2):360–6.

66. Matsui O, Kobayashi S, Sanada J, et al. Hepatocelluar nodules in liver cirrhosis: hemodynamic evaluation (angiography-assisted CT) with special reference to multi-step hepatocarcinogenesis. Abdom Imaging 2011;36(3):264–72.

67. Forner A, Vilana R, Ayuso C, et al. Diagnosis of hepatic nodules 20 mm or smaller in cirrhosis: prospective validation of the noninvasive diagnostic criteria for hepatocellular carcinoma. Hepatology 2008;47(1):97–104.

68. Fowler KJ, Karimova EJ, Arauz AR, et al. Validation of Organ Procurement and Transplant Network (OPTN)/United Network for Organ Sharing (UNOS) criteria for imaging diagnosis of hepatocellular carcinoma. Transplantation 2013;95(12):1506–11.

69. Sangiovanni A, Manini MA, Iavarone M, et al. The diagnostic and economic impact of contrast imaging techniques in the diagnosis of small hepatocellular carcinoma in cirrhosis. Gut 2010;59(5):638–44.

70. Serste T, Barrau V, Ozenne V, et al. Accuracy and disagreement of computed tomography and magnetic resonance imaging for the diagnosis of small hepatocellular carcinoma and dysplastic nodules: role of biopsy. Hepatology 2012;55(3):800–6.

71. Kim TK, Lee KH, Jang HJ, et al. Analysis of gadobenate dimeglumine-enhanced MR findings for characterizing small (1-2-cm) hepatic nodules in patients at high risk for hepatocellular carcinoma. Radiology 2011;259(3):730–8.

72. Jang HJ, Kim TK, Khalili K, et al. Characterization of 1- to 2-cm liver nodules detected on HCC surveillance ultrasound according to the criteria of the American Association for the Study of Liver Disease: is quadriphasic CT necessary? AJR Am J Roentgenol 2013;201(2):314–21.

73. Bolondi L, Gaiani S, Celli N, et al. Characterization of small nodules in cirrhosis by assessment of vascularity: the problem of hypovascular hepatocellular carcinoma. Hepatology 2005;42(1):27–34.

74. Yacoub JH, Miller FH. Understanding LI-RADS, its relationship to AASLD and OPTN, and the challenges of its adoption. Curr Hepatol Rep 2017;16(1):72–80.

75. Burke LM, Sofue K, Alagiyawanna M, et al. Natural history of Liver Imaging Reporting and Data System category 4 nodules in MRI. Abdom Radiol (NY) 2016; 41(9):1758–66.

76. Choi JY, Cho HC, Sun M, et al. Indeterminate observations (Liver Imaging Reporting and Data System category 3) on MRI in the cirrhotic liver: fate and clinical implications. AJR Am J Roentgenol 2013;201(5):993–1001.

77. Tanabe M, Kanki A, Wolfson T, et al. Imaging outcomes of Liver Imaging Reporting and Data System version 2014 category 2, 3, and 4 observations detected at CT and MR imaging. Radiology 2016;281(1):129–39.

78. Lyshchik A, Kono Y, Dietrich CF, et al. Contrast-enhanced ultrasound of the liver: technical and lexicon recommendations from the ACR CEUS LI-RADS working group. Abdom Radiol (NY) 2018;43(4):861–79.

79. Wilson SR, Lyshchik A, Piscaglia F, et al. CEUS LI-RADS: algorithm, implementation, and key differences from CT/MRI. Abdom Radiol (NY) 2018;43(1):127–42.

80. Deng H, Shi H, Lei J, et al. A meta-analysis of contrast-enhanced ultrasound for small hepatocellular carcinoma diagnosis. J Cancer Res Ther 2016; 12(Supplement):C274–6.

81. Forner A, Vilana R, Bianchi L, et al. Lack of arterial hypervascularity at contrast-enhanced ultrasound should not define the priority for diagnostic work-up of nodules <2 cm. J Hepatol 2015;62(1):150–5.

82. Giorgio A, Montesarchio L, Gatti P, et al. Contrast-enhanced ultrasound: a simple and effective tool in defining a rapid diagnostic work-up for small nodules detected in cirrhotic patients during surveillance. J Gastrointestin Liver Dis 2016; 25(2):205–11.

83. Guang Y, Xie L, Ding H, et al. Diagnosis value of focal liver lesions with SonoVue(R)-enhanced ultrasound compared with contrast-enhanced computed tomography and contrast-enhanced MRI: a meta-analysis. J Cancer Res Clin Oncol 2011;137(11):1595–605.

84. Leoni S, Piscaglia F, Granito A, et al. Characterization of primary and recurrent nodules in liver cirrhosis using contrast-enhanced ultrasound: which vascular criteria should be adopted? Ultraschall Med 2013;34(3):280–7.

85. Roberts LR, Sirlin CB, Zaiem F, et al. Imaging for the diagnosis of hepatocellular carcinoma: a systematic review and meta-analysis. Hepatology 2018;67(1): 401–21.

86. Hanna RF, Miloushev VZ, Tang A, et al. Comparative 13-year meta-analysis of the sensitivity and positive predictive value of ultrasound, CT, and MRI for detecting hepatocellular carcinoma. Abdom Radiol (NY) 2016;41(1):71–90.

87. Xie L, Guang Y, Ding H, et al. Diagnostic value of contrast-enhanced ultrasound, computed tomography and magnetic resonance imaging for focal liver lesions: a meta-analysis. Ultrasound Med Biol 2011;37(6):854–61.

88. Friedrich-Rust M, Klopffleisch T, Nierhoff J, et al. Contrast-enhanced ultrasound for the differentiation of benign and malignant focal liver lesions: a meta-analysis. Liver Int 2013;33(5):739–55.

89. Liu GJ, Wang W, Lu MD, et al. Contrast-enhanced ultrasound for the characterization of hepatocellular carcinoma and intrahepatic cholangiocarcinoma. Liver Cancer 2015;4(4):241–52.

90. Wildner D, Bernatik T, Greis C, et al. CEUS in hepatocellular carcinoma and intrahepatic cholangiocellular carcinoma in 320 patients—early or late washout matters: a subanalysis of the DEGUM multicenter trial. Ultraschall Med 2015;36(2): 132–9.

91. Wildner D, Pfeifer L, Goertz RS, et al. Dynamic contrast-enhanced ultrasound (DCE-US) for the characterization of hepatocellular carcinoma and cholangiocellular carcinoma. Ultraschall Med 2014;35(6):522–7.

Imaging in Autoimmune Pancreatitis and Immunoglobulin G4–Related Disease of the Abdomen

Kumaresan Sandrasegaran, MD[a],*, Christine O. Menias, MD[b]

KEYWORDS

- Autoimmune pancreatitis • Systemic IgG4 disease • IgG4 sclerosing cholangitis
- Pancreas cancer • Cholangiocarcinoma • Primary sclerosing cholangitis

KEY POINTS

- Autoimmune pancreatitis (AIP) is classified into type I, which is associated with systemic immunoglobulin (Ig)G4 disease, and type 2, which is localized to the pancreas.
- AIP may present as diffuse, segmental, or focal disease of pancreas.
- Fecal AIP may mimic pancreas cancer, although in many cases imaging features help to differentiate the 2 entities.
- IgG4 sclerosing cholangitis usually presents with a tapering or funnel-shaped biliary ductal stricture, whereas cholangiocarcinoma typically presents with an abrupt stricture.

INTRODUCTION

Autoimmune pancreatitis (AIP) is a benign fibroinflammatory disease. This disease was initially reported in 1995[1] and its association with immunoglobulin G subclass 4 (IgG4)-related autoimmunity was recognized between 2001 and 2003 by Japanese researchers.[2,3] Since then, IgG4 disease has been reported to affect almost all organ systems, including the liver, biliary tree, kidneys, prostate gland, testicles, the peritoneum and the retroperitoneum, salivary and lacrimal glands, orbital tissues, pituitary gland, thyroid gland, lungs, lymph nodes, breasts, and vascular structures. In 2004, a new version of AIP (AIP type 2) without IgG4 disease, but with histologic features of a granulocytic epithelial lesion, was described.[4] Diagnosis of AIP requires the combination of clinical, serologic, imaging, and pathologic findings, as well as a good

Disclosure: The authors have nothing to disclose.
[a] Department of Radiology, Indiana University School of Medicine, 550 North University Boulevard, UH0279, Indianapolis, IN 46202, USA; [b] Department of Radiology, Mayo Clinic School of Medicine, Mayo Clinic Hospital, 5777 East Mayo Boulevard, Phoenix, AZ 85054, USA
* Corresponding author.
E-mail address: ksandras@iupui.edu

Gastroenterol Clin N Am 47 (2018) 603–619
https://doi.org/10.1016/j.gtc.2018.04.007
0889-8553/18/© 2018 Elsevier Inc. All rights reserved.

gastro.theclinics.com

response to corticosteroids. In this article, we highlight the imaging features of AIP and the spectrum of other abdominal IgG4 disease.

EPIDEMIOLOGY AND SUBTYPES

It is difficult to estimate the prevalence of AIP, because many cases are undiagnosed. Most reports of AIP come from Japan, where the incidence is estimated to be approximately 1 per 100,000 and AIP accounts for 5% to 6% of patients with chronic pancreatitis.[5] Studies in the United States have reported that 2% to 3% of pancreatic resections show autoimmune pancreatitis at pathologic analysis.[6]

AIP is now classified into types 1 and 2 (**Table 1**). Type 1 AIP is predominantly an IgG4-mediated disease and can affect virtually every organ system in the body (**Table 2**). Nevertheless, IgG4 may not be the only underlying cause of the disease. Type 1 AIP typically affects older, male patients. This type accounts for nearly all cases of AIP in Japan and Korea and 60% to 80% of cases in the United States.[7–9] Type 2 AIP is usually confined to the pancreas and there is an association with inflammatory bowel disease but no association with elevated IgG4 levels. Type 2 subtype is seen more often in Europe than in the United States.[6] The imaging findings of both type 1 and 2 are similar with minor differences, as discussed in this article.

CLINICAL PRESENTATION

The typical presentation of type 1 AIP is an elderly man with painless obstructive jaundice (up to 75% cases).[8] Thus, clinical differentiation from pancreas cancer may be difficult and the diagnosis is often made on imaging. Other clinical features include unexplained chronic abdominal pain, weight loss, and steatorrhea.[10] Exocrine functional abnormalities are seen in up to 80% of patients.[6] Type 2 diabetes mellitus may predate or present synchronously in up to 80% of patients with AIP. Surprisingly, in some patients with AIP, diabetes may improve with steroid therapy.[11] Type 2 AIP presents in younger patients, with roughly equal gender distribution. As with type 1 AIP, the most common presentation of type 2 AIP is painless jaundice. Presentation with acute pancreatitis is more commonly seen in patients with type 2 disease who have concurrent inflammatory bowel disease.[12]

Table 1
Differences between types 1 and 2 autoimmune pancreatitis (AIP)

	Type 1 AIP	Type 2 AIP
Synonyms	Lymphoplasmocytic sclerosing pancreatitis	Idiopathic duct-centric chronic pancreatitis
Mean age, y	Elderly: 64	Middle aged: 43
Male:female ratio	5:1	1:1
Incidence	Japan >> US, EU	EU > US > Japan
Obstructive jaundice, %	50	<5
Acute pancreatitis, %	15	33
Extrapancreatic disease	IgG4-systemic disease	Chronic ulcerative colitis in 30%
Serum IgG4	80% have elevated (>140 mg/dL)	Normal
Response to steroids	Good response (90%) but relapse ≈ 30%–40%	Good (90%) response and relapse <10%

Abbreviation: EU, European Union.
Data from Refs.[6,12,24,32]

Table 2
Organs affected by immunoglobulin G4 disease

Organ	Clinicopathologic Features	Incidence, %
Pancreas	Lymphoplasmacytic sclerosing pancreatitis (type 1 autoimmune pancreatitis)	40–60
Bile duct	Sclerosing cholangitis	20–40
Gall bladder	Acalculous sclerosing cholecystitis	
Liver	Sclerosing cholangitis, inflammatory pseudotumor, lobular hepatitis	5
Colon	Ulcerative colitis	5, type 1; 15–30, type 2
Kidney/Ureter	Tubulointerstitial nephritis, membranous glomerulopathy, inflammatory pseudotumor	10–30
Retroperitoneum/ Mesentery	Retroperitoneal fibrosis, sclerosing mesenteritis	10–20
Prostate gland	Prostatitis	
Central nervous system	Hypophysitis, sclerosing pachymeningitis	
Lacrimal glands/Orbit	Chronic sclerosing dacryoadenitis, inflammatory pseudotumor	20–30
Salivary glands	Chronic sclerosing sialadenitis (Kuttner tumor), Mikulicz disease	40–50
Thyroid	Riedel thyroiditis	
Lung	Inflammatory pseudotumor, interstitial pneumonia	10–30
Cardiovascular/Aorta	Periaortitis, abdominal aortic aneurysm	2–10
Mediastinum	Sclerosing mediastinitis	
Breast	Sclerosing mastitis	
Lymph node	Lymphadenopathy without or with Castleman disease–like features	25–60

The ranges of incidence reflect whether the quoted series evaluated patients with autoimmune pancreatitis or those with systemic immunoglobulin G4 disease. In addition, percentages varied on whether the series was primarily based on imaging or on histology.
Data from Refs.[6,24,32–35]

SEROLOGIC MARKERS

Type 1 AIP is associated with elevated titers of γ-globulin ($\geq$2.0 g/dL), IgG ($\geq$1800 mg/dL) and its subset IgG4 ($\geq$140 mg/dL), and rheumatoid factor.[6] Serum IgG4 levels greater than 140 mg/dL are considered to be 86% sensitive, 96% specific, and 91% accurate for the diagnosis of AIP.[13] It should be noted that type 2 AIP accounts for 20% to 40% of all AIP cases in the United States, and will not have elevated IgG4 levels.[6,14] There are no serologic markers for type 2 disease.

PATHOLOGY

The pathologic hallmarks of type 1 AIP are dense infiltration by plasma cells and lymphocytes, swirling (or storiform) fibrosis, and obliterative phlebitis.[15] Increased IgG4-positive plasma cell infiltrate in the pancreas is a helpful marker for AIP, but may not be entirely specific. Moderately increased IgG4-positive plasma cell infiltrate in the pancreas (>10 cells per high-powered field) may be seen in 75% of AIP but also may be seen in 10% of patients with alcoholic chronic pancreatitis and 12% of patients with pancreatic adenocarcinoma.[6,16] IgG4 immunostaining should be interpreted cautiously when the tissue sample is small (as in a core biopsy) or if IgG4 plasma cell positivity is limited to fewer than 10 cells per high-powered field.[15]

Type 2 AIP shows predominantly neutrophil infiltration in the ductal lumen, walls, and in acini of the pancreas.[6] Plasma cells are present in limited numbers. Obliterative phlebitis is also not a common feature. In common with type 1 AIP, there is periductal inflammation and storiform fibrosis.[17]

CLASSIFICATION SYSTEMS

Diagnosis of AIP may be difficult because the clinical presentation is nonspecific, and AIP is a relatively uncommon disease, compared with diseases it mimics, such as pancreatic cancer or acute or chronic pancreatitis. In the first decade of 2000, separate classification systems were described by researchers in Japan, Korea, Germany, Italy, and the United States.[18] To unify these approaches, in 2011 an international panel of experts developed the International Consensus Diagnostic Criteria for AIP. This complex classification system uses imaging features of the pancreatic parenchyma and pancreatic ducts, serologic findings, evidence of other organ involvement by IgG4 disease, histology of pancreas, and response to steroids.[6,18]

IMAGING OF AUTOIMMUNE PANCREATITIS AND IMMUNOGLOBULIN G4 DISEASE

Table 2 gives the distribution of IgG4-related diseases. The exact frequency depends on whether the series evaluated systemic disease or the disease focused on a specific presentation, such as AIP. AIP is the most common single-organ manifestation of IgG4 disease.

Pancreatic Parenchymal Disease

Parenchymal involvement may be diffuse, regional, or focal in AIP (**Box 1**). Diffuse disease typically presents with sausage-shaped enlargement of the gland with loss of fat clefts (**Figs. 1** and **2**). Glandular necrosis, peripancreatic collections, or pseudocysts are rare findings. The gland typically enhances less than expected in the arterial phase with increased enhancement on the delayed phases.[6] A specific finding is a

---

Box 1
Imaging features of autoimmune pancreatitis (AIP)

Diffuse glandular enlargement (50%–70%)

Focal masses (30%: up to 80% in type 2 AIP)

Segmental disease (30%–40%)

Tail truncation (up to 40% in type 2 AIP)

Delayed enhancement (90%)

Soft tissue rim around pancreas with delayed enhancement (15%–40%)

Peripancreatic fluid collections, pseudocysts (rare)

Ductal or parenchymal calculi (rare, except in type 2 AIP with colitis)

Peripancreatic lymphadenopathy (20%)

Reduced apparent diffusion coefficient ($<1.0 \times 10^{-3}$ mm^2/s)

Data from Refs.[6,12,19,24,32,35,36]

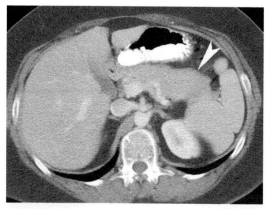

Fig. 1. A 45-year-old woman with abdominal pain. Axial CT shows a featureless swollen pancreas (*arrowhead*) with loss of the normal fat clefts. AIP was suggested and confirmed on biopsy.

hypoenhancing soft tissue rim around the gland (**Figs. 3** and **4**) made of cellular infiltrate and fibrosis. This finding is seen in approximately 15% to 40% of AIP and may be better discerned on MRI than computed tomography (CT), as a hypointense capsule on T1-weighted and T2-weighted scans.[19] Subtle delayed enhancement of the capsule may be seen. It should be noted that a normal-appearing pancreas on CT or MRI does not rule out AIP.[12] The main differential for a nonacute patient with diffusely swollen poorly enhancing pancreas is pancreatic lymphoma. Differentiation of imaging may be difficult (**Fig. 5**), although moderate volume adenopathy (>1.5 cm short axis) should suggest lymphoma.

The segmental form of the disease affects an entire part of the gland, for example, tail or body. On MRI, the affected gland may show relative hypointensity on T1-weighting and mild hyperintensity on T2-weighting. Poor early enhancement and more intense delayed enhancement is the typical pattern (**Fig. 6**). There is usually a sharp demarcation between the affected and nonaffected pancreas.

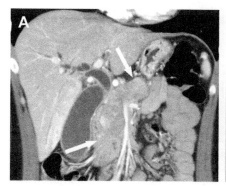
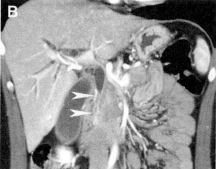

Fig. 2. A 54-year-old man with painless jaundice. (*A*) Coronal CT reformation shows a swollen hypoenhancing pancreas (*arrows*) (*B*). Coronal CT reformation shows a stricture of the distal CBD with a thick, enhancing wall (*arrowheads*). The appearances are characteristic of type 1 AIP with IgG4 SC.

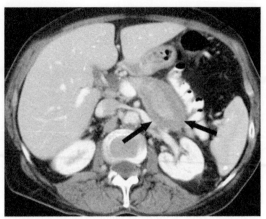

Fig. 3. A 58-year-old man with abdominal pain. There is a soft tissue hypoenhancing rim (*arrows*) around the pancreas that is a classic finding of AIP.

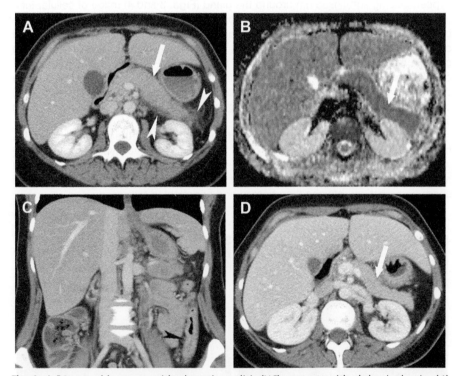

Fig. 4. A 34-year-old woman with ulcerative colitis (UC) presents with abdominal pain. (*A*) Axial CT shows a swollen pancreas (*arrow*) and hypoenhancing capsule (*white arrowheads*). (*B*) ADC map shows a hypointense pancreas (*arrow*) consistent with restricted diffusion from cellular infiltrate. ADC was 0.78×10^{-3} mm^2/s. (*C*) Coronal CT reformation shows a thickened left colon (*black arrowhead*) in keeping with UC. Given the patient's age and the presence of UC, type 2 AIP was considered and proven on biopsy. (*D*) Axial CT after steroid therapy shows atrophy of the pancreas (*arrow*).

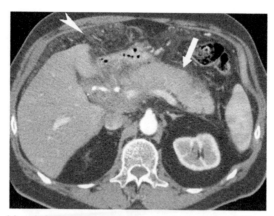

Fig. 5. A 75-year-old with fever and weight loss. Axial CT shows a diffusely swollen hypoen-hancing pancreas (*arrow*) and omental nodularity (*arrowhead*). AIP was reported on CT, but biopsy showed B-cell non-Hodgkin lymphoma. Constitutional symptoms, such as fever, should raise possibility of lymphoma rather than AIP.

Nodular disease presents with 1 or more masses in the pancreas (**Fig. 7**). This sub-type is seen more commonly in type 2 AIP (35%–80% incidence)[6,12] and the imaging features are discussed later under Autoimmune Pancreatitis versus Pancreas Cancer. These masses may mimic pancreas cancer. A characteristic finding seen in up to 40% of type 2 AIP is complete atrophy of the pancreatic tail (tail truncation sign).[6]

AIP type 1 may be diagnosed primarily using imaging criteria. If there are typical im-aging findings, such as diffuse pancreatic swelling or an enhancing rim of soft tissue, 1 of the following 3 criteria is required for diagnosis: (1) elevated serum IgG4, (2) evi-dence of extrapancreatic disease on imaging, or (3) positive biopsy of the duodenal papilla on endoscopy. When atypical findings such as segmental pancreatic enhance-ment are seen, at least 2 of the criteria and evidence of pancreatic ductal disease are required for diagnosis. Type 1 AIP also may be confirmed in the absence of imaging findings if the histologic findings on core biopsy or glandular resection are diagnostic. Type 2 AIP usually requires biopsy confirmation, because elevated IgG4 levels and

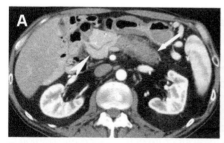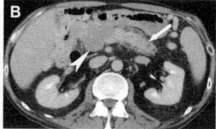

Fig. 6. A 57-year-old man with abdominal pain. Arterial phase (*A*) and 5-minute delayed (*B*) postcontrast phases show decreased early enhancement and more intense delayed enhance-ment of the tail of pancreas (*arrows*). The normal head of the pancreas (*arrowheads*) shows the opposite enhancement pattern. The appearances are of segmental AIP of the tail. There is sharp demarcation of affected and nonaffected gland. Small peripancreatic fluid pockets are present. This patient probably had type 2 AIP because acute pancreatitis changes are more common with this type.

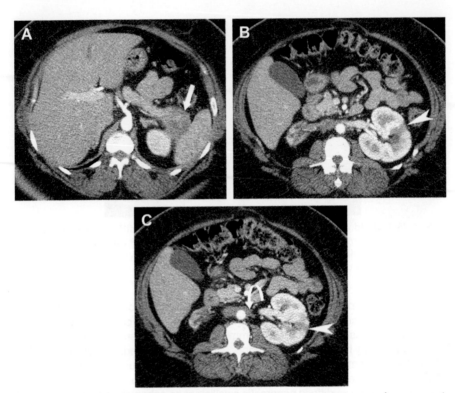

Fig. 7. A 42-year-old woman with back and abdominal pain. Axial CT images show a mass in the tail of pancreas (*arrow*) (*A*), which was reported as highly worrisome for pancreatic cancer. There were hypoenhancing wedge-shaped peripheral cortical defects (*arrowheads*) (*B, C*) and retroperitoneal fibrosis (*curved arrow*) (*C*) that should have indicated that AIP was the cause of the pancreatic mass. Biopsy confirmed type 1 AIP. It is important to look for extrapancreatic organ disease whenever AIP is suspected.

extrapancreatic disease are not typically seen in this subtype. Compression, encasement, or thrombosis of splenic and mesenteric veins is reported in 25% to 50% of AIP cases.[6,10] Uptake of fluorine-18-deoxyglucose is seen in 90% to 100% of cases of AIP, in contrast to approximately 10% of cases of chronic pancreatitis.[20,21]

Pancreatic Ductal Disease

Typical ductal features on magnetic resonance cholangiopancreatography (MRCP) or endoscopic retrograde cholangiopancreatography (ERCP) are long (ie, greater than one-third of the length of duct) or multiple strictures without upstream duct dilation (duct caliber <5 mm) (**Fig. 8**). Dilated main duct is uncommon in AIP and, if present, an alternate diagnosis, such as pancreatic cancer, should be considered. Side branch dilation may be seen at sites of strictures. A focal stricture of the pancreatic portion of the common bile duct (CBD) may be found, usually signifying associated IgG4-related sclerosing cholangitis (see later in this article).

Ductal calculi are rare at presentation, but may occur in approximately 7% of patients with type 1 AIP on follow-up.[22] Risk factors for pancreatic calculi include excessive alcohol consumption and recurrent AIP relapses. Ductal calculi are not considered to be common in type 2 AIP.

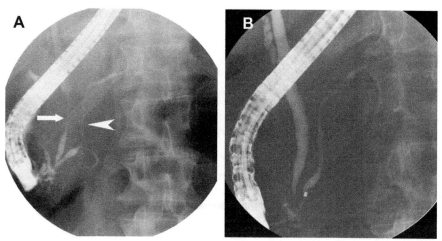

Fig. 8. A 72-year-old man with obstructive jaundice. ERCP images before (*A*) and 6 weeks after start of steroid therapy (*B*) show that the CBD (*arrow*) and pancreatic ductal (*arrowhead*) strictures have substantially improved after treatment.

Autoimmune Pancreatitis Versus Pancreatic Cancer

When a mass is seen in the pancreas, pancreatic cancer (ductal adenocarcinoma) is usually the main consideration. There is moderate overlap in the findings of pancreas cancer and focal AIP, including a hypodense mass, double duct sign, perivascular soft tissue cuffing, omental nodules, and local adenopathy. **Table 3** gives a list of features that support either diagnosis. A single abrupt duct cutoff, with upstream duct dilation and atrophy of tail at presentation is highly diagnostic of pancreatic cancer. The focal

Table 3
Differentiating autoimmune pancreatitis (AIP) from pancreas cancer

AIP	Pancreas Cancer
Diffuse pancreatic enlargement	Atrophy of body and/or tail
Ill-defined mass	Well-defined mass with reduced enhancement
Long segment (>1/3 length) MPD stricture	Short segment stricture
MPD dilatation <5 mm	MPD dilation >5 mm
Multiple sites of MPD stricture	Single site of MPD stricture: abrupt cut off
"Capsule" sign	No capsule sign
Duct-penetrating sign	No duct-penetrating sign
Side branch dilation at site of MPD stricture	No side branches seen at MPD stricture
ADC value <1.0 × 10^{-3} mm²/s	ADC values typically >1.0 × 10^{-3} mm²/s
Renal cortical hypoenhancing lesions	Liver metastases but no renal masses
CBD stricture with thick (>1 cm) enhancing wall	CBD stricture but no wall thickening
Responds to short steroid course	Nonresponsive to steroids

Abbreviations: ADC, apparent diffusion coefficient; CBD, common bile duct; MPD, main pancreatic duct.
Data from Refs.[12,32,37–39]

mass also will be more clearly defined than in AIP. Clearly, the presence of hepatic metastases favors cancer.

Multiple pancreatic masses, multiple or long-segment pancreatic ductal strictures without dilation more than 5 mm, diffusely swollen gland, distal CBD stricture with thickened and intensely enhancing wall, and renal cortical hypoenhancing lesions are suggestive of AIP (see **Fig. 7**; **Fig. 9**). The duct-penetrating sign (**Fig. 10**) is seen in benign strictures with a specificity of approximately 94% and sensitivity of 85%.[23] When these findings are present, it may be best practice to raise the diagnosis of AIP, so that serum IgG4 and if necessary pancreatic biopsy may be performed.

Immunoglobulin G4–Related Hepatobiliary Disease

Biliary tract involvement (IgG4-related sclerosing cholangitis) is seen in 60% to 80% of patients with type 1 AIP.[24] The typical clinical presentation is painless jaundice. Biliary tract disease may be seen rarely without pancreatic disease.

Extrahepatic duct involvement is more common than intrahepatic disease. Extrahepatic disease usually affects the distal CBD in the pancreatic head. Its main differential diagnosis is cholangiocarcinoma. There are some clues on imaging that may suggest a benign stricture, such as funnel-shaped narrowing, intense and homogeneous wall enhancement, and the presence of remote pancreatic ductal abnormalities (**Figs. 11** and **12**, **Table 4**).[25,26] Nevertheless, the diagnosis may be difficult on imaging, and endoscopic cytologic brushing with fluorescence in situ hybridization techniques or cholangioscopy (Spyglass DS; Boston Scientific, Marlborough, MA) may help.

Intrahepatic IgG4 sclerosing cholangitis (IgG4 SC) mimics primary sclerosing cholangitis (PSC) on imaging. Both diseases show irregular multiple strictures with intervening normal or mildly dilated ducts. Severe ductal dilation is uncommon. Pathologically, the 2 entities are different, with onion-skin–type concentric periductal fibrosis (which is a hallmark of PSC) not seen in IgG4 SC. PSC is an unremitting fibrotic disease that progresses to cirrhosis with liver failure on average in 12 years, whereas IgG4-related sclerosing cholangitis responds well to steroid therapy in most cases. Differences between IgG4 SC and PSC are given in **Table 5**.[25,27]

The gallbladder may be involved in approximately 25% of patients with AIP. Imaging features are nonspecific, and the diagnosis is usually made on surgical pathology. Gallstones are less common in IgG4 cholecystitis compared with acute cholecystitis. Hepatic involvement is also seen in patients with type 1 AIP. The most common

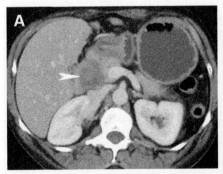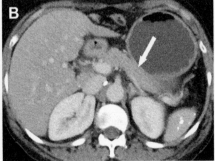

Fig. 9. A 48-year-old woman with painless jaundice. (*A*) Axial CT shows a mass in the pancreatic head (*arrowhead*) that was reported as pancreatic cancer. However, the absence of upstream ductal dilation or glandular atrophy (*arrow* in *B*) makes cancer less likely. Patient underwent the Whipple procedure and AIP was diagnosed on resected specimen.

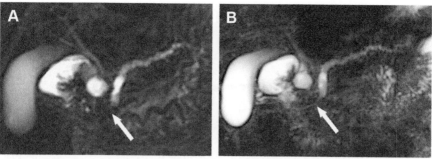

Fig. 10. A 71-year-old man with abdominal pain. (*A*) MRCP shows an abrupt pancreatic duct cutoff (*arrow*), which is worrisome for cancer. (*B*) Secretin-enhanced MRCP shows a narrow duct (*arrow*) passing beyond the stricture. This is the "duct-penetrating" sign, which is highly specific for a benign stricture. Surgical pathology showed AIP. Intravenous secretin increases pancreatic secretions and improves the visualization of the main pancreatic duct, especially in patients with chronic pancreatitis.

presentation is a mass lesion, often referred to as an inflammatory pseudotumor, in the hepatic hilum. Such lesions cause biliary obstruction and may mimic hilar cholangiocarcinoma. The radiologist should consider the possibility of IgG4 disease so that unnecessary major hepatic resection is avoided (**Fig. 13**).

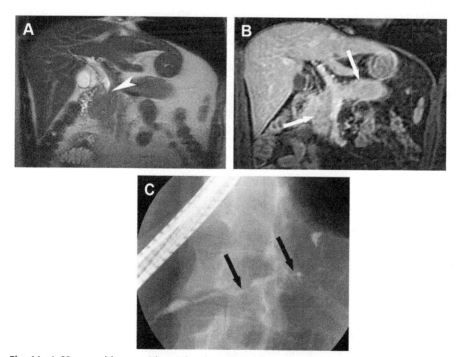

Fig. 11. A 60-year-old man with painless jaundice. (*A*) Coronal T2-weighted turbo spin echo (HASTE) shows a tapered stricture of the distal CBD (*arrowhead*). (*B*) Postcontrast MRI shows a swollen, hypoenhancing pancreas (*white arrows*). (*C*) Subsequent ERCP shows multiple main pancreatic ductal strictures (*black arrows*) remote from the CBD stricture. The conglomeration of findings should suggest type 1 AIP with IgG4 SC.

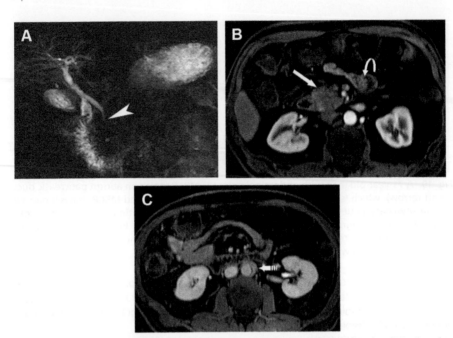

Fig. 12. A 74-year-old man with painless jaundice. (*A*) Coronal T2-weighted turbo spin echo (HASTE) shows a funnel-shaped stricture of the distal CBD (*arrowhead*). (*B*) Postcontrast MRI shows a hypoenhancing pancreas (*white arrow*). There is ill-defined soft tissue (*curved arrow*) in the mesentery, consistent with sclerosing mesenteritis. (*C*) There is eccentric soft tissue surrounding the aorta (*dashed arrow*) in keeping with inflammatory periaortitis. The conglomeration of findings is highly typical of IgG4 SC and associated diseases.

Immunoglobulin G4–Related Renal Disease

IgG4 renal disease may be seen in up to 35% of patients with type 1 AIP.[6] Renal disease may present with elevated creatinine (70%), proteinuria, or, less commonly, hematuria. The most common histologic finding is tubulointerstitial nephritis. Five patterns of disease have been described[6,28–30]: (1) bilateral rounded or wedge-shaped peripheral cortical hypoenhancing defects, which is the most common finding;

Table 4
Differentiation of immunoglobulin G4 sclerosing cholangitis (IgG4 SC) from cholangiocarcinoma

	IgG4 SC	Extrahepatic Cholangiocarcinoma
Appearance of stricture	Tapered or funnel-shaped stricture	Shelf with abrupt cut off
CBD wall thickness	>1 cm	Usually <1 cm
CBD enhancement in parenchymal phase	Homogeneous enhancement	Heterogeneous enhancement with less-enhancing outer wall
MPD	Remote MPD stricture	Double duct sign but no remote MPD stricture
Pancreatic swelling	Often seen (80%)	Not seen

Abbreviation: MPD, main pancreatic duct.
Data from Refs.[25–27]

Table 5
Differentiation of intrahepatic immunoglobulin G4 sclerosing cholangitis (IgG4 SC) from primary sclerosing cholangitis (PSC)

	IgG4 SC	PSC
Male:Female ratio	7:1	1.5:1.0
Age, y	Older (>50)	Younger (<40)
Serum IgG4	IgG4 >200 mg/dL 97% specific for IgG4 SC	Not elevated
Presentation	Acute: obstructive jaundice	Chronic: abnormal LFTs
Findings of cirrhosis	Not seen	Often present
Ulcerative colitis, %	<5	80
IgG4-positive plasma cells in major papilla biopsy, %	50–80	0
Pancreatic changes of AIP, %	90	<5
Response to steroids, %	90	Rare

Data from Refs.[25,27,40]

(2) ill-defined diffuse hypoenhancement of kidneys; (3) rim of soft tissue around the kidney; (4) bilateral hypoenhancing foci in the renal sinuses; and (5) diffuse wall thickening of the renal pelvis (see **Fig. 7**; **Fig. 14**). The enhancement pattern of IgG4-related renal lesions is like that of AIP, with poor initial enhancement followed by more intense delayed enhancement. The differential diagnosis includes renal infarction, pyelonephritis, or metastases.

Immunoglobulin G4–Related Retroperitoneal Disease

Retroperitoneal fibrosis is a chronic fibro-inflammatory condition that may result from infection, radiotherapy, drugs, malignancy, or trauma. Approximately 20% of patients

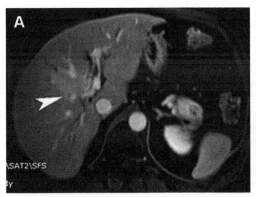
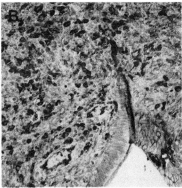

Fig. 13. A 66-year-old man with jaundice. (A) Five-minute post-gadolinium axial MRI shows a 5.5-cm enhancing mass (*arrowhead*). The mass did not enhance on the arterial or venous phases. There is dilation of bile ducts peripheral to the mass. Cholangiocarcinoma was diagnosed, and the patient underwent extended right hepatectomy. (B) Immunohistochemical stain for IgG4 of resected specimen shows 30 to 40 IgG4-positive plasma cells (*gold color stain*) per high-power field, characteristic of IgG4-related inflammatory pseudotumor of the liver. The imaging appearance of IgG4-related liver mass is similar to that of hilar cholangiocarcinoma. Differentiation on imaging may be impossible if there is no evidence of IgG4-related disease in other organs. (H&E, original magnification ×600).

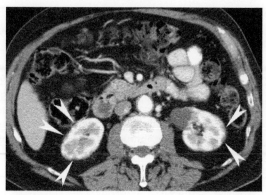

Fig. 14. An 81-year-old man with proteinuria. Axial CT shows several peripheral cortical hypoenhancing foci (*arrowheads*), which is a typical pattern of IgG4-related renal disease. There was no evidence of AIP.

with type 1 AIP have retroperitoneal fibrosis, with IgG4-positive plasma cell infiltration on biopsy. On imaging, IgG4-related retroperitoneal fibrosis presents as a soft tissue mass surrounding the aorta and the inferior vena cava (see **Fig. 7**). Abdominal aortic branches traverse the mass without occlusion. Ureteric obstruction is often seen, and requires stent placement. Steroid response is common.

Inflammatory periaortitis presents as eccentric soft tissue in and around the aortic wall (see **Fig. 12**). An aneurysm may or may not be present. In the absence of a known cause for periaortitis, for example, large vessel vasculitis or sarcoidosis, it is useful to raise the possibility of IgG4-related periaortitis, so that the appropriate immunostains may be performed on the biopsy specimen.

TREATMENT AND OUTCOMES OF AUTOIMMUNE PANCREATITIS

Response to steroid therapy is seen in 90% to 95% of both type 1 and 2 AIP. The glandular swelling decreases and the lobularity of the pancreatic contour become visible. Morphologic changes may be seen as early as 2 months after commencement of therapy (see **Fig. 4**). Atrophy of the gland is often seen. Peripancreatic stranding and the hypodense halo may resolve. The enhancement pattern returns to normal. Altered signal on T1-weighted and T2-wieghted scans also returns to normal.

Ductal irregularities and strictures tend to disappear, leaving a nearly normal duct (see **Fig. 8**). Apparent diffusion coefficient (ADC) values normalize and return to more than 1.0×10^{-3} mm^2/s. Persistently low ADC is associated of increased risk of recurrence.

Three-year relapse rates of type 1 AIP are reported to be as high as 60%, compared with fewer than 5% of type 2 AIP.[19] Risk factors for recurrence include extrapancreatic disease in type 1 AIP, a persistent focal mass after resolution of diffuse pancreatic swelling, and ductal stricture.[31] There is no clear association of AIP with cancers, although lymphoma and pancreas and other cancers have been reported to occur in patients with AIP. It is thought that AIP does not substantially shorten life span.[32]

SUMMARY

AIP is a rare type of chronic pancreatitis that mimics more common diseases, such as pancreatic cancer and cholangiocarcinoma. In this article, we covered the imaging differential features of AIP and IgG4 SC from malignancies. A heightened awareness allows the radiologists to raise the possible diagnosis of AIP or IgG4 disease so that appropriate tests are performed, obviating need for major surgery.

REFERENCES

1. Yoshida K, Toki F, Takeuchi T, et al. Chronic pancreatitis caused by an autoimmune abnormality. Proposal of the concept of autoimmune pancreatitis. Dig Dis Sci 1995;40(7):1561–8.
2. Hamano H, Kawa S, Horiuchi A, et al. High serum IgG4 concentrations in patients with sclerosing pancreatitis. N Engl J Med 2001;344(10):732–8.
3. Kamisawa T, Funata N, Hayashi Y, et al. A new clinicopathological entity of IgG4-related autoimmune disease. J Gastroenterol 2003;38(10):982–4.
4. Zamboni G, Luttges J, Capelli P, et al. Histopathological features of diagnostic and clinical relevance in autoimmune pancreatitis: a study on 53 resection specimens and 9 biopsy specimens. Virchows Arch 2004;445(6):552–63.
5. Nishimori I, Tamakoshi A, Otsuki M, et al. Prevalence of autoimmune pancreatitis in Japan from a nationwide survey in 2002. J Gastroenterol 2007;42(Suppl 18):6–8.
6. Khandelwal A, Shanbhogue AK, Takahashi N, et al. Recent advances in the diagnosis and management of autoimmune pancreatitis. AJR Am J Roentgenol 2014;202(5):1007–21.
7. Sah RP, Chari ST. Autoimmune pancreatitis: an update on classification, diagnosis, natural history and management. Curr Gastroenterol Rep 2012;14(2):95–105.
8. Kamisawa T, Chari ST, Giday SA, et al. Clinical profile of autoimmune pancreatitis and its histological subtypes: an international multicenter survey. Pancreas 2011;40(6):809–14.
9. Sugumar A, Kloppel G, Chari ST. Autoimmune pancreatitis: pathologic subtypes and their implications for its diagnosis. Am J Gastroenterol 2009;104(9):2308–10 [quiz: 2311].
10. Raina A, Yadav D, Krasinskas AM, et al. Evaluation and management of autoimmune pancreatitis: experience at a large US center. Am J Gastroenterol 2009;104(9):2295–306.
11. Nishimori I, Tamakoshi A, Kawa S, et al. Influence of steroid therapy on the course of diabetes mellitus in patients with autoimmune pancreatitis: findings from a nationwide survey in Japan. Pancreas 2006;32(3):244–8.
12. Majumder S, Takahashi N, Chari ST. Autoimmune pancreatitis. Dig Dis Sci 2017;62(7):1762–9.
13. Choi EK, Kim MH, Lee TY, et al. The sensitivity and specificity of serum immunoglobulin G and immunoglobulin G4 levels in the diagnosis of autoimmune chronic pancreatitis: Korean experience. Pancreas 2007;35(2):156–61.
14. Sah RP, Chari ST, Pannala R, et al. Differences in clinical profile and relapse rate of type 1 versus type 2 autoimmune pancreatitis. Gastroenterology 2010;139(1):140–8 [quiz: e112–43].
15. Zhang L, Smyrk TC. Autoimmune pancreatitis and IgG4-related systemic diseases. Int J Clin Exp Pathol 2010;3(5):491–504.
16. Ghazale A, Chari ST, Smyrk TC, et al. Value of serum IgG4 in the diagnosis of autoimmune pancreatitis and in distinguishing it from pancreatic cancer. Am J Gastroenterol 2007;102(8):1646–53.

17. Cai O, Tan S. From pathogenesis, clinical manifestation, and diagnosis to treatment: an overview on autoimmune pancreatitis. Gastroenterol Res Pract 2017; 2017:3246459.

18. Shimosegawa T, Chari ST, Frulloni L, et al. International consensus diagnostic criteria for autoimmune pancreatitis: guidelines of the International Association of Pancreatology. Pancreas 2011;40(3):352–8.

19. Crosara S, D'Onofrio M, De Robertis R, et al. Autoimmune pancreatitis: multimodality non-invasive imaging diagnosis. World J Gastroenterol 2014;20(45): 16881–90.

20. Lee TY, Kim MH, Park DH, et al. Utility of 18F-FDG PET/CT for differentiation of autoimmune pancreatitis with atypical pancreatic imaging findings from pancreatic cancer. AJR Am J Roentgenol 2009;193(2):343–8.

21. Zhang J, Shao C, Wang J, et al. Autoimmune pancreatitis: whole-body 18F-FDG PET/CT findings. Abdom Imaging 2013;38(3):543–9.

22. Ikeura T, Miyoshi H, Shimatani M, et al. Long-term outcomes of autoimmune pancreatitis. World J Gastroenterol 2016;22(34):7760–6.

23. Ichikawa T, Sou H, Araki T, et al. Duct-penetrating sign at MRCP: usefulness for differentiating inflammatory pancreatic mass from pancreatic carcinomas. Radiology 2001;221(1):107–16.

24. Martinez-de-Alegria A, Baleato-Gonzalez S, Garcia-Figueiras R, et al. IgG4-related disease from head to toe. Radiographics 2015;35(7):2007–25.

25. Joshi D, Webster GJ. Biliary and hepatic involvement in IgG4-related disease. Aliment Pharmacol Ther 2014;40(11–12):1251–61.

26. Yata M, Suzuki K, Furuhashi N, et al. Comparison of the multidetector-row computed tomography findings of IgG4-related sclerosing cholangitis and extrahepatic cholangiocarcinoma. Clin Radiol 2016;71(3):203–10.

27. Gardner CS, Bashir MR, Marin D, et al. Diagnostic performance of imaging criteria for distinguishing autoimmune cholangiopathy from primary sclerosing cholangitis and bile duct malignancy. Abdom Imaging 2015;40(8):3052–61.

28. Khalili K, Doyle DJ, Chawla TP, et al. Renal cortical lesions in patients with autoimmune pancreatitis: a clue to differentiation from pancreatic malignancy. Eur J Radiol 2008;67(2):329–35.

29. Takahashi N, Kawashima A, Fletcher JG, et al. Renal involvement in patients with autoimmune pancreatitis: CT and MR imaging findings. Radiology 2007;242(3): 791–801.

30. Triantopoulou C, Malachias G, Maniatis P, et al. Renal lesions associated with autoimmune pancreatitis: CT findings. Acta Radiol 2010;51(6):702–7.

31. Madhani K, Farrell JJ. Autoimmune pancreatitis: an update on diagnosis and management. Gastroenterol Clin North Am 2016;45(1):29–43.

32. Morse B, Centeno B, Vignesh S. Autoimmune pancreatitis: updated concepts of a challenging diagnosis. Am J Med 2014;127(10):1010.e1-9.

33. Divatia M, Kim SA, Ro JY. IgG4-related sclerosing disease, an emerging entity: a review of a multi-system disease. Yonsei Med J 2012;53(1):15–34.

34. Brito-Zeron P, Ramos-Casals M, Bosch X, et al. The clinical spectrum of IgG4-related disease. Autoimmun Rev 2014;13(12):1203–10.

35. Vlachou PA, Khalili K, Jang HJ, et al. IgG4-related sclerosing disease: autoimmune pancreatitis and extrapancreatic manifestations. Radiographics 2011; 31(5):1379–402.

36. Kozoriz MG, Chandler TM, Patel R, et al. Pancreatic and extrapancreatic features in autoimmune pancreatitis. Can Assoc Radiol J 2015;66(3):252–8.

37. Shin JU, Lee JK, Kim KM, et al. The differentiation of autoimmune pancreatitis and pancreatic cancer using imaging findings. Hepatogastroenterology 2013; 60(125):1174–81.

38. Sugumar A, Takahashi N, Chari ST. Distinguishing pancreatic cancer from auto-immune pancreatitis. Curr Gastroenterol Rep 2010;12(2):91–7.

39. Takahashi N, Fletcher JG, Fidler JL, et al. Dual-phase CT of autoimmune pancre-atitis: a multireader study. AJR Am J Roentgenol 2008;190(2):280–6.

40. Okazaki K, Uchida K, Koyabu M, et al. IgG4 cholangiopathy: current concept, diagnosis, and pathogenesis. J Hepatol 2014;61(3):690–5.

Percutaneous Biliary Interventions

Rocio Perez-Johnston, MD[a], Amy R. Deipolyi, MD, PhD[b], Anne M. Covey, MD[b],*

KEYWORDS

- Percutaneous • Biliary • Interventions

KEY POINTS

- Many types of percutaneous biliary procedures are performed by interventional radiologists.
- Indications and specific treatment options for percutaneous biliary intervention in the setting of benign and malignant disease are discussed.
- Preprocedure evaluation, including review of imaging and symptoms related to biliary obstruction, are discussed.
- When a percutaneous approach versus endoscopic or surgical intervention is indicated is reviewed.

INTRODUCTION

Biliary obstruction can result from benign or malignant etiologies. As a result of biliary obstruction, patients may present with jaundice, pruritus, or with cholangitis if there has been prior biliary intervention. The indications for intervention and ultimate management of benign and malignant biliary obstruction are different, and it is important for the patient, caregiver, and operator to have a clear and common understanding of the goals of intervention.

Commonly performed percutaneous biliary interventions include cholangiography, external or internal/external biliary drainage, stent placement, biliary stone retrieval and bile duct biopsy. Well-accepted indications for percutaneous biliary intervention include diagnosis and decompression of a stricture, access to remove bile duct stones, diversion of bile in the setting of a bile leak, to lower the bilirubin to allow for chemotherapy, and to treat pruritus or cholangitis. A general list of possible procedures and their indications is provided in **Table 1**.

Disclosure: A.M. Covey is a shareholder of Amgen and a consultant at Accurate Medical. A.R. Deipolyi and R. Perez-Johnston have nothing to disclose.
[a] Memorial Sloan Kettering Cancer Center, 1275 York Avenue, H-118, New York, NY 10065, USA; [b] Memorial Sloan Kettering Cancer Center, Weill Cornell Medical Center, 1275 York Avenue, H-118, New York, NY 10065, USA
* Corresponding author.
E-mail address: coveya@mskcc.org

Gastroenterol Clin N Am 47 (2018) 621–641
https://doi.org/10.1016/j.gtc.2018.04.008
0889-8553/18/© 2018 Elsevier Inc. All rights reserved.

gastro.theclinics.com

Table 1
Percutaneous biliary interventions

Procedure	Indication	Relative Contraindications
PTC	Anatomic characterization	Coagulopathy Allergy to iodinated contrast Ascites
PTBD	Cholangitis Pruritus Symptoms related to jaundice (anorexia, nausea) Decrease serum bilirubin for chemotherapy Preoperative optimization Bile leak	Same as PTC Multiple segmental or subsegmental isolations (in which case drainage is unlikely to provide palliation except of pruritus)
Percutaneous balloon dilatation	Definitive treatment of benign strictures	Same as PTBD Sepsis, cholangitis
Percutaneous metallic stent placement	Definitive treatment of benign or malignant strictures Exclude bile leak	Same as PTBD Sepsis, cholangitis Surgical candidate
Percutaneous transcatheter brush biopsy	Diagnose cause of biliary stricture	Sepsis, cholangitis Coagulopathy

Abbreviations: PC, percutaneous cholangiography; PTDB, percutaneous biliary drainage.

TECHNICAL CONSIDERATIONS
Preprocedural Planning

Before any biliary intervention, a detailed clinical history of prior biliary intervention and recent high-quality cross-sectional computed tomography (CT) scan or magnetic resonance imaging (MRI) should be reviewed. Careful review of imaging helps to define the bile duct anatomy, evaluate for parenchymal atrophy and portal vein patency, and for the presence of ascites. With good quality imaging, the presence of segmental or lobar isolation of bile ducts can often be predicted. By following the bile ducts in an orderly fashion, segment by segment, from the periphery to the hilus, a mental 3-dimensional model of the biliary tree can be constructed to plan intervention. This information is critical, not only for procedure planning, but to adequately inform the patient and referring team about the likelihood of success and realistic outcomes, including the possibility of having an external catheter versus an internal stent.

Preprocedure cross-sectional imaging can sometimes also define the nature of the obstruction. Magnetic resonance cholangiopancreatography (MRCP) has a diagnostic accuracy of more than 90%, with benign strictures showing regular, symmetric, and short segment narrowing; malignant strictures, in contrast, tend to be irregular, asymmetric, and long segment.[1] When distinction between benign and malignant cannot be made on cross-sectional imaging, a biopsy may be warranted.

The level of obstruction can be defined as high or low. Low bile duct obstruction involves the common bile duct, below the insertion of the cystic duct. Typically, low bile duct obstruction is best managed endoscopically because the placement of a single (plastic or metal) stent can effectively drain the entire biliary tree. If an endoscopic approach is not possible, for example, because of prior surgery, or not successful, a percutaneous approach can be considered.

High bile duct obstruction occurs at or above the common hepatic duct. The Bismuth-Corlette classification describes types of high bile duct obstruction from cholangiocarcinoma (**Fig. 1**). Obstruction is considered complete when isolated ducts are not opacified on cholangiography (**Fig. 2**). Effective isolation is when isolated ducts are opacified with contrast during cholangiography, but do not drain effectively (**Fig. 3**). Impending isolation occurs when bile ducts are opacified and drain but are compromised by duct narrowing likely to occlude in the near future (**Fig. 4**). Because of potential contamination of these ducts during cholangiography, impending and effectively isolated ducts are prone to developing cholangitis.

A percutaneous approach is preferred in high bile duct obstruction for several reasons. First, unlike endoscopy, a specific duct can be targeted to maximize biliary drainage. In addition, for high obstruction percutaneous access and definitive treatment (ie, stent) can be accomplished without disrupting the ampulla, thereby preserving the function of the sphincter and sterility of the biliary tree. This approach minimizes the introduction of enteric flora into the biliary tree, decreasing the risk of subsequent cholangitis.

Cholangitis is largely an iatrogenic disease, the result of contamination of the biliary tree from prior endoscopic, percutaneous, or operative procedures. When the indication for intervention is cholangitis, close attention to prior intervention and imaging is important to identify the segments of the liver that were previously contaminated. Based on that information, an informed decision can be made about what portion of the biliary tree is most likely to be infected and, therefore, to require drainage.

The combination of biliary obstruction and portal vein occlusion ultimately results in atrophy of the affected liver segments.[2] This has the appearance of crowded, dilated bile ducts with little intervening hepatic parenchyma (**Fig. 5**). Drainage of atrophic segments should be avoided unless there is refractory cholangitis, because it is unlikely to provide benefit in terms of recovering liver function.

Ascites is common in multiple disease states. Large ascites can displace the liver from the abdominal wall, increasing the technical difficulty of percutaneous intervention. In addition, patients are likely to have pericatheter leakage of ascites causing skin breakdown and psychological distress. Preprocedural paracentesis is an effective but temporary solution. Because ascites is predominantly dependent in the abdomen, a left-sided approach (anterior epigastric) can decrease the risk and volume of pericatheter leakage in the setting of ascites.

Antibiotics

Biliary intervention is at best a clean contaminated procedure according to the National Academy of Sciences.[3] Therefore, the Society of Interventional Radiology

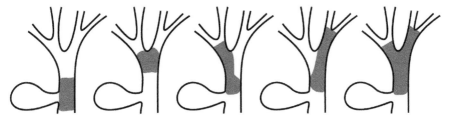

Fig. 1. Bismuth classification of hilar obstruction. Type I involves only the common bile duct, below the level of the confluence of the right and left ducts. Type II involves the confluence of right and left hepatic ducts. Type IIIa extends into the bifurcation or the right hepatic duct. Type IIIb extends to the bifurcation of the left hepatic duct. Type IV extends to the bifurcation of both the right and left hepatic ducts or multifocal involvement.

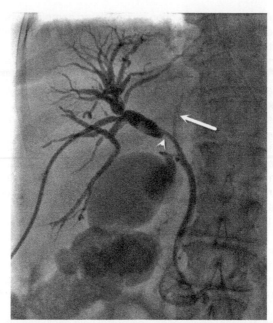

Fig. 2. Complete isolation. Catheter cholangiogram in a 79-year-old woman with cholangio-carcinoma opacifies only right bile ducts owing to an obstructing hilar mass (*arrowhead*). No contrast enters the left biliary ducts, previously drained by an endoscopic plastic stent placed (*arrow*).

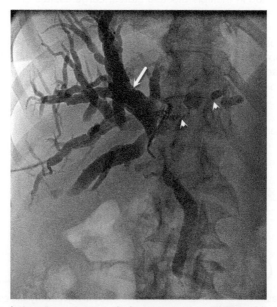

Fig. 3. Effective isolation. Percutaneous cholangiogram in a 73-year-old woman with meta-static appendiceal carcinoid tumor demonstrates a hilar mass which isolates the right biliary ducts (*arrow*) from the left biliary ducts (*arrowheads*). Some left biliary ducts fill with contrast but do not empty.

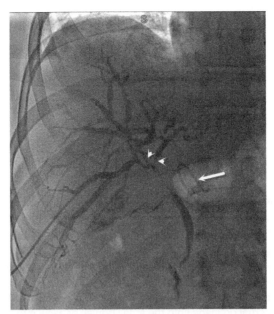

Fig. 4. Impending isolation. Percutaneous cholangiogram in a 50-year-old man with metastatic colon cancer demonstrates narrowing of the central right and left hepatic ducts (*arrowheads*); contrast filled the left-sided ducts and emptied. A hepatic artery infusion pump catheter (*arrow*) is noted.

guidelines recommend prophylactic antibiotics in all patients undergoing percutaneous transhepatic biliary drainage.[4] There is no consensus in the first-choice agent, but frequent pathogens include *Enterococcus*, *Escherichia coli*, and *Klebsiella*; thus, a beta-lactam such as ampicillin/sulbactam or piperacillin/tazobactam or a third-generation cephalosporin such as ceftriaxone are commonly used.

Access

Under fluoroscopic or ultrasound guidance, a 21-G styleted needle is used to access a peripheral bile duct. A 0.018-inch guidewire is then advanced through the needle into

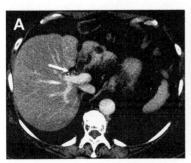
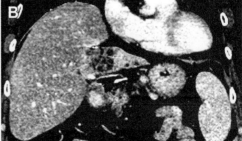

Fig. 5. Hepatic atrophy owing to malignant biliary and portal venous obstruction. (*A*) Axial image from a contrast-enhanced computed tomography scan in a 72-year-old man with hilar cholangiocarcinoma demonstrates left biliary dilation and portal vein occlusion owing to a hilar tumor (*arrow*). (*B*) Coronal image demonstrates resultant atrophy of the left hemiliver, with compensatory hypertrophy of the right hemiliver.

the biliary tree and the needle exchanged for a coaxial set (eg, Neff introducer, Cook Medical, Bloomington, IN) that is advanced into the biliary tree. With secure access, diagnostic cholangiography can be performed. In the setting of cholangitis, the volume of contrast injected for cholangiography should be limited to decrease the risk of bacterial translocation into the bloodstream.

Drainage Catheters

The external biliary drain (EBD) is a catheter that terminates in the bile duct and drains bile externally into a bag. Therefore, in most situations, it cannot be capped. It is also less stable and more prone to dislodgement than an internal/EBD (IEBD). EBDs are typically placed in 3 clinical settings:

1. The obstruction cannot be crossed at the time of drainage;
2. The patient has cholangitis and an EBD requires less manipulation than IEBD; or
3. The biliary obstruction has been relieved (eg, stent, treatment of lymphoma, surgical bypass) and a catheter is in place for a trial of physiologic internal drainage.

An IEBD is a catheter with multiple side holes above and below the obstruction to allow for both internal and external drainage, and a locking loop positioned in the bowel or distal to the obstruction without crossing the ampulla (**Fig. 6**). Side holes placed both above and below the obstruction allow for the exteriorized portion of the catheter to be capped to force internal drainage (into the small bowel) or allow it to be connected to a drainage bag for external drainage. The advantages of the IEBD are improved catheter stability compared with EBD owing to its length, and the versatility of drainage options (internal or external) allowing the option of forcing internal drainage, simulating normal physiology. One disadvantage of external drainage is that substantial fluid loss can occur, leading to hypovolemia and electrolyte imbalance. Scenarios in which IEBD and EBD may be used are summarized in **Table 2**.

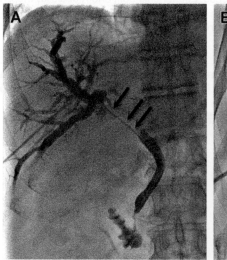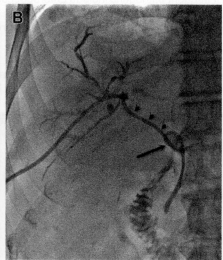

Fig. 6. Functional internal–external biliary drain. (*A*) Catheter cholangiogram in a 79-year-old man with extrahepatic cholangiocarcinoma demonstrates occlusion of the common bile duct (*arrows*). (*B*) A functional internal–external drainage catheter is in place with side holes above and below the occlusion (*arrowheads*), and the locking pigtail (*arrow*) positioned above the ampulla to prevent biliary contamination with bowel flora.

Table 2 Indications for biliary drainage	
Internal-External Biliary Drainage	**External Biliary Drainage**
• Initial drainage of obstructed bile ducts when diagnosis is unknown • Preoperative drainage • Before internalization, to decrease bilirubin to certain endpoint • Duodenal disease (likely to preclude adequate stent function) • Occluded metallic stent • Access for brachydynamic or photodynamic therapy	• Biliary obstruction cannot be crossed • Need to drain 2 separately isolated portions of liver using a single catheter • Septic patients (minimize manipulation) • Preserve access after stent placement "safety" catheter

Metallic Stents

In general, metallic biliary stents are indicated for patients with active malignancy and limited life expectancy, or for patients with no other good option. Stents may be bare or covered. In the setting of malignancy, bare stents with narrow interstices (eg, Wallstent, Boston Scientific, Marlborough, MA) are typically used because they limit tumor ingrowth, minimize stent migration, and minimize obstruction of the cystic, pancreatic, or other bile ducts. When stents are indicated for the treatment of benign strictures, covered metallic stents may be preferred because, unlike bare metal stents, covered stents can be removed or exchanged.[5]

Percutaneous biliary stenting can be performed as a primary biliary stent (PS) or as staged percutaneous biliary stent (SS). In the 1-stage procedure, the stent is placed across the obstructed duct in a single procedure. After PS, access tract embolization with Gelfoam pledgets is routinely performed in our institution to avoid postprocedure bile leak. In the staged procedure, the first step is percutaneous external or internal–external biliary drainage, followed by conversion to a stent in a second procedure, typically several weeks later.

During PS or SS stent deployment, if there is inadequate flow through the stent or into the bowel, a "safety" catheter can be left in place for a few days to preserve access. The catheter can be capped to test stent function. Abdominal pain, fever, or leakage around the capped catheter indicates that there is inadequate flow through the stent and the catheter can be uncapped to allow external drainage. The catheter can also be used for subsequent contrast study to demonstrate possible causes of stent failure, including inadequate stent expansion, papillary dysfunction, or inadequate bowel peristalsis. In our experience, approximately 75% of the safety catheters are removed within 24 hours.[6]

PS should be considered for nonsurgical candidates, patients with ascites who might otherwise suffer from pericatheter leakage of peritoneal fluid, and in patients with high bile duct obstruction when biliary access accomplishes drainage of the intended volume of liver. Compared with PS, SS has a higher rate of major complications, including hemobilia, cholangitis, and sepsis,[7] suggesting that PS may be safer, although differences may be due to selection bias. PS and SS do not differ in stent patency and patient survival.[8] The mean stent patency for malignant obstruction is 8.5 months. In our experience, with well-selected patients, PS improves overall quality of life and affords more than 90% of patients catheter-free survival.[6,9]

There is controversy as to what volume of liver needs to be drained in malignant obstruction. In patients with type IV bismuth strictures, superior patency rates, clinical outcomes, and survival have been reported when drainages are performed bilaterally.[10,11] Two stent configurations have been described for bilateral stenting: "T" and "Y." Y refers to the placement of side-by-side right and left stents (**Fig. 7**) that are parallel below the hepatic confluence. In a "T" configuration, 2 stents are placed from a single access, one side-to-side (eg, right-to-left) and the second stent is placed "down" into the common duct or across the ampulla.[12] Patients who present with occluded stents may require additional drainage. This may be accomplished with a drainage catheter or additional stent placement. In some cases, a new stent may be placed through the interstices of an occluded stent (**Fig. 8**).

Complications

Major complications of biliary drainage include sepsis, hemorrhage, pleural transgression, and death. Complications rates range from 3% to 10% and procedural mortality

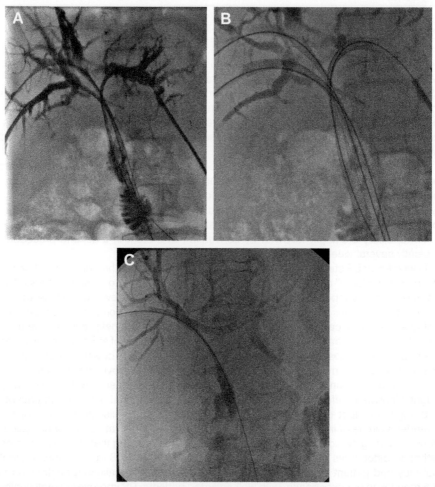

Fig. 7. Y and T biliary stent configuration. (*A*) Sheath cholangiogram during metallic stent deployment in a 54-year-old woman with intrahepatic cholangiocarcinoma demonstrates hilar obstruction with isolation of the anterior and posterior right and left bile ducts. (*B*) Final image demonstrates bilateral stents in a Y configuration. (*C*) Stents in a T configuration are positioned from right-to-left and right common bile duct providing bilateral drainage from a single access.

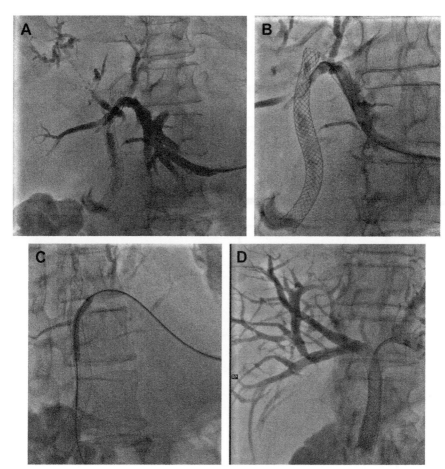

Fig. 8. Stent-in-stent placement. (*A*) Initial sheath cholangiogram in a 66-year-old man with metastatic rectal cancer demonstrates left biliary ductal dilation with effective isolation from the right biliary ducts, which were previously stented. (*B*) A wire and catheter are manipulated through the interstices of the preexisting stent into the stent and into the bowel. (*C*) A noncompliant balloon is used to dilate open the interstices. (*D*) A second stent is deployed such that the ends terminate in the left bile duct and the preexisting stent.

ranges from 0.1% to 0.8%. The most frequent major complications are sepsis and hemorrhage, with an incidence of 2.5%.[13]

Although all patients undergoing biliary intervention receive prophylactic antibiotics, transient bacteremia has been reported in 1.8%.[14] If the patient develops chills, fever, tachycardia, or hypotension, immediate management with intravenous fluids and antibiotics is warranted. If the infection does not respond to these measures, additional drainage may be required to address incompletely drained or isolated ducts.[15]

Hemobilia is common immediately after the procedure and usually clears within 24 hours. Persistent hemobilia may be due to a side hole positioned in a portal or hepatic vein branch. This complication can be diagnosed by a contrast catheter study and treated by repositioning and/or upsizing the catheter to provide tamponade. Pericatheter bleeding with or without hemobilia in our experience is most likely due to a hepatic artery injury. At angiography, the injury is usually near where the catheter crosses an arterial branch. Findings include pseudoaneurysm, arteriobiliary fistula, or most subtly, a narrow vessel in spasm, all of which are treated with coil embolization.

CLINICAL INDICATIONS FOR BILIARY INTERVENTIONS
Malignant Biliary Tract Obstruction

Malignant biliary obstruction occurs when a neoplasm within or adjacent to a bile duct blocks the flow of bile from the liver into the small bowel. The most frequent causes of malignant bile duct obstruction are cholangiocarcinoma, gallbladder cancer, pancreatic cancer, and metastatic disease. Cholestasis then leads to jaundice, hyperbilirubinemia, pruritus, choluria and acholic stool, resulting in significant morbidity and mortality, and negatively impacting quality of life[16] (**Fig. 9**).

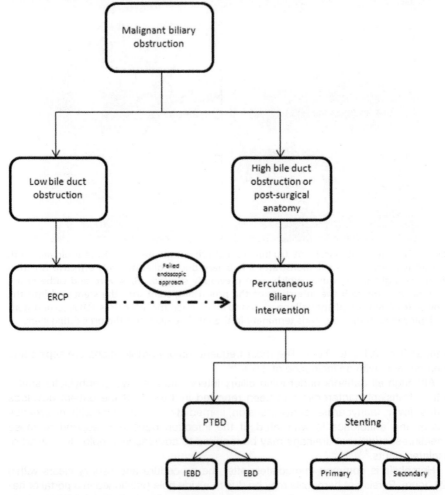

Fig. 9. Management algorithm for malignant biliary obstruction. EBD, external biliary drain; ERCP, endoscopic retrograde cholangiopancreatography; IEBD, internal/external biliary drain.

Preoperative drainage

The role of biliary drainage in patients without cholangitis who are candidates for curative surgical resection has been a controversial topic over the last 3 decades. Some surgeons believe that preoperative drainage improves liver function, decreases inflammation, and results in fewer postoperative complications and improved outcomes.[17] In contrast, a prospective randomized trial of 75 patients with a serum bilirubin of greater than 10 mg/dL showed no difference in 30-day mortality between patients who underwent preoperative percutaneous biliary drainage (PTBD) and those who did not (8.1% vs 5.3%, respectively), although patients drained preoperatively had a significantly longer postoperative duration of hospital stay.[18] A Cochrane Group systematic review of all randomized clinical trials on preoperative biliary drainage in 2012 concluded that there was a higher rate of serious adverse events in patients preoperatively drained, such that drainage should only be considered in the context of a clinical trial to generate more data.[19] When preoperative drainage is performed, a 2017 metaanalysis demonstrated a lower rate of procedural-related morbidity after PTBD compared with endoscopic drainage.[20]

In addition to the usual risks of bleeding and infection, there is a risk of tumor seeding along the course of the biliary catheter, reported in as many as 3.8% of patients with PBD tract after R0 resection[21] (**Fig. 10**).

Inoperable malignancy

In patients with unresectable malignancy, palliative options include surgical bypass, percutaneous external drainage/stenting, or endoscopic stenting. Surgical bypass is the most durable among the 3 options and early reports demonstrated improved survival in the palliative surgical bypass group compared with PTBD.[22] However, surgical morbidity and mortality are relatively high and many of these patients are near the end of life, so a less invasive/shorter hospital stay procedure is often preferable.

In Bismuth I and II, endoscopic drainage is preferred given its less invasive nature. For patients with high bile duct obstruction (Bismuth III and IV) there is consensus that PTBD is preferred,[23–25] to reduce the risk of cholangitis. In this clinical scenario, PTBD has a higher rate of success compared with endoscopic drainage, with a lower risk of cholangitis, and no significant difference in pancreatitis, overall complications, or 30-day mortality.[26]

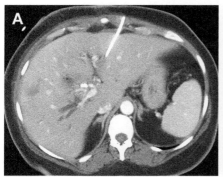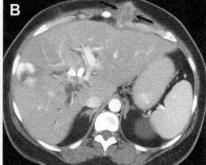

Fig. 10. Tumor seeding after percutaneous biliary intervention. (*A*) Contrast-enhanced computed tomography (CT) scanning demonstrates a left biliary catheter in a 39-year-old woman with gallbladder adenocarcinoma. (*B*) Subsequent CT demonstrates tumor along the prior biliary drain track (*arrows*), consistent with tumor seeding.

Bile duct biopsy

Benign and malignant strictures can be indistinguishable by cross-sectional imaging or cholangiography, and bile duct biopsy may be required to establish the diagnosis. There are several possible techniques, including sending bile for cytology, brush biopsy, and forceps biopsy.

Intraluminal tumors such as cholangiocarcinoma or intraductal metastases can be diagnosed by brush or forceps biopsy (**Fig. 11**). Because the sensitivity of either technique is in the 40% to 70% range, a negative biopsy does not exclude the possibility of malignancy.[27] Alternatively, when bile duct strictures are not associated with a mass lesion, percutaneous fine needle aspiration biopsy can be performed under cholangiographic guidance using a notched needle directed to the stricture (**Fig. 12**). In our experience, sensitivity is higher for percutaneous fine needle aspiration biopsy (77%) compared with brush biopsy (44%).[28] The main concern in percutaneous fluoroscopic approach is advancing the needle potentially traversing critical structures resulting in complications. However, our recent study including 34 percutaneous fine needle aspiration biopsies reported no complications, suggesting it is a safe

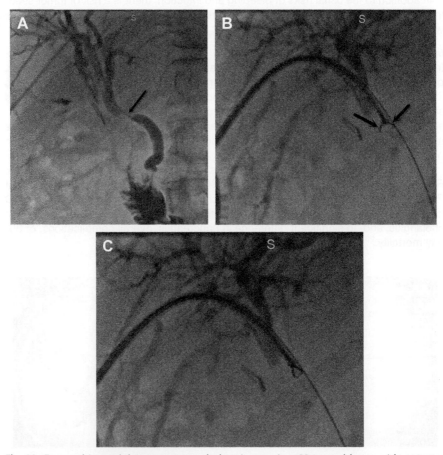

Fig. 11. Forceps biopsy. (*A*) Percutaneous cholangiogram in a 68-year-old man with metastatic gastric cancer demonstrates a focal mid-common bile duct obstruction (*arrow*). (*B*) Through the sheath, a forceps is advanced and opened (*arrows*) at the level of the obstruction. (*C*) The forceps is closed to obtain tissue.

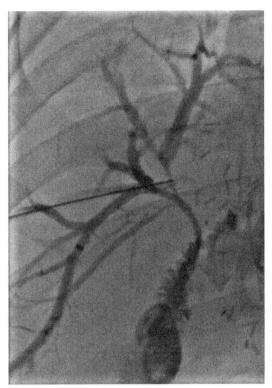

Fig. 12. Percutaneous fine needle aspiration. Catheter cholangiogram demonstrates a hilar stricture in a 68-year-old woman with cholangiocarcinoma. A 20- or 22-G needle is advanced using fluoroscopic guidance toward the obstruction.

approach, increasing the diagnostic accuracy when brush biopsy has been inconclusive.[28]

Benign Biliary Disease

Benign bile duct stricture

Most benign biliary strictures result from prior biliary tract surgery.[29] Initial management is focused on relieving the obstruction through biliary drainage. First-line treatment is endoscopic balloon dilatation and stent placement in low bile duct obstruction. High bile duct strictures and patients with bilioenteric anastomosis are usually treated percutaneously.

If the stricture involves a major bile duct, balloon dilatation is the first treatment option. Short segment strictures respond to balloon dilatation with short-term patency rates up to 90% and long-term patency rate of up to 74%.[30–32] To obtain adequate dilatation of the stricture, the balloon diameter is oversized by 15% to 20% compared with the diameter of the bile duct.[33]

Long segment, multifocal strictures and postsurgical anastomotic edema are less likely to respond to dilatation, and other management strategies should be considered.[29]

Biliary stones

Endoscopic retrograde cholangiopancreatography is the first line of management for biliary duct stones; however, it may not be feasible in patients with previous gastrointestinal surgeries (eg, Billroth II, bilioenteric anastomosis), or in patients with anatomic anomalies such as duodenal periampullary diverticulum. If the stones are in the intrahepatic ducts, or there are large impacted stones, a percutaneous approach is generally preferred.[34]

Intraductal stones that form in the setting of stasis owing to distal obstruction are usually pigment or "brown" stones and not calcified like typical gallstones.[35] Treatment of this type of stone may be accomplished by balloon maceration, retrieval by basket or choledochoscope, or sweeping of the duct after dilation of the offending stricture. Calcified cholesterol stones that form in the gallbladder may also pass into the common bile duct. Removal of these stones is more challenging because they cannot be macerated easily. Calcified stones smaller than 5 mm can be swept into the duodenum after angioplasty of a distal obstruction. Stones measuring 5 to 10 mm usually require papillotomy, which can be performed from a percutaneous approach using an angioplasty ballon.[36] Larger stones may require lithotripsy performed with a flexible ureteroscope with holmium laser fiber. By focusing the laser on the stone, plasma composed of a gaseous mixture of free electrons and ions is produced and though oscillation of these plasma bubbles, fragmentation of large stones is achieved.[34,37]

Percutaneous removal of stones has a success rate of more than 90% for common bile duct stones and approximately 60% for intrahepatolithiasis (**Fig. 13**). Clearance of large or multiple stones usually requires multiple treatment sessions.[38] The most common causes of procedure failure are impaction of stones, intrahepatic duct strictures, and inability to fragment the stones. Complications include cholangitis and subcapsular bilomas in 6.8% of patients.[39]

Primary sclerosing cholangitis

Primary sclerosing cholangitis (PSC) is a chronic progressive disease that affects both the intrahepatic and extrahepatic bile ducts.[40,41] Approximately one-half of patients

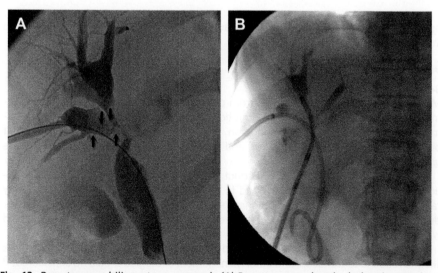

Fig. 13. Percutaneous biliary stone removal. (A) Percutaneous sheath cholangiogram in a 64-year-old woman with recurrent pyogenic cholangiohepatitis demonstrates multiple filling defects consistent with stones (arrows). (B) A choledochoscope was placed through a T-tube tract for stone removal.

with PSC develop a dominant stricture during the course of the disease. Dominant strictures could represent cholangiocarcinoma or the sequela of ascending cholangitis and stone disease, and establishing the diagnosis of a dominant stricture is critical in management.[40] MRCP has largely replaced conventional cholangiography in detecting dominant strictures. Patients who require intervention for treatment are usually treated endoscopically, with percutaneous approaches reserved for patients with failed endoscopic intervention (**Fig. 14**).

Chemotherapy-induced biliary sclerosis

Patients with liver metastasis from colorectal and other cancers may be treated with hepatic arterial infusion pump chemotherapy. Over the course of treatment, some patients develop jaundice owing to chemotherapy-induced biliary sclerosis.[42,43] This entity is diagnosed after exclusion of tumor as a cause of obstruction. With current treatment regimens, the incidence of chemotherapy-induced biliary sclerosis in patients with hepatic arterial infusion pump chemotherapy is less than 5%.[44]

It is unclear whether biliary sclerosis results from direct toxicity to the bile ducts themselves or ischemia from hepatic arteriolar injury. The common bile duct is usually spared, perhaps owing to its separate blood supply from branches of the gastroduodenal artery.[45] On cholangiography, flamelike segmental narrowing or obstruction of the common hepatic duct near, and often involving the confluence of the right and left hepatic ducts is seen[46] (**Fig. 15**). The presence of fat stranding in the hepatoduodenal ligament, enhancing thickening of the bile duct wall, narrow stenosis, and periductal edema support the diagnosis.[43]

Once biliary sclerosis has developed, therapeutic approaches are limited to reducing intraarterial chemotherapy, and/or endoscopic or PTBD.[47] When adequately treated with stenting or dilatation, chemotherapy-induced biliary sclerosis does not negatively impact survival.[44] Balloon dilation alone may be effective, but often patients require placement of biliary drains or, in the setting of active malignancy, stent placement.[45]

Posttransplant biliary complications

Biliary complications occur in 22% to 33% of patients after liver transplantation, the most common being strictures and leaks. Biliary strictures occur in 15% to 18% and are classified as anastomotic or nonanastomotic.[48,49]

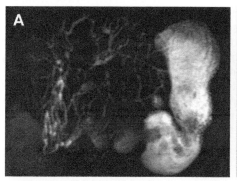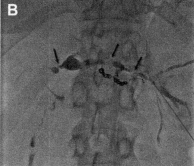

Fig. 14. Primary sclerosing cholangitis (PSC). (*A*) Coronal image from a T2-weighted MR cholangiogram in a 58-year-old woman with colon cancer and PSC demonstrates multifocal alternating intrahepatic strictures and dilations consistent with PSC. (*B*) These multifocal strictures (*arrows*) are clearly demonstrated on percutaneous cholangiogram.

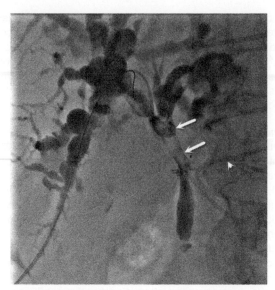

Fig. 15. Chemotherapy-induced biliary sclerosis. Catheter cholangiogram in a 76-year-old woman with intrahepatic cholangiocarcinoma and a hepatic arterial infusion pump (*arrowhead*) demonstrates a high bile duct obstruction with a flamelike appearance of the hilar filling defect (*arrows*). There is impending isolation of the left from right and the anterior from posterior right bile ducts.

Anastomotic strictures may be due to tension at the surgical anastomosis, ischemia or size mismatch between the donor and recipient. Nonanastomotic strictures are usually multifocal and are associated with compromised hepatic artery flow (stenosis or thrombosis), cold ischemia before transplantation, infection, rejection, or recurrent PSC.[50]

MRCP is used for diagnosis because of the high sensitivity of 96% and specificity of 94% compared with ultrasound examination, which has a reported sensitivity of 71%.[51] Management options include balloon dilatation and stent placement. Percutaneous management is generally performed when endoscopic retrograde cholangiopancreatography is not feasible, most commonly because of a Roux-en-Y enteric anastomosis. In patients who have undergone bilioplasty and/or stent, the overall primary patency rates at 1 and 3 years were 94% and 45%, respectively, and better results were found in nonischemic compared with ischemic strictures. The primary patency of stents at 1 and 2 years was 100% and 71%, respectively. Thus, the percutaneous approach is highly effective in treating posttransplant biliary strictures, with better outcomes for nonischemic etiologies.[52]

In treating posttransplant biliary obstruction, it is important to know what type of anastomosis was performed. For instance, patients with native biliary tract disease such as PSC or severe donor–recipient mismatch may require a Roux-en-Y choledochojejunostomy instead of a duct-to-duct anastomosis limiting endoscopic options.[53]

Iatrogenic bile duct injuries

Bile duct injuries are an infrequent but serious complication of hepatobiliary surgery or abdominal trauma.[54] A multidisciplinary approach is needed for optimal management of these patients. Diagnostic imaging and interventional radiology play important roles in detecting, classifying, and treating these injuries.

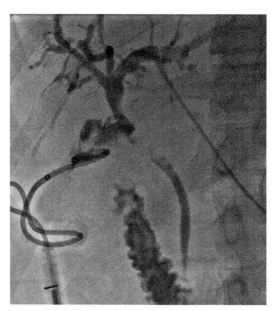

Fig. 16. Postoperative biliary leak. A 60-year-old woman underwent cholecystectomy and developed a postoperative fluid collection in the gallbladder bed. Injection of the left bile ducts demonstrates extravasation into the collection.

The most common locations for leaks is the cystic duct remnant or ducts of Luschka (accessory subvesical bile duct) in postcholecystectomy patients, the biliary anastomosis in transplant recipients, and in the surgical bed after partial hepatectomy with extended left hepatectomy and caudate lobe resection.[55] On cross-sectional imaging, biliary leaks appear as perihepatic fluid collections. Delayed contrast-enhanced MRI with a hepatobiliary contrast agent can be used to depict site of the leak.[56]

Small leaks may resolve with conservative management. Larger leaks can be treated with a combination of drainage of the biloma and biliary diversion. This procedure is often performed in a staged manner: first the collection is drained for control of symptoms or infection and once the biloma is controlled, biliary diversion is performed. Biliary drainage may be technically easier when the biloma cavity has decreased in size and contrast injection into the drain opacifies the offending bile duct. In this manner, the correct duct can be selected for drainage and drainage of the nondilated duct is facilitated because it is opacified with contrast (**Fig. 16**). In some patients with intractable leakage owing to an isolated bile duct, the culprit duct may be sclerosed either with either ethanol or cyanoacrylate.[57]

SUMMARY

PTBD is an important part of the care of patients with malignant and benign biliary disease. Careful preprocedural assessment is important to determine which patients are likely to benefit from intervention. Setting accurate expectations regarding likely outcomes and the possibility of multiple interventions is key to ensuring satisfaction.

REFERENCES

1. Suthar M, Purohit S, Bhargav V, et al. Role of MRCP in differentiation of benign and malignant causes of biliary obstruction. J Clin Diagn Res 2015; 9:TC8–12.
2. Hann LE, Getrajdman GI, Brown KT, et al. Hepatic lobar atrophy: association with ipsilateral portal vein obstruction. AJR Am J Roentgenol 1996;167(4): 1017–21.
3. Berard F, Gandon J. Postoperative wound infections: the influence of ultraviolet irradiation of the operating room and of various other factors. Ann Surg 1964; 160:1–192.
4. Burke DR, Lewis CA, Cardella JF, et al, Society of Interventional Radiology Standards of Practice Committee. Quality improvement guidelines for percutaneous transhepatic cholangiography and biliary drainage. J Vasc Interv Radiol 2003; 14:S243–6.
5. Venbrux AC, Osterman FA. Percutaneous management of benign biliary strictures. Tech Vasc Interv Radiol 2001;3:141–6.
6. Thornton RH, Frank BS, Covey AM, et al. Catheter-free survival after primary percutaneous stenting of malignant bile duct obstruction. AJR Am J Roentgenol 2011;197:W514–8.
7. Chatzis N, Pfiffner R, Glenck M, et al. Comparing percutaneous primary and secondary biliary stenting for malignant biliary obstruction: a retrospective clinical analysis. Indian J Radiol Imaging 2013;23:38–45.
8. Inal M, Aksungur E, Akgül E, et al. Percutaneous placement of metallic stents in malignant biliary obstruction: one-stage or two-stage procedure? Pre-dilate or not? Cardiovasc Intervent Radiol 2003;26:40–5.
9. Maybody M, Brown KT, Brody LA, et al. Primary patency of Wallstents in malignant bile duct obstruction: single vs. two or more non coaxial stents. Cardiovasc Intervent Radiol 2009;32:707–13.
10. Inal M, Akgül E, Aksungur E, et al. Percutaneous placement of biliary metallic stents in patients with malignant hilar obstruction: unilobar versus bilobar drainage. J Vasc Interv Radiol 2003;14:1409–16.
11. Chang WH, Kortan P, Haber GB. Outcome in patients with bifurcation tumors who undergo unilateral versus bilateral hepatic duct drainage. Gastrointest Endosc 1998;47:354–62.
12. Karnabatidis D, Spiliopoulos S, Katsakiori P, et al. Percutaneous trans-hepatic bilateral biliary stenting in Birmuth IV malignant obstruction. World J Hepatol 2013;5:114–9.
13. Weber A, Gaa J, Rosca B, et al. Complications of percutaneous transhepatic biliary drainage in patients with dilated and nondilated intrahepatic bile ducts. Eur J Radiol 2009;72:412–7.
14. Winick AB, Waybill PN, Venbrux AC. Complications of percutaneous transhepatic biliary interventions. Tech Vasc Interv Radiol 2001;4:200–6.
15. Yarmohammadi H, Covey A. Percutaneous biliary interventions and complications in malignant bile duct obstruction. Chin Clin Oncol 2016;5:68.
16. Sauvanet A, Boher JM, Paye F, et al. Severe jaundice increases early severe morbidity and decreases long-term survival after pancreaticoduodenectomy for pancreatic adenocarcinoma. J AM Coll Surg 2015;221:380–9.
17. Dennin D, Ellinson EC, Carey LC. Preoperative percutaneous transhepatic biliary decompression lower operative morbidity in patients with obstructive jaundice. Am J Surg 1981;141:61–5.

18. Pitt HA, Gomes AS, Lois JF, et al. Does preoperative percutaneous biliary drainage reduce operative risk or increase hospital cost? Ann Surg 1985;201: 545–53.

19. Fang YI, Gurusamy KS, Wang Q, et al. Pre-operative biliary drainage for obstructive jaundice. Cochrane Database Syst Rev 2012;(9):CD005444.

20. Al Mahjoub A, Menaham B, Fohlen A, et al. Preoperative biliary drainage in patients with resectable perihilar cholangiocarcinoma; is percutaneous transhepatic biliary drainage safer and more effective than endoscopic biliary drainage? A meta-analysis. J Vasc Interv Radiol 2017;28:576–82.

21. Kim KM, Park JW, Lee JK, et al. A comparison of perioperative biliary drainage methods for perihilar cholangiocarcinoma: endoscopic versus percutaneous transhepatic biliary drainage. Gut liver 2015;9:791–9.

22. Wongkonkitsin N, Phugkhem A, Jenwitheesuk K, et al. Palliative surgical bypass versus percutaneous transhepatic biliary drainage on unresectable hilar cholangiocarcinoma. J Med Assoc Thai 2006;89:1890–5.

23. Mansour JC, Aloia TA, Crane CH, et al. Hilar cholangiocarcinoma: expert consensus statement. HPB (Oxford) 2015;17:691–9.

24. Rerknimitr R, Angsuwatcharakon P, Ratanachu-ek T, et al. Asia-Pacific consensus recommendations for endoscopic and interventional management of hilar cholangiocarcinoma. J Gastroenterol Hepatol 2013;28:593–607.

25. Choi J, Ryu JK, Lee SH, et al. Biliary drainage for obstructive jaundice caused by unresectable hepatocellular carcinoma: the endoscopic versus percutaneous approach. Hepatobiliary Pancreat Dis Int 2012;11:636–42.

26. Moole H, Dharmapuri S, Duvuri A, et al. Endoscopic versus percutaneous biliary drainage in palliation of advanced malignant hilar obstruction: a meta-analysis and systematic review. Can J Gastroenterol Hepatol 2016;2016: 4726078.

27. Tapping CT, Byass OR, Cas JE. Cytologic sampling versus forceps biopsy during percutaneous transhepatic biliary drainage and analysis of factors predicting success. Cardiovasc Intervent Radiol 2012;35:883–9.

28. Gonzalez-Aguirre A, Covey AM, Erinjeri JP, et al. Comparison of biliary brush biopsy and fine needle biopsy in the diagnosis of biliary strictures. Minim Invasive Ther Allied Technol 2018;(1):1–6.

29. Fidelman N. Benign Biliary strictures: evaluation and approaches to percutaneous treatment. Tech Vasc Interv Radiol 2015;18:210–7.

30. Kocher M, Cerna M, Havlik R, et al. Percutaneous treatment of benign bile duct strictures. Eur J Radiol 2007;62:170–4.

31. Cantwell CP, Pena CS, Gervais DA, et al. Thirty years' experience with balloon dilation of benign postoperative biliary strictures: long- term outcomes. Radiology 2008;249:1050–7.

32. Janssen JJ, van Delden OM, van Lienden KP, et al. Percutaneous balloon dilatation and long-term drainage as treatment of anastomotic and non-anastomotic benign biliary strictures. Cardiovasc Intervent Radiol 2014;37: 1559–67.

33. Zajko AB, Sheng R, Zetti GM, et al. Transhepatic balloon dilation of biliary strictures in liver transplant patients: a 10-year experience. J Vasc Interv Radiol 1995;6:79–83.

34. Copelan A, Kapoor B. Choledocolitiasis diagnosis and management. Tech Vasc Interv Radiol 2015;18:244–55.

35. Carey MC. Pathogenesis of gallstones. Recent Prog Med 1992;83:379–91.

36. Stokes KR, Clouse ME. Biliary duct stones: percutaneous transhepatic removal. Cardiovasc Intervent Radiol 1990;13:240–4.
37. Rimon U, Kleinmann N, Bensaid P, et al. Percutaneous transhepatic endoscopic holmium laser lithotripsy for intrahepatic and choledochal biliary stones. Cardiovasc Intervent Radiol 2011;34:1262–6.
38. Zuckerman A, Malloy PC. Nonsurgical management of biliary stones, in society of cardiovascular and interventional radiology (ed): Biliary Interventions (SCVIR Syllabus). Philadelphia (PA): Lippincott Williams & Wilkins; 1995. p. 202–19.
39. Ozcan N, Kahriman G, Mavili E. Percutaneous transhepatic removal of bile duct stones: results of 261 patients. Cardiovasc Intervent Radiol 2012;35:621–7.
40. Chapman R, Fevery J, Kalloo A, et al. Diagnosis and management of primary sclerosing cholangitis. Hepatology 2010;51:660–78.
41. Tischendorf JJ, Hecker H, Krüger M, et al. Characterization, outcome, and prognosis in 273 patients with primary sclerosing cholangitis: a single center study. Am J Gastroenterol 2007;102:107–14.
42. Torrisi JM, Schwartz LH, Gollub MJ, et al. CT findings of chemotherapy induced toxicity: what radiologists need to know about the clinical and radiologic manifestations of chemotherapy toxicity. Radiology 2011;258(1):41–56.
43. Phongkitkarun S, Kobayashi S, Varavithya V, et al. Bile duct complications of hepatic arterial infusion chemotherapy evaluated by helical CT. Clin Radiol 2005;60: 700–9.
44. Ito K, Ito H, Kemeny NE, et al. Biliary sclerosis after hepatic arterial infusion pump chemotherapy for patients with colorectal cancer liver metastasis: incidence, clinical features, and risk factors. Ann Surg Oncol 2012;19:1609–17.
45. Sandrasegaran K, Alazmi WM, Tann M, et al. Chemotherapy-induced sclerosing cholangitis. Clin Radiol 2006;61:670–8.
46. Botet JF, Watson RC, Kemeny N, et al. Cholangitis complicating intraarterial chemotherapy in liver metastasis. Radiology 1985;156:335–7.
47. Alazmi WM, McHenry L, Watkins JL, et al. Chemotherapy-induced sclerosing cholangitis: long term response to endoscopic therapy. J Clin Gastroenterol 2006;40:353–7.
48. Lladó L, Fabregat J, Baliellas C, et al. Surgical treatment of biliary tract complications after liver transplantation. Transplant Proc 2012;44(6):1557–9.
49. Gunawansa N, McCall JL, Holden A, et al. Biliary complications following orthotopic liver transplantation: a 10-year audit. HPB (Oxford) 2011;13(6):391–9.
50. Buis CI, Verdonk RC, Van der Jagt EJ, et al. Nonanastomotic biliary strictures after liver transplantation, part 1: radiological features and risk factors for early vs. late presentation. Liver Transpl 2007;13(5):708–18.
51. Jorgensen JE, Waljee AK, Volk ML, et al. Is MRCP equivalent to ERCP for diagnosing biliary obstruction in orthotopic liver transplant recipients? A meta-analysis. Gastrointest Endosc 2011;73(5):955–62.
52. Giampalma E, Renzulli M, Mosconi C, et al. Outcome of post-liver transplant ischemic and nonischemic biliary stenoses treated with percutaneous interventions: the Bologna experience. Liver Transpl 2012;18:177–87.
53. Lladó L, Figueras J. Techniques of orthotopic liver transplantation. HPB (Oxford) 2004;6(2):69–75.
54. Flum DR, Cheadle A, Prela C, et al. Bile duct injury during cholecystectomy and survival in Medicare beneficiaries. JAMA 2003;290:2168–73.
55. Sakamoto K, Tamesa R, Yukio T, et al. Risk factors and management of bile leakage after hepatectomy. World J Surg 2016;40:182–9.

56. Camacho JC, Coursey-Moreno C, Telleria JC, et al. Non vascular post-liver transplantation complications: from US screening to cross sectional and interventional imaging. Radiographics 2015;35:87–104.
57. Carrafiello G, Lerardi AM, Piacentino F, et al. Percutaneous transhepatic embolization of biliary leakage with N-butyl cyanoacrylate. Indian J Radiol Imaging 2012;22:19–22.

Splenomegaly

A Combined Clinical and Radiologic Approach to the Differential Diagnosis

Brett P. Sjoberg, MD[a], Christine O. Menias, MD[b],
Meghan G. Lubner, MD[a], Vincent M. Mellnick, MD[c],
Perry J. Pickhardt, MD[a],*

KEYWORDS

- Spleen • Splenomegaly • CT

KEY POINTS

- Splenomegaly is commonly encountered at clinical imaging, whether due to a known condition, an incidental finding, or an undiagnosed condition leading to symptomatic evaluation.
- The differential diagnosis for splenomegaly is broad but can be grouped into discrete categories based on pathophysiology.
- The differential diagnosis for splenomegaly can be narrowed by incorporating all relevant clinical and radiologic data.

INTRODUCTION

An enlarged spleen is a common imaging finding. Splenomegaly may be an incidental imaging finding, an expected finding based on a known clinical entity, or related to the underlying cause of a patient's symptoms or clinical presentation.[1] The broad physiologic functions of the spleen make it susceptible to involvement by a variety of pathophysiologic processes. Understanding the pathophysiology of splenomegaly allows for the formation of a limited differential diagnosis. By incorporating all relevant clinical and radiologic data, the differential diagnosis may be narrowed even further. This article provides an overview of splenomegaly, including a general categorization method of splenomegaly based on the pathophysiology and associated imaging findings.

Disclosures: Dr P.J. Pickhardt is co-founder of VirtuoCTC; advisor to Check-Cap and Bracco; and shareholder in SHINE, Elucent, and Cellectar Biosciences.
[a] Department of Radiology, University of Wisconsin School of Medicine and Public Health, Madison, WI, USA; [b] Department of Radiology, Mayo Clinic Scottsdale, Scottsdale, AZ, USA; [c] Department of Radiology, Mallinckrodt Institute of Radiology, St Louis, MO, USA
* Corresponding author.
E-mail address: ppickhardt2@uwhealth.org

Gastroenterol Clin N Am 47 (2018) 643–666
https://doi.org/10.1016/j.gtc.2018.04.009
0889-8553/18/© 2018 Elsevier Inc. All rights reserved.

ANATOMY AND FUNCTION

A mesodermal derivative in the dorsal mesogastrium, the spleen migrates to the left upper quadrant during embryogenesis, where it connects to the stomach and the left kidney via the gastrosplenic and splenorenal ligaments, respectively. The celiac artery supplies the spleen via the splenic artery, which enters the spleen along with lymphatics and nerves at the splenic hilum. The splenic artery supplies end arteries that branch into small arterioles. The lack of collateral flow between the end arteries makes the spleen susceptible to infarction from branch occlusion. Small central end arterioles are surrounded by red pulp, consisting of pulp sinuses and pulp cords, and white pulp, which consists of B-cell follicles, marginal zones surrounding follicles, and T-cell lymphoid tissue surrounding the arterioles. A fraction of blood goes from the arterioles to capillaries, through the splenic veins, and out the spleen, but the larger percentage of blood enters the macrophage-lined sinuses and cords. The cords are blind-ending structures with very small openings through which red blood cells (RBCs) must traverse to re-enter the sinusoids and systemic circulation. RBCs that are damaged cannot squeeze through these slits[2] and are then destroyed and recycled. Venous drainage of the spleen is via the splenic vein, which drains into the portal vein. If the splenic vein is obstructed, collateral perigastric veins or a splenic vein to renal vein shunt can form.

The unique structure of the spleen allows for its participation in the body's adaptation to hostile circumstances. As a reticuloendothelial organ with hematopoietic capabilities, the normal physiologic roles of the spleen include erythrocyte quality control via removal of abnormal RBCs, antibody synthesis, and removal of bacteria and blood cells coated by antibodies. Additionally, the spleen is able to undergo hematopoiesis as a normal physiologic response during gestation.[2] These normal physiologic roles allow the spleen to assist in clearing bacteria and particulates from the blood, generating immune responses, and generating blood cells if the marrow is unable to meet the body's needs.

Interpreting the normal spleen size depends on the interpreter's desired position on the receiver operating characteristic curve. There is a normative distribution and wide variety of normal splenic volumes. Although volumetric assessment of the spleen is most accurate, this has generally not yet been practical. In attempting to determine a single maximum splenic length to accurately diagnose splenomegaly, Bezerra and colleagues[3] suggest that a 9.8-cm craniocaudal dimension corresponds with a volume of greater than 314.5 cm³, which has previously been suggested as the upper volume limit of the normal spleen.[4] Other studies have suggested that a maximal diameter of 13 cm or greater on imaging is abnormal.[5,6] Given the variation in gender-specific normal spleen sizes and volumes (**Fig. 1**), the authors believe that a maximal craniocaudal dimension of 13 cm is a reasonable marker of splenomegaly, with automated volumetric assessment most optimal in the (near) future.

PATHOPHYSIOLOGY

Pathologic splenomegaly can best be considered as the result of any combination of 3 general pathophysiologic mechanisms: (1) hyperplasia or hypertrophy of normal splenic components, (2) passive congestion, and (3) infiltrative diseases. Alternative categorization systems based on the type of pathologic condition affecting the spleen have also been proposed,[1] with a general classification system, including (1) hematologic, (2) infectious, (3) congestive, (4) inflammatory, (5) neoplastic, and (6) infiltrative

Normal Splenic Volume Distribution

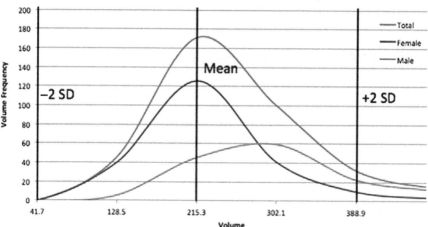

Fig. 1. Gender-specific distribution of splenic volumes in adults based on semiautomated CT measurement in approximately 40 asymptomatic healthy adults. Note the wider variation in men, with a general shift toward larger sizes.

etiologies. Although either of these can serve as general classification systems, many disease processes do not fit perfectly into 1 category, and, in many cases, the presence of splenomegaly results from a combination of pathophysiologic mechanisms.

A retrospective study by O'Reilly[7] identified the most common causes of splenomegaly in a single large university setting: (1) liver disease (33%), (2) hematologic malignancy (27%), (3) infection (23%), (4) congestion or inflammation (8%), (5) primary splenic disease (4%), and other or unknown causes (5%). This article discusses common and rare causes of splenomegaly based on a combination of the aforementioned categorical systems, with emphasis on radiologic imaging.

RETICULOENDOTHELIAL SYSTEM HYPERPLASIA

Hyperplasia of the reticuloendothelial system occurs when a disease process results in increased removal of defective erythrocytes. This leads to splenic engorgement and can occur secondary to hemoglobinopathies, such as sickle cell anemia (early), thalassemia major, spherocytosis, ovalocytosis, paroxysmal nocturnal hemoglobinemia, and pernicious anemia. These conditions result in defective blood cells that obstruct or are removed by the reticuloendothelial system of the spleen. Secondary to the resulting anemia, extramedullary hematopoiesis can also lead to splenomegaly. For example, sickle cell anemia affects the spleen via multiple mechanisms. The slow tortuous microcirculation of the spleen makes it susceptible to vascular occlusion by the abnormal sickle-shaped RBCs, leading to ischemia and infarction (**Fig. 2**). Sequestration syndrome (splenic sequestration crisis) is an acute, life-threatening complication where a large percentage of intravascular blood is sequestered in the spleen as the abnormal cells are occluded in the capillaries and venules.[8,9] Ultrasound (US) shows patency of the larger splenic veins but no flow within the spleen, consistent with obstruction at the level of smaller intrasplenic veins or within sinusoids.[10] As the sickle cell disease progresses, decreased splenic size and calcification are typical (autoinfarction).

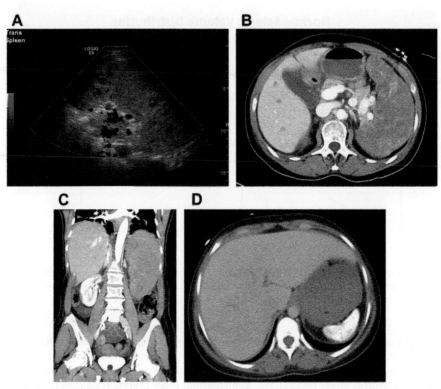

Fig. 2. Sickle cell disease: marked splenomegaly (A–C) and heterogeneity in a patient with sickle cell disease and acute splenic infarctions. Color Doppler US (A) demonstrates the absence of splenic flow, despite the patency of splenic hilar vessels as seen on CT (B). Contrast-enhanced CT (B, C) shows decreased enhancement of the spleen despite the portal venous phase. Chronic recurrent infarctions in a different patient (D) led to eventual autosplenectomy with fibrosis and dense calcification of the small remaining spleen (D), a typical appearance.

IMMUNE SYSTEM HYPERPLASIA—INFECTIOUS

Hyperplasia of the immune system during systemic infection affects spleen size because the splenic immune response includes increased antibody synthesis and clearance of bacteria and particulates from the blood. Although the spleen can enlarge secondary to a systemic response, the spleen can also be a focal site of infection via hematogenous or contiguous spread. The infectious agents affecting the spleen include viral, bacterial, fungal, and parasitic pathogens (**Box 1**). Infection is a known cause of atraumatic splenic rupture (**Fig. 3**), identified in one literature review as the second most common etiology (27% of cases).[11]

The infectious agent can often be predicted based on the clinical context. Infectious mononucleosis–induced splenomegaly should be considered in a young adult who presents with viral pharyngitis, fever, and lymphadenopathy. The most common infectious agent in this setting is Epstein-Barr virus, which infects the reticuloendothelial system via circulating B cells (see **Fig. 3**). Splenic microabscesses (**Fig. 4**) typically occur in immunocompromised patients. These are most commonly fungal infections (eg, candidiasis), an important distinction, because adequate treatment requires antifungal therapy.[12] A host of other infectious agents may affect immunocompromised or

> **Box 1**
> **Causes of infectious splenomegaly**
>
> Mononucleosis (Epstein-Barr virus most common)
>
> Fungal microabscesses (candida most common)
>
> Viral hepatitis
>
> HIV/AIDS
>
> Cytomegalovirus
>
> Malaria
>
> Toxoplasmosis
>
> Pyogenic abscess (bacterial endocarditis)
>
> Tuberculosis (and *Mycobacterium avium–intracellulare* infection)
>
> Syphilis
>
> Histoplasmosis
>
> Echinococcosis
>
> Actinomycosis
>
> Typhoid
>
> Ehrlichiosis
>
> Schistosomiasis
>
> Leishmaniasis
>
> Brucellosis

immunocompetent individuals (**Fig. 5**). Bacterial splenic abscesses are associated with endocarditis, and their appearance may be confused with infarcts on CT.[13] The most common infecting organisms in bacterial abscesses from endocarditis include streptococcus, enterococcus, and staphylococcus.[14]

Although the appearance of splenic infection is often nonspecific on imaging, including splenomegaly with or without associated focal lesions/abscesses, there may be associated imaging findings that help narrow the differential diagnosis (see **Fig. 5**).

IMMUNE SYSTEM HYPERPLASIA—INFLAMMATION AND ABNORMAL IMMUNOREGULATION

As the spleen that participates in both the innate and adaptive immune response, noninfectious splenic hyperplasia can occur in the setting of disordered immune-regulation or an overactive immune system. Examples include processes, such as autoimmune hemolytic anemia (AIHA), immune-mediated thrombocytopenia, systemic lupus erythematosus, Felty syndrome (rheumatoid arthritis) (**Fig. 6**), granulomatosis with polyangiitis (see **Fig. 6**), serum sickness, collagen vascular disease, drug reactions, sarcoidosis, thyrotoxicosis, and interleukin 2 therapy.

AIHA exemplifies the multifactorial causes of splenomegaly seen in many conditions. AIHA occurs when autoantibodies attack RBCs and cell removal or hemolysis results. IgG-coated RBCs are partially ingested by splenic and liver macrophages, and the abnormal cell remnants are removed by the reticuloendothelial system.[15] The resultant anemia can also lead to extramedullary hematopoiesis. If enough hemolysis occurs in the spleen, hypersplenism can occur (**Fig. 7**) and splenectomy may be performed for treatment.

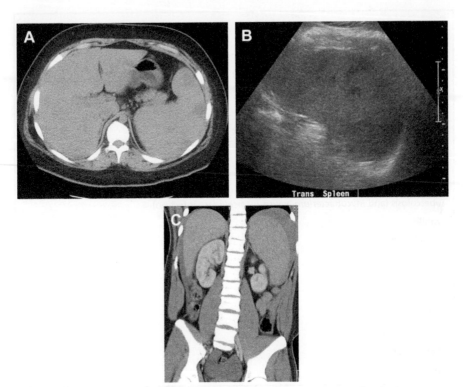

Fig. 3. Mononucleosis: 2 different patients with infectious mononucleosis demonstrate marked splenomegaly and the associated complications of infarction (*A*, *B*) and splenic rupture with hematoma (*C*). Infarcts manifest as peripheral wedge-shaped areas of hypoattenuation on CT (*A*) and hypoechogenicity on US (*B*). Infection is a common cause of atraumatic spontaneous rupture, as seen in this patient (*C*) with a perisplenic hematoma in the setting of mononucleosis.

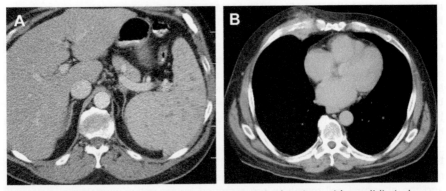

Fig. 4. Candidiasis: CT images in an immunocompromised patient with candidiasis demonstrating multiple very small hypoattenuating lesions within the enlarged spleen (*A*), consistent with fungal microabscesses. A trans-spatial abscess is also present in the right anterior chest wall (*B*).

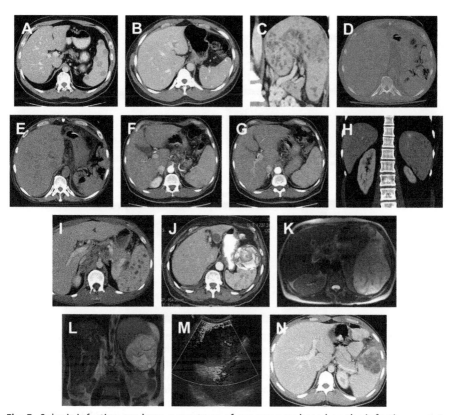

Fig. 5. Splenic infection can have a spectrum of appearances based on the infectious agent. (*A, B*) Histoplasmosis: multiple small abscesses on CT (*A*). The remote sequelae of infection include calcifications within healed granulomas (*B*). (*C*) Actinomycosis: coronal CT image shows multiple small hypoattenuating microabscesses in the setting of diffuse splenic enlargement. (*D, E*) Mucormycosis: an aggressive infection associated with diabetes and immunocompromised states,[34] disseminated mucormycosis on noncontrast CT demonstrates splenomegaly with extensive gas throughout the spleen. (*F, G*) Malaria parasite (plasmodium): splenomegaly is induced via inciting and altering the splenic immune response and by increasing the reticuloendothelial system removal of RBCs.[35] The altered architecture and circulatory occlusion can result in loss of the normal splenic arciform arterial enhancement pattern, as depicted on arterial-phase CT images in this patient with malarial infection. (*H, I*) Mycobacterial infections: contrast-enhanced CT images from 2 different immunocompromised patients show low-attenuation microabscesses related to tuberculosis (*H*) and mycobacterium avium complex (*I*). (*J–N*) Hydatid disease: produced by the larval stage of the Echinococcus tapeworm, hematogenous dissemination can result in multiorgan involvement. Splenic involvement can occur from hematogenous or intraperitoneal spread, and splenic cysts are typically solitary with imaging features similar to liver hydatid cysts.[36] Three different patients with splenic hydatid disease (*J–N*) demonstrate the common imaging features. CT (*J*) shows dense peripheral and internal calcifications, with undulating internal membranes. T2-weighted single shot fast spin echo MR images (*K, L*) in a second patient with splenic hydatid involvement show a complex cystic lesion with undulating internal membranes and small peripheral daughter cysts. Images from a third patient with splenic hydatid disease (*M, N*) show a complex cystic lesion on US with vascularity of a thick septation (*M*); CT shows a multiloculated cystic lesion in the enlarged spleen (*N*).

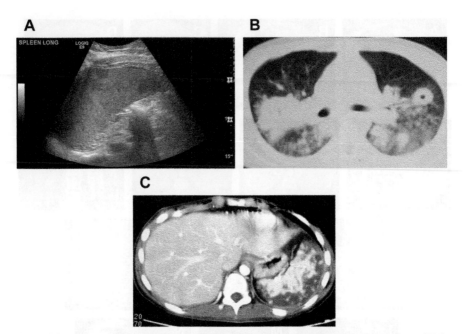

Fig. 6. (*A*) Felty syndrome: US shows splenomegaly and small infarcts in the setting of Felty syndrome, characterized by the triad of rheumatoid arthritis, splenomegaly, and neutropenia. Felty syndrome occurs in less than 1% of rheumatoid arthritis and splenectomy results in immediate improvement of the neutropenia.[37] (*B, C*) Granulomatosis with polyangiitis: cavitary lesions and confluent lung opacities (*B*) in granulomatosis with polyangiitis with marked heterogeneity and granuloma formation in the spleen (*C*).

Sarcoidosis is a systemic inflammatory disease that is hypothesized to occur due to triggering of an exaggerated cellular immune response, which results in the formation of noncaseating granulomas. Splenomegaly can occur in up to 60% of patients, and multifocal hypoattenuating splenic nodules are fairly common on CT.[16] When typical findings of sarcoidosis are present in other organ systems, or if a diagnosis of sarcoidosis is known, the focal splenic lesions (with or without splenomegaly) can be confidently attributed to sarcoidosis (**Fig. 8**).

HYPERPLASIA—EXTRAMEDULLARY HEMATOPOIESIS

Splenic hyperplasia and splenomegaly may also occur in the setting of marrow dysfunction leading to extramedullary hematopoiesis, as can be seen with myelofibrosis, marrow infiltration, and marrow toxicity. Any process insulting the bone marrow, the primary hematopoietic organ in the body, can lead to profound anemia. Extramedullary sites of hematopoietic potential can then attempt to compensate, with common sites including the spleen, liver, and lymph nodes.[17]

Myelofibrosis is a myeloproliferative process that affects erythropoietic elements of the bone marrow. Myelofibrosis occurs as primary and secondary forms, with the secondary forms occurring in the setting of polycythemia vera or essential thrombocytopenia. Deposition of reticulin and collagen fibers leads to progressive fibrosis and profound anemia and cytopenia.[18] Extramedullary hematopoiesis compensates, with the resulting splenomegaly leading to debilitating signs and symptoms, which may require palliative splenectomy[19] (**Fig. 9**).

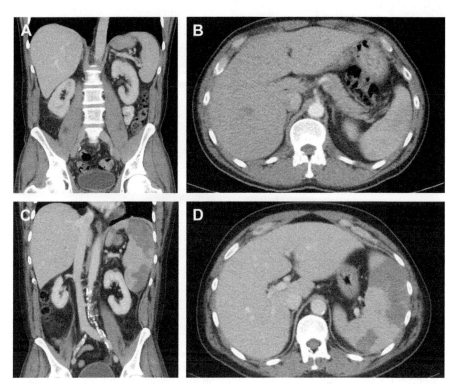

Fig. 7. Evans syndrome: sequential CT scans in a patient with Evans syndrome, which includes AIHA and immune-mediated thrombocytopenia. Initial scans (*A, B*) show a normal spleen. CT scan 3 months later (*C, D*), on onset of the acute illness, shows the rapid development of splenomegaly with multiple splenic infarcts.

PASSIVE CONGESTION

The most common cause of splenomegaly encountered by the radiologist on a daily basis is passive congestion. Any cause of decreased venous outflow from the spleen can lead to congestion and splenomegaly, including splenic vein obstruction (**Fig. 10**), but passive congestion of the spleen is most often caused by portal hypertension (**Fig. 11**). Causes include cirrhosis, congestive heart failure, portal or hepatic vein obstruction, and hepatic schistosomiasis. Portal hypertension–induced siderotic microhemorrhages, known as Gandy-Gamna bodies, can occur in the splenic follicles and manifest as hypointense foci on T2 and gradient-echo MRI sequences.

Splenic peliosis is a rare, benign entity characterized by multiple blood-filled cavities. Isolated splenic involvement is rare and usually incidental. When the liver is involved, the abnormal blood filled spaces may result from obstruction at the level of the hepatic sinusoids, sinusoidal breakdown, and/or cell necrosis.[20] The resulting cavities can resemble cysts, and their lack of a normal endothelial lining increases the risk of atraumatic splenic rupture and hemorrhage (**Fig. 12**). Associations include HIV, anabolic steroids, oral contraceptives, tuberculosis, hematological disorders, and malignancy.[21]

INFILTRATIVE—HEMATOLOGIC MALIGNANCY

As the largest lymphoid organ in the body, the spleen is susceptible to involvement by many hematologic malignancies, including lymphomas, leukemias, and other

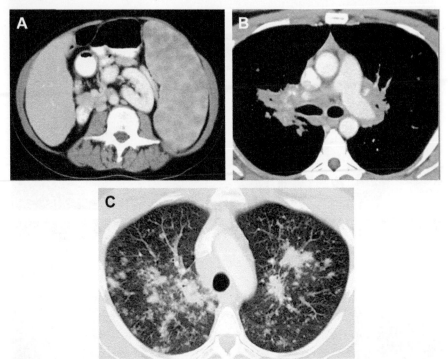

Fig. 8. Sarcoidosis: CT shows splenomegaly and multiple uniform low attenuation lesions in the spleen (*A*). Peripherally calcified lymph nodes (*B*) and confluent perilymphatic lung micronodules (*C*) are present in the chest, confirming the clinical suspicion for sarcoidosis.

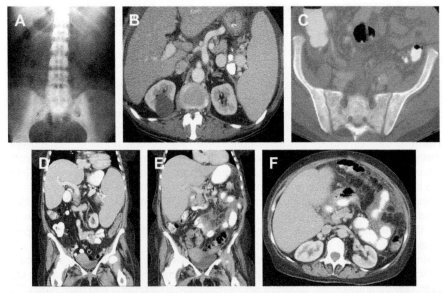

Fig. 9. Myelofibrosis: as marrow space fibrosis occurs in the setting of myelofibrosis, the axial skeleton appears densely sclerotic (*A*); note also splenomegaly. CT redemonstrates splenomegaly (*B*) and osteosclerosis (*C*). As the bones become fibrotic, extramedullary hematopoiesis occurs in the spleen, as well as the liver and lymph nodes. Palliative splenectomy is often performed (*D–F*). In this patient, the preoperative CT scan (*D*) shows marked splenomegaly. After splenectomy, new sites of extramedullary hematopoiesis developed in the liver and peritoneum (*E, F*).

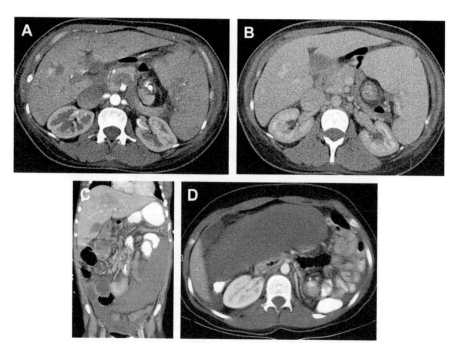

Fig. 10. Splenic torsion: obstruction of splenic outflow from torsion can result in splenomegaly. (*A, B*) In this postpartum woman with abdominal pain, contrast-enhanced CT in the arterial (*A*) and portal venous phase (*B*) demonstrates swirling and torsion of the splenic hilar vessels, resulting in splenomegaly from outlet obstruction. (*C, D*) Wandering spleen occurs when abnormal or absent splenic suspensory ligaments allows splenic migration into the abdomen or pelvis. The spleen is then susceptible to vascular pedicle torsion and infarction. CT images in 2 additional patients show malpositioning of the spleen in the left lower quadrant (*C*) and right midabdomen (*D*) with torsion of the vascular pedicles and resulting splenic infarction.

hematologic malignancies[22] (**Figs. 13–16**). Although lymphoma may involve the spleen as a primary malignancy, secondary involvement of the spleen is much more common. Non-Hodgkin lymphoma is the most common hematological malignancy to affect the spleen, with splenic involvement at presentation in 30% to 40%.[22] Hodgkin lymphoma involves the spleen in up to one-third of cases.[22] Primary lymphoma in the spleen is rare and is most commonly due to diffuse large B-cell lymphoma. Saboo and colleagues[22] describe 4 imaging patterns of the spleen in lymphoma. From most common to least frequent (see **Fig. 13**), they are (1) splenomegaly without a focal lesion, (2) infiltration by small, sub–5-mm lesions, (3) multiple focal nodules between 1 cm and 10 cm in size, and (4) large solitary mass.

Lymphoma is an example of splenomegaly whereby the etiology can be inferred based on associated imaging and clinical findings, specifically, by the presence of lymphadenopathy and abnormal hematologic studies. The absence of splenomegaly, however, does not rule out lymphomatous involvement, and the presence of splenomegaly does not necessarily confirm lymphomatous involvement. Fluorodeoxyglucose (FDG) PET/CT is useful for staging and assessing treatment response because splenic involvement shows FDG-avid nodules (see **Fig. 15**).

Leukemia can also involve the spleen, with nonspecific imaging features similar to lymphoma (see **Fig. 16**). In addition to splenomegaly, the most common imaging features include miliary nodules, which can be difficult to differentiate from

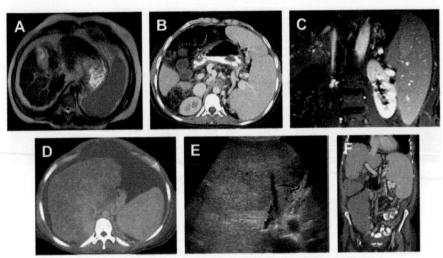

Fig. 11. Portal hypertension: chronic liver disease is the most common cause of splenomegaly. (*A*, *B*) T2-weighted MR demonstrates a nodular liver contour with marked splenomegaly (*A*). Contrast-enhanced CT of a different patient (*B*) shows multiple portosystemic varices with splenomagaly. (*C*) Splenomegaly secondary to liver involvement in α1-antitrypsin deficiency as depicted on contrast-enhanced T1-weighted MR with fat saturation. (*D*, *E*) Budd-Chiari syndrome demonstrating splenomegaly and heterogeneous liver enhancement on CT (*D*) with earlier enhancement in the caudate region. Color Doppler US (*E*) shows absence of flow in the hepatic veins. (*F*) Cystic fibrosis with fatty atrophy of the pancreas, biliary cirrhosis, and splenomegaly.

microabscesses in the setting of immunoceompromise (see **Fig. 16**A), and associated lymphadenopathy.

INFILTRATIVE—DEPOSITION/CELLULAR PROLIFERATION

Infiltration of the spleen and splenomegaly can occur via abnormal intracellular or extracellular deposition of substances or cellular proliferation, such as can be seen with amyloidosis, glycogen storage disease, Langerhans cell histiocytosis, Gaucher disease, mastocytosis, mucopolysaccharidoses, Niemann-Pick disease, tangier disease, and paraproteinemia.

Splenomegaly due to mastocytosis is difficult to classify in regard to the pathophysiology (**Fig. 17**). A disorder of mast cell proliferation, systemic mastocytosis could be considered both a cellular infiltrative process and a hematologic neoplastic process. In this condition, mast cells proliferate and infiltrate 1 or multiple organs, including the skin, gastrointestinal tract, bone marrow, spleen, and lymph nodes.[23] Symptoms occur secondary to the release of mast cell mediators, such as histamine, and mast cell infiltration of the involved organs. In the spleen, the mast cells infiltrate the paratrabecular compartments.[24]

Primary systemic amyloidosis frequently infiltrates the spleen by depositing amyloid fibrils in the red pulp or blood vessels[25] (**Fig. 18**). Splenic involvement and splenomegaly in the setting of primary systemic amyloidosis is less common than hyposplenism, with splenomegaly reported in 4% to 13% of cases.[26] Amyloidosis-induced atraumatic splenic rupture has been described, noting a possible contribution by granulocyte colony-stimulating factor treatment-induced hematopoiesis in the spleen.[26]

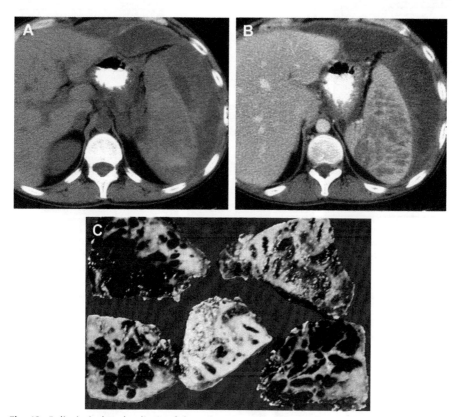

Fig. 12. Peliosis: isolated peliosis of the spleen is rare and typically incidental. The abnormal blood-filled cavities preferentially involve the parafollicular areas of the spleen, and the distorted architecture increases the risk for splenic rupture. CT images without (A) and with (B) contrast show hypoattenuating, multiloculated lesions, with a subtle hematocrit level on the noncontrast images (A). On more delayed imaging, these lesions typically enhance and become less defined. In this case, splenic rupture has occurred with a large perisplenic hematoma and hemoperitoneum. Surgical specimen (C) demonstrates the abnormal blood-filled cavities.

Gaucher disease is an autosomal recessive lysosomal storage disease in which an enzyme deficiency results in the accumulation of glucosylceramide in macrophages of the reticuloendothelial system.[27] These enlarged macrophages, termed Gaucher cells, can accumulate in multiple organs, including the bone marrow, liver, and spleen. Multifactorial splenomegaly can occur both due to extramedullary hematopoiesis/sequestration and from the accumulation of Gaucher cells. Conglomerations of Gaucher cells can also manifest as focal splenic nodules and masses (**Fig. 19**).

NEOPLASTIC—BENIGN MASSES

A majority of focal splenic lesions are benign, especially in the absence of a known malignancy. Benign neoplastic masses in the spleen include splenic cysts, hemangiomas, hamartomas, littoral cell angiomas, lymphangiomas, and sclerosing angiomatoid nodular transformation (SANT).

Cystic lesions in the spleen are rare and can be generally categorized as congenital, inflammatory, vascular, posttraumatic or neoplastic.[28] In general, the use of the term,

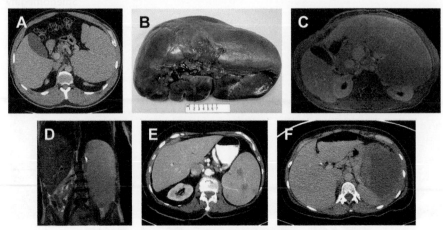

Fig. 13. Lymphoma: lymphoma in the spleen can present as 4 general imaging patterns. (*A, B*) Splenomegaly without a focal lesion. Contrast-enhanced CT shows marked splenomegaly in a patient with large cell lymphoma, with gross specimen (*B*). (*C, D*) Splenomegaly with infiltration by small, sub–5-mm lesions. T1-weighted MR with contrast (*C*) and coronal T2-weighted MR (*D*) images show multiple sub-5-mm hypoenhancing, T2 hypointense nodules in a patient with primary marginal zone lymphoma. (*E*) Splenomegaly with multiple focal nodules between 1 cm and 10 cm in size. Contrast-enhanced CT in a patient with a large cell lymphoma shows multiple hypoenhancing lesions. (*F*) Large solitary mass. Patient with diffuse large cell lymphoma with a contrast-enhanced CT showing a large heterogeneous mass in the enlarged spleen.

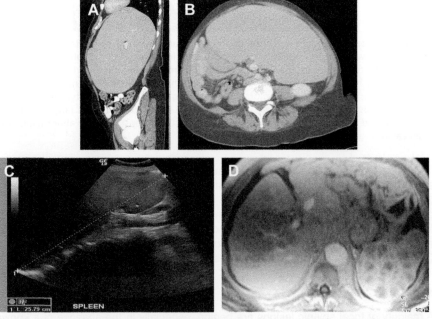

Fig. 14. Myeloproliferative and lymphoproliferative disorders (*A–C*). Polycythemia vera–induced splenomegaly might best be considered both a hyperplastic hematopoietic process and an infiltrative hematologic malignancy, because clonal cells stimulate the unregulated production of normal blood elements. Massive splenomegaly can result as depicted on CT (*A, B*) and US (*C*). (*D*) Contrast-enhanced MR shows abnormal enhancement patterns of the liver and spleen after solid organ transplantation, secondary to post-transplant lymphoproliferative disease.

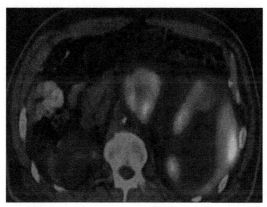

Fig. 15. Lymphoma: FDG PET-CT demonstrates marked increased FDG avidity surrounding a necrotic lesion in the spleen as well as FDG-avid retroperitoneal lymphadenopathy.

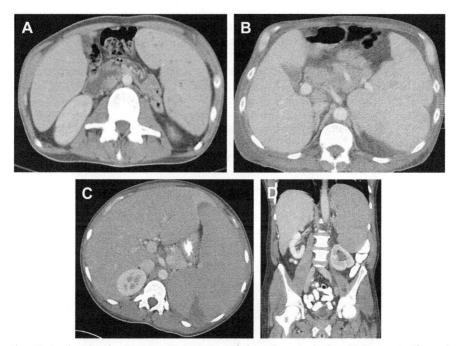

Fig. 16. Leukemia: the imaging appearance of the spleen in leukemia is nonspecific and appears similar to lymphoma. (*A*) Patient with chronic myelogenous leukemia with spleno-megaly and multiple low-attenuating miliary lesions in the spleen seen on CECT. Although unable to differentiate between leukemia or lymphoma, these lesions actually represented microabscesses from candida in the setting of neutropenic fever. (*B*) Marked splenomegaly and lymphadenopathy seen on CT in patient with chronic lymphocytic leukemia. (*C*) Compli-cations of massive splenomegaly include acute infarction, which manifests as a peripheral wedge-shaped area of hypoenhancement on CT, as seen in this patient with chronic myelog-enous leukemia. (*D*) Hairy cell leukemia is a known cause of massive splenomegaly and can present as spontaneous splenic rupture (not depicted). (*Data from* Grever M. How I treat hairy cell leukemia. Blood 2010;115(1):21–8.)

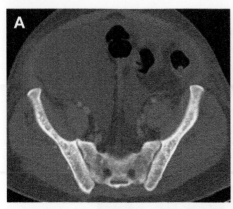
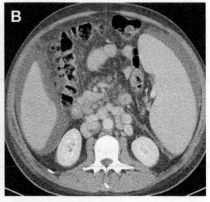

Fig. 17. Mastocytosis: mastocytosis occurs when mast cells proliferate and infiltrate the skin, liver, gastrointestinal tract, bone marrow (*A*), spleen (*B*), and lymph nodes (*B*). Marrow involvement can result in osteolysis or osteosclerosis (*A*) in the axial skeleton. (*Data from* Carter MC, Metcalfe DD, Komarow HD. Mastocytosis. Immunol Allergy Clin North Am 2014;34(1):181–96.)

splenic cyst, is used to refer to both true congenital cysts and false pseudocysts, with the distinction based on the presence or absence of a cellular lining. Benign cysts of the spleen include epidermoid cysts (true cysts), pseudocysts (false cysts), and lymphovascular cysts (**Fig. 20**).

The most common benign solid tumors in the spleen include hemangiomas and hamartomas. Hemangiomas are the most common benign neoplasm of the spleen with a reported prevalence between 0.3% and 14%.[29] Hemangiomas arise from sinusoidal epithelium and contain proliferated vascular channels. They may be small and incidental or large with resulting symptomatic splenomegaly. The imaging appearance is nonspecific and ranges from cystic to solid, with the typical hemangioma presenting as a solid mass with cystic spaces (**Fig. 21**). Calcifications may be present and avid contrast enhancement is typical. Hamartomas are typically incidental but may result in splenomegaly. A non-neoplastic malformation composed of splenic red pulp elements, hamartomas are difficult to distinguish from hemangiomas by pathology.[29] Imaging features most commonly include well-defined homogeneous and hypervascular solid masses, with isoattenuation to the spleen before and after intravenous contrast (**Fig. 22**). Overall, the imaging appearance is less typical compared with hepatic cavernous hemangiomas.

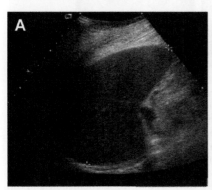
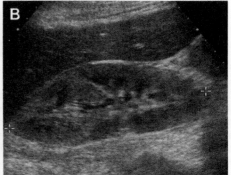

Fig. 18. Amyloidosis: US gray-scale images in systemic amyloidosis show splenomegaly (*A*) and an enlarged, echogenic kidney (*B*), secondary to the deposition of amyloid fibrils.

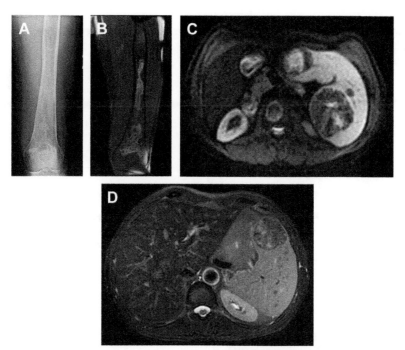

Fig. 19. Gaucher disease: Gaucher cells, glucosylceramide-engorged macrophages, deposit in the marrow (*A*, *B*) and spleen (*C*, *D*). Radiograph (*A*) and short T1 inversion recovery (STIR) MRI (*B*) of the femur show infiltration of the marrow and a serpigenous lesion consistent with bone infarct. The Gaucher cells in the spleen can accumulate into focal splenic masses, as shown on diffusion-weighted imaging (DWI) (*C*) and T2-weighted (*D*) MRI.

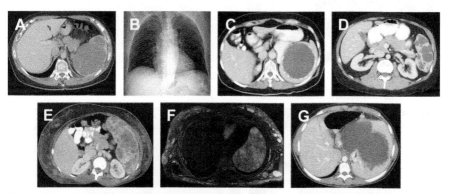

Fig. 20. Benign splenic cysts: (*A*) epidermoid squamous cysts are true cysts with a cellular lining. These may contain thin septations but otherwise appear well-circumscribed and homogeneous. (*B*, *C*) Splenic pseudocysts are false cysts that occur after trauma, likely the end result of an intrasplenic hematoma, and account for up to 80% of all splenic cysts in the West.[28] Pseudocysts often contain dystrophic calcifications within a thick fibrous wall, as seen on radiograph (*B*) and CECT (*C*). (*D–F*) Lymphovascular cysts, also known as lymphangiomas, are a lymphovascular malformation that can present as a solitary or multiple cystic lesions (*D*) or as diffuse lymphangiomatosis.[29] Proteus syndrome is a rare multifocal overgrowth syndrome which can include extensive lymphatic and vascular lesions, including splenic lymphangiomatosis, as seen on contrast-enhanced CT (*E*) and T2-weighted MR (*F*), where multiple thin-walled lymhangiomas infiltrate the spleen.[38] Note the vascular malformations in the superficial soft tissues. (*G*) Epithelial cysts are also benign true cysts, which contains an epithelial lining.

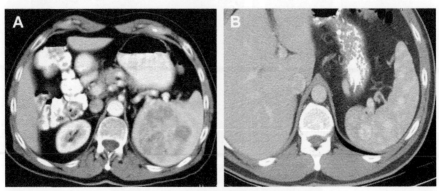

Fig. 21. Hemangiomas: as seen on CECT, hemangiomas may be solitary (*A*) or multifocal (*B*) and variably present as solid lesions with heterogeneous (*A*) or more uniform (*B*) enhancement. Splenic hemangiomas can but often do not show the same classic enhancement characteristics of hepatic hemangiomas.

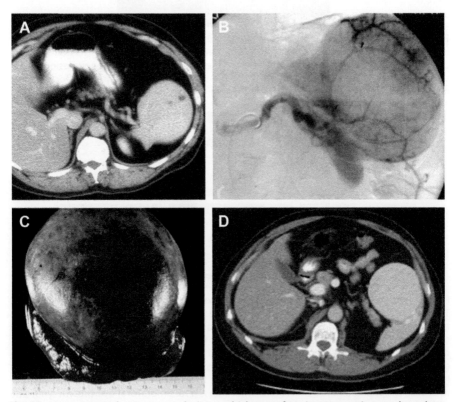

Fig. 22. Hamartomas: homogenous lesions, which are often isoattenuating to the spleen, hamartomas can result in contour deformities, as shown on CECT (*A*, *D*). Conventional angiogram (*B*) shows hypervascularity with areas of blush within the lesion. Gross specimen (*C*) demonstrates the vascular appearance of the tumor.

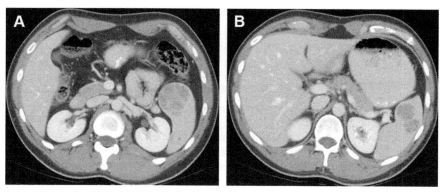

Fig. 23. Littoral cell angiomas: these vascular lesions have a nonspecific imaging appearance, with hypoattenuating, heterogeneous enhancing masses on CECT (*A*, *B*). These can become isoattenuating to the spleen on delayed phases.

Littoral cell angioma is a rare, benign vascular neoplasm of the spleen composed of multiple nodules of varying sizes.[30] CT findings include multiple hypoattenuating nodules, which become isoattenuating to the background spleen on delayed phases. This appearance is nonspecific, however, and does not allow differentiation from other splenic lesions (**Fig. 23**). MRI shows low signal intensity on both T1-weighted and T2-weighted images due to the presence of hemosiderin.[30]

Another benign vascular splenic lesion is SANT (**Fig. 24**), in which multiple vascular nodules surround a dense fibrous stroma.[31] Although benign and typically incidental, an association with malignancy has been suggested. Imaging findings include peripheral enhancing radiating lines, progressive heterogeneous enhancement in the delayed phase, and low signal on T2-weighted images due to hemosiderin deposition.[31]

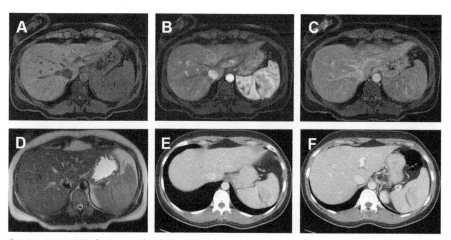

Fig. 24. SANT: MR features of SANT, as shown on precontrast (*A*), arterial phase (*B*), delayed phase (*C*), and T2-weighted (*D*) images, include peripheral enhancement and scar, with progressive enhancement on delayed phases. Typical T2 hypointensity is not seen in this case. CECT also shows peripheral enhancement with a nonenhancing scar (*E*, *F*).

NEOPLASTIC—MALIGNANT MASSES

Lymphoma is the most common malignant mass in the spleen and is discussed elsewhere. Metastatic lesions are the next most common malignancy but are overall rare, with splenic involvement ranging from 2% to 10% in large cancer populations; the prevalence increases with the presence of multiorgan metastases.[32] The most common primary lesions to metastasize to the spleen include breast, lung, ovarian, colorectal, gastric, and melanoma. The imaging features vary based on the underlying primary malignancy (**Fig. 25**).

Angiosarcoma is a rare primary splenic malignancy that is often metastatic to other organs at the time of diagnosis (**Fig. 26**). Splenomegaly is common, and imaging features include diffuse infiltration, large masses, or multiple discrete masses.[33]

MASSIVE SPLENOMEGALY

Massive splenomegaly is not precisely defined radiologically, but its specific presence suggests a more limited differential diagnosis. Clinically, massive splenomegaly is palpable more than 8 cm below the left costal margin. From an imaging perspective, massive splenomegaly is often confirmed as a gestalt. The main differential considerations include lymphoma, leukemia, sarcoidosis, diffuse splenic hemangiomatosis, AIHA, Gaucher disease, polycythemia vera, myelofibrosis, kala-azar (visceral leishmaniasis), β-thalassemia major, and AIDS with mycobacterium avium complex (**Fig. 27**).

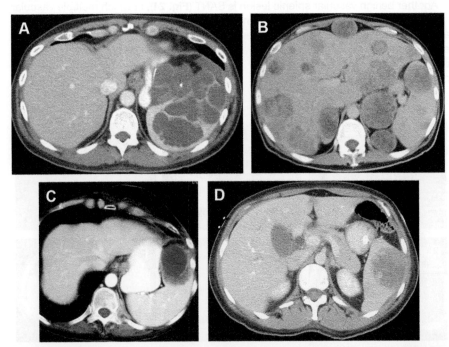

Fig. 25. Metastases: metastatic lesions to the spleen and are typically present in the setting of multi-organ metastatic disease. CT images in multiple patients show splenic metastases involving enlarged spleens, including appendiceal mucinous adenocarcinoma (*A*), breast cancer (*B*), melanoma (*C*), and choriocarcinoma (*D*).

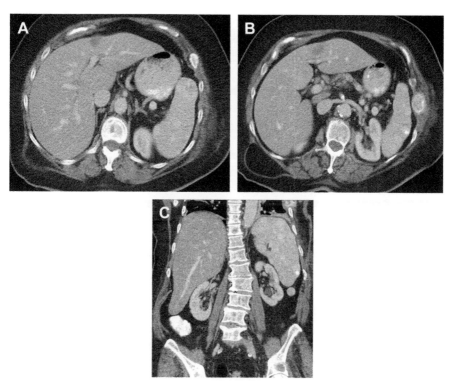

Fig. 26. Angiosarcoma: often metastatic at presentation, CT images of splenic angiosarcoma show multiple enhancing splenic lesions (*A–C*) as well as hepatic and osseous metastatic disease (*A, B*).

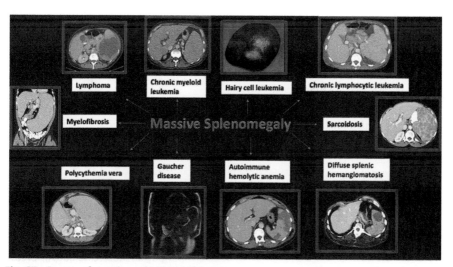

Fig. 27. Causes of massive splenomegaly.

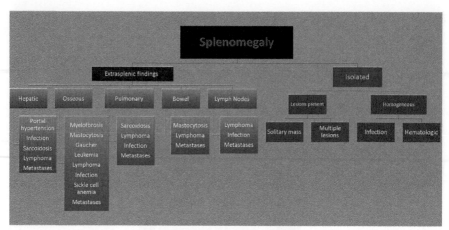

Fig. 28. Differential diagnosis of splenomegaly: the presence or absence of associated findings with splenomegaly can help limit the differential diagnosis.

SUMMARY

Splenomegaly is a common imaging finding with a spectrum of pathophysiologic mechanisms and disease associations. By incorporating clinical data and associated imaging findings (**Fig. 28**), the significance of the imaging findings can be elucidated and a more narrow differential diagnosis can help direct management.

REFERENCES

1. Pozo AL, Godfrey EM, Bowles KM. Splenomegaly: investigation, diagnosis and management. Blood Rev 2009;23(3):105–11.

2. Lymphadenopathy and Splenomegaly. In: Longo DL, Fauci AS, Kasper DL, et al, editors. Harrison's principles of internal medicine. 18th edition. vols. 59. New York: McGraw-Hill; 2014. p. 465–71.

3. Bezerra AS, D'Ippolito G, Faintuch S, et al. Determination of splenomegaly by CT: is there a place for a single measurement? AJR Am J Roentgenol 2005;184(5): 1510–3.

4. Prassopoulos P, Daskalogiannaki M, Raissaki M, et al. Determination of normal splenic volume on computed tomography in relation to age, gender and body habitus. Eur Radiol 1997;7(2):246–8.

5. Tamayo SG, Rickman LS, Mathews WC, et al. Examiner dependence on physical diagnostic tests for the detection of splenomegaly: a prospective study with multiple observers. J Gen Intern Med 1993;8(2):69–75.

6. Arkles LB, Gill GD, Molan MP. A palpable spleen is not necessarily enlarged or pathological. Med J Aust 1986;145(1):15–7.

7. O'Reilly RA. Splenomegaly in 2,505 patients at a large university medical center from 1913 to 1995. 1963 to 1995: 449 patients. West J Med 1998;169(2):88–97.

8. Lonergan GJ, Cline DB, Abbondanzo SL. Sickle cell anemia. Radiographics 2001;21(4):971–94.

9. Sheth S, Ruzal-Shapiro C, Piomelli S, et al. CT imaging of splenic sequestration in sickle cell disease. Pediatr Radiol 2000;30(12):830–3.

10. Roshkow JE, Sanders LM. Acute splenic sequestration crisis in two adults with sickle cell disease: US, CT, and MR imaging findings. Radiology 1990;177(3): 723–5.

11. Renzulli P, Hostettler A, Schoepfer AM, et al. Systematic review of atraumatic splenic rupture. Br J Surg 2009;96(10):1114–21.

12. Hatley RM, Donaldson JS, Raffensperger JG. Splenic microabscesses in the immune-compromised patient. J Pediatr Surg 1989;24(7):697–9 [discussion: 701–2].

13. Robinson SL, Saxe JM, Lucas CE, et al. Splenic abscess associated with endo-carditis. Surgery 1992;112(4):781–6 [discussion: 786–7].

14. Johnson JD, Raff MJ, Barnwell PA, et al. Splenic abscess complicating infectious endocarditis. Arch Intern Med 1983;143(5):906–12.

15. Dhaliwal G, Cornett PA, Tierney LM Jr. Hemolytic anemia. Am Fam Physician 2004;69(11):2599–606.

16. Warshauer DM, Lee JK. Imaging manifestations of abdominal sarcoidosis. AJR Am J Roentgenol 2004;182(1):15–28.

17. Yassin MA, Nashwan A, Mohamed S. Extramedullary hematopoiesis in patients with primary myelofibrosis rare and serious complications. Blood 2016;128(22).

18. Zahr AA, Salama ME, Carreau N, et al. Bone marrow fibrosis in myelofibrosis: pathogenesis, prognosis and targeted strategies. Haematologica 2016;101(6): 660–71.

19. Randhawa J, Ostojic A, Vrhovac R, et al. Splenomegaly in myelofibrosis–new options for therapy and the therapeutic potential of Janus kinase 2 inhibitors. J Hematol Oncol 2012;5:43.

20. Iannaccone R, Federle MP, Brancatelli G, et al. Peliosis hepatis: spectrum of im-aging findings. AJR Am J Roentgenol 2006;187(1):W43–52.

21. Davidson J, Tung K. Splenic peliosis: an unusual entity. Br J Radiol 2010;83(990): e126–8.

22. Saboo SS, Krajewski KM, O'Regan KN, et al. Spleen in haematological malig-nancies: spectrum of imaging findings. Br J Radiol 2012;85(1009):81–92.

23. Horny HP. Mastocytosis: an unusual clonal disorder of bone marrow-derived he-matopoietic progenitor cells. Am J Clin Pathol 2009;132(3):438–47.

24. Travis WD, Li CY. Pathology of the lymph node and spleen in systemic mast cell disease. Mod Pathol 1988;1(1):4–14.

25. Mainenti PP, D'Agostino L, Soscia E, et al. Hepatic and splenic amyloidosis: dual-phase spiral CT findings. Abdom Imaging 2003;28(5):688–90.

26. Oran B, Wright DG, Seldin DC, et al. Spontaneous rupture of the spleen in AL amyloidosis. Am J Hematol 2003;74(2):131–5.

27. Simpson WL, Hermann G, Balwani M. Imaging of Gaucher disease. World J Ra-diol 2014;6(9):657–68.

28. Urrutia M, Mergo PJ, Ros LH, et al. Cystic masses of the spleen: radiologic-pathologic correlation. Radiographics 1996;16(1):107–29.

29. Abbott RM, Levy AD, Aguilera NS, et al. From the archives of the AFIP: primary vascular neoplasms of the spleen: radiologic-pathologic correlation. Radio-graphics 2004;24(4):1137–63.

30. Bhatt S, Huang J, Dogra V. Littoral cell angioma of the spleen. AJR Am J Roent-genol 2007;188(5):1365–6.

31. Lewis RB, Lattin GE Jr, Nandedkar M, et al. Sclerosing angiomatoid nodular transformation of the spleen: CT and MRI features with pathologic correlation. AJR Am J Roentgenol 2013;200(4):W353–60.

32. Comperat E, Bardier-Dupas A, Camparo P, et al. Splenic metastases: clinicopathologic presentation, differential diagnosis, and pathogenesis. Arch Pathol Lab Med 2007;131(6):965–9.

33. Thompson WM, Levy AD, Aguilera NS, et al. Angiosarcoma of the spleen: imaging characteristics in 12 patients. Radiology 2005;235(1):106–15.

34. Sugar AM. Mucormycosis. Clin Infect Dis 1992;14(Suppl 1):S126–9.

35. Del Portillo HA, Ferrer M, Brugat T, et al. The role of the spleen in malaria. Cell Microbiol 2012;14(3):343–55.

36. Pedrosa I, Saiz A, Arrazola J, et al. Hydatid disease: radiologic and pathologic features and complications. Radiographics 2000;20(3):795–817.

37. Balint GP, Balint PV. Felty's syndrome. Best Pract Res Clin Rheumatol 2004;18(5):631–45.

38. Jamis-Dow CA, Turner J, Biesecker LG, et al. Radiologic manifestations of Proteus syndrome. Radiographics 2004;24(4):1051–68.

MRI of the Nontraumatic Acute Abdomen

Description of Findings and Multimodality Correlation

Bryan Dustin Pooler, MD[a],*, Michael D. Repplinger, MD, PhD[a,b],
Scott B. Reeder, MD, PhD[a,b,c,d,e], Perry J. Pickhardt, MD[a]

KEYWORDS

- Abdomen • Magnetic resonance • Computed tomography • Appendicitis
- Abdominal pain

KEY POINTS

- Imaging plays a critical role in evaluation of the acute abdomen; the signs and symptoms of disease processes causing acute abdomen have a high degree of overlap.
- Although computed tomography and ultrasound are first-line imaging tests for the acute abdomen, MRI offers comparable diagnostic performance for many disease entities.
- MRI may be considered for evaluation of the nontraumatic acute abdomen when other modalities are equivocal, suboptimal, or contraindicated.
- In some patient populations with certain indications, MRI may be appropriate as the first-line imaging test.

Disclosures: Dr P.J. Pickhardt is co-founder of VirtuoCTC; advisor to Check-Cap and Bracco; and shareholder in SHINE, Elucent Medical, and Cellectar Biosciences. Dr S.B. Reeder is co-founder of Calimetrix and shareholder in Elucent Medical and Cellectar Biosciences. The other authors have no disclosures.
[a] Department of Radiology, University of Wisconsin School of Medicine and Public Health, E3/311 Clinical Science Center, 600 Highland Avenue, Madison, WI 53792-3252, USA; [b] Department of Emergency Medicine, University of Wisconsin School of Medicine and Public Health, University Bay Office Building, Suite 310, 800 University Bay Drive, Madison, WI 53705, USA; [c] Department of Medical Physics, University of Wisconsin School of Medicine and Public Health, Wisconsin Institutes for Medical Research, Room 1005, 1111 Highland Avenue, Madison, WI 53705, USA; [d] Department of Medicine, University of Wisconsin School of Medicine and Public Health, Medical Foundation Centennial Building, Room 5158, 1685 Highland Avenue, Madison, WI 53705, USA; [e] Department Biomedical Engineering, University of Wisconsin School of Medicine and Public Health, Engineering Centers Building, Room 2120, 1550 Engineering Drive, Madison, WI 53706, USA
* Corresponding author.
E-mail address: bpooler@uwhealth.org

INTRODUCTION

The diagnosis of a specific etiology of nontraumatic acute abdominal pain presents a continual clinical challenge. This is particularly true for the so-called acute abdomen, referring to a severe, progressively worsening abdominal pain that often represents a true medical emergency. The abdomen and pelvis contain multiple organ systems, any of which can be home to a disease process presenting as acute abdominal pain. Chief among these is the gastrointestinal system, but the vascular system, genitourinary system, and—especially in women—the reproductive system are frequent sources of an acute abdomen presentation.[1,2]

Numerous factors contribute to the challenge of clinical diagnosis of the acute abdomen. Symptoms, including pain location, pain quality, guarding, rebound tenderness, abdominal fullness, nausea, vomiting, and diarrhea, often overlap considerably among specific disease entities, and often no specific cause for pain is ever found.[3] For example, the exact location of pain in acute appendicitis can vary based on the variable location of the appendix within the abdomen.[4] Acute diverticulitis, which is often thought of as a disease principally of the sigmoid colon (left lower quadrant pain), can occur anywhere along the large bowel.[5] Laboratory studies, including white blood cell count and other inflammatory markers such as C-reactive protein, are elevated in many different processes.[6] Furthermore, patients may have other comorbidities or may have difficulty relaying history, which complicates the overall clinical picture.

Fortunately, over the last 25 years, the role of imaging in cases of acute abdominal pain has expanded greatly; imaging tests are now routine standard of care for many suspected abdominal diagnoses.[3] This has led to far more accurate and timely diagnoses of acute abdomen presentations. For most suspected abdominal diagnoses, computed tomography (CT) of the abdomen and pelvis with or without intravenous contrast (depending on the leading differential diagnosis consideration) is widely considered to be the first-line imaging study.[7–10] Ultrasound examination is preferred for select indications, most notably evaluation of the gallbladder,[11] female pelvis,[12] and appendicitis in young children.[10]

However, there are a number of cases where CT or ultrasound examination may be contraindicated or suboptimal. Radiation exposure, although generally not problematic at the typical doses used for diagnostic CT, is always a consideration and is more of a concern in younger patients and pregnant women. In patients with an allergy to iodinated contrast agents or with poor renal function, CT may be of limited usefulness. For ultrasound imaging, anatomic considerations—including body habitus—and technical factors may limit the examination. In these patients, MRI is emerging as a viable alternative, allowing for conclusive diagnosis of a wide variety of etiologies for an acute abdomen.[13–20]

In this article, we first present a brief general discussion of imaging options for acute abdominal pain and a description of our institutional MRI protocol used to image patients with emergently presenting acute abdominal pain. We follow this with a discussion of the MRI findings of a number of common etiologies of nontraumatic acute abdominal pain, including direct correlation with CT and, where relevant, ultrasound and nuclear scintigraphy studies as well. Direct MRI–CT correlation for the illustrated cases was afforded by a prospective trial where patients underwent both examinations.[21] As we will discuss, MRI is often complimentary to other modalities in the setting of acute abdominal pain, with a number of comparative advantages and disadvantages depending on the specific pathology and organ of interest.

GENERAL MODALITY COMPARISON

CT remains the workhorse modality for evaluation of the abdomen.[22] CT relies on differences in x-ray attenuation (density) among structures for visualization. Advantages of CT include speed (images acquired in a matter of seconds), high spatial resolution (on the order of 0.5–1.0 mm),[23] excellent visualization of bone and gas-containing structures, and good tissue contrast when iodinated intravenous contrast agents are administered. Positive, or radiodense, oral contrast may be given to opacify bowel loops, improving visualization and enabling distinction of bowel from other structures (eg, fluid collections), which may be of similar density. An ionizing radiation dose occurs, although this is generally small and far outweighed by the diagnostic information obtained by the study. Disadvantages of CT include poor visualization of structures which may be similar in density (eg, seeing gallstones in a background of bile) or when structures are pressed close together with little intervening fat (eg, the organs of the female pelvis). CT scans may also be limited if intravenous contrast is not administered.

Ultrasound examination is the preferred modality for evaluation of the gallbladder[11] (transabdominal) and female pelvis[12] (transabdominal/transvaginal), which are comparative weaknesses for CT scans. Ultrasound imaging relies on reflected sound waves to produce images, and consequently depends on interfaces between different tissue types which reflect the sound beam back toward the transducer. With ultrasound imaging, there is a tradeoff between resolution and penetration: high-frequency transducers offer excellent resolution but are limited to superficial structures, whereas lower frequency transducers can image deeper structures, but with less resolution. Although generally excellent for the evaluation of soft tissues and fluid-containing structures, the ultrasound beam cannot penetrate gas-containing structures (eg, lungs, stomach, bowel, colon) or bone. Penetration of the ultrasound beam decreases with depth and, consequently, ultrasound may be limited in larger patients or for the evaluation of deeper anatomic structures. Ultrasound imaging is also susceptible to a number of artifacts,[24] and although many of these degrade the image quality, some have definite diagnostic usefulness.

MRI has both advantages and disadvantages when compared with CT and ultrasound examination. MRI does not use ionizing radiation. The MR signal relies on the excitation and relaxation of the hydrogen atoms of water and fat molecules within a strong magnetic field to produce and detect radiofrequency signal, which may be translated into images. MRI depend on the presence of water and/or fat within tissue to generate signal, and the signal varies based on the local molecular environment of that tissue. Consequently, the primary advantage of MRI when compared with CT or ultrasound imaging is superior soft tissue contrast, even in the absence of intravenous contrast, and with it the ability to use multiple contrast mechanisms to better characterize tissue. Furthermore, the safety profile of gadolinium-based contrast agents is generally considered superior to iodinated agents, without any nephrotoxicity and a much lower rate of adverse reactions. The main disadvantages of MRI include a slightly lower spatial resolution (typically on the order of 1–4 mm voxel dimensions)[23] and some susceptibility to motion, depending on the type of acquisition. Furthermore, the presence of gas or, more severely, metal, in or around a structure can lead to susceptibility-related artifacts. In routine imaging of the abdomen, evaluation of the small bowel and colon has historically been limited owing to the presence of intraluminal gas and peristaltic motion. However, motion-resistant single-shot methods are less sensitive to both gas and motion. Similar to ultrasound imaging, MRI offers excellent evaluation of the gallbladder and biliary system, and is generally considered to be the noninvasive reference standard for nonemergent imaging of the female reproductive organs.

Additionally, there are other disadvantages of MRI specific to the emergency setting, which may preclude its use as the first-line imaging test in some situations. Historically, the availability of MRI in emergency departments has been limited, particularly during evening and night hours, although this is no longer the case in some larger medical centers. Longer protocol times (typically 30–45 minutes compared with seconds for a routine abdominal CT scan) have also historically been a factor in the decision to use MRI in the emergency setting, although in recent years these protocol times have become shorter. In general, MRI examinations are more costly than CT scans—generally on the order of 20% to 40% more[25]—for a comparable examination, but this expense can vary greatly based on insurance coverage and examination type. Claustrophobia, which limits patient tolerance of the examination, has been reported in up to 30% of patients undergoing MRI,[26] although design changes in newer scanners have resulted in improvements in patient tolerance.[27] Finally, there are specific examination contraindications, including metallic implants and electronic devices (with accompanying screening process, which is more onerous than for CT scans), which may preclude imaging by MRI.

MRI PROTOCOL FOR THE EMERGENTLY PRESENTING ACUTE ABDOMINAL PAIN

The MRI protocol used at our institution[28] for patients presenting to the emergency department with acute abdominal pain is specifically tailored to efficiently acquire a comprehensive set of images of the abdomen and pelvis that is both sensitive and specific for a number of common disease entities. The protocol requires approximately 15 to 20 minutes of table time and involves the use of an intravenous gadolinium-based contrast agent (except in pregnant patients, where the administration of gadolinium-based contrast agents is contraindicated[29]). Of note, the agent currently used by our institution, gadobenate dimeglumine (MultiHance, Bracco Diagnostics, Melville, NY), has not been associated with the development of nephrogenic systemic fibrosis[30,31] and in may be safely administered in patients with relatively poor renal function where CT imaging may be suboptimal.

Specific MRI sequences acquired during the protocol include the following.

- Three plane localizer to establish imaging planes and verify coil coverage;
- Coronal and axial T2-weighted single shot fast spin echo to provide high-resolution motion resistant evaluation of normal anatomy, fluid collections and inflammatory changes;
- Axial T2-weighted single shot fast spin echo with fat suppression to characterize fat-containing lesions;

- Precontrast axial T1-weighted spoiled gradient echo with fat suppression as a basis of comparison for postcontrast images;
- Postcontrast coronal T1-weighted spoiled gradient echo with fat suppression at 90 seconds after contrast administration and postcontrast axial T1-weighted spoiled gradient echo with fat suppression at 3 minutes after contrast administration to evaluate for regions of enhancement; and
- Axial diffusion-weighted imaging with an apparent diffusion coefficient map to provide a survey of inflammatory changes in the abdomen.

This protocol allows for efficient imaging of the abdomen in at least 2 different planes, and allows the radiologist to simultaneously evaluate a number of MRI characteristics of the structures of the abdomen and pelvis, including inherent T1 and T2 signal intensity, the presence of fat, the presence of fluid collections and inflammatory changes, the presence and degree of contrast enhancement, and the presence and degree of diffusion restriction. These imaging characteristics may be used in combination to diagnose a wide range of inflammatory, infectious, and neoplastic etiologies of acute abdominal pain.

MRI FINDINGS OF SPECIFIC PATHOLOGIC ENTITIES
Gastrointestinal System

Acute appendicitis
Acute appendicitis (**Fig. 1**) represents the most common indication for emergent abdominal surgery in the United States, affecting more than 250,000 people each

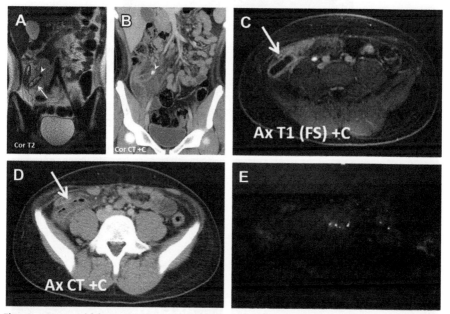

Fig. 1. 14-year-old boy with uncomplicated acute appendicitis. (*A*) Coronal T2-weighted image demonstrates appendiceal dilation and wall thickening (*arrow*). Note the presence of an appendicolith in the appendiceal tip (*arrowhead*), which appears on T2-weighted MRI as a round, intensely hypointense focus. (*B*) MRI findings are confirmed on a computed tomography (CT) scan, with the appendicolith easily seen as a round hyperdense focus (*arrowhead*). (*C, D*) Axial T1-weighted fat-suppressed postcontrast image additionally demonstrates appendiceal wall hyperenhancement (*arrow*), which is confirmed at CT. (*E*) The appendix was shown to be grossly inflamed but not perforated at laparoscopic appendectomy.

year.[32] Approximately 1 in 7 people will be diagnosed with acute appendicitis in their lifetime, with a mean age at the time of diagnosis of 22 years.[33,34] Although CT remains the imaging test of choice when acute appendicitis is suspected,[10,35] recent metaanalyses suggest that MRI has comparable diagnostic performance to CT scans.[36,37] Indeed, noncontrast MRI is commonly used as the first-line imaging study in pregnant patients with suspected acute appendicitis, with excellent diagnostic performance.[38–40] In nonpregnant patients, the use of intravenous contrast may further improve MRI performance.[21] Common imaging findings in acute appendicitis include dilation of the appendix, fluid distension of the appendix, appendiceal wall thickening, appendiceal wall hyperenhancement, and periappendiceal inflammation. The visualization of an appendicolith can be a helpful imaging finding, although this finding is more challenging with MRI. Imaging findings of perforated appendicitis (**Fig. 2**) may also include a visible defect in the appendiceal wall, extraluminal gas, or the presence of an organizing periappendiceal fluid collection.

Acute diverticulitis

Acute diverticulitis of the colon (**Fig. 3**) classically presents with left lower quadrant pain.[41] Imaging features of uncomplicated acute diverticulitis typically include inflammation associated with a colonic diverticulum and associated focal colonic wall thickening. A small focus of gas may also be present, either within the diverticulum itself or

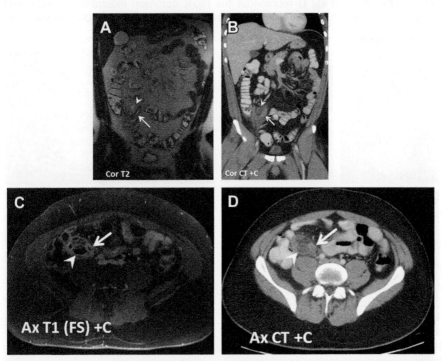

Fig. 2. A 27-year-old man with a perforated acute appendicitis. (*A, B*) Coronal T2-weighted image demonstrates a dilated appendix with a thickened wall (*arrow*) in addition to a mildly hyperintense fluid collection with a thin wall (*arrowhead*); these findings are confirmed on a computed tomography (CT) scan. (*C*) Axial T1-weighted fat-suppressed postcontrast image demonstrates appendiceal wall hyperenhancement (*arrow*) with rim enhancement of the adjacent fluid collection (*arrowhead*). (*D*) Findings are again confirmed on CT scanning.

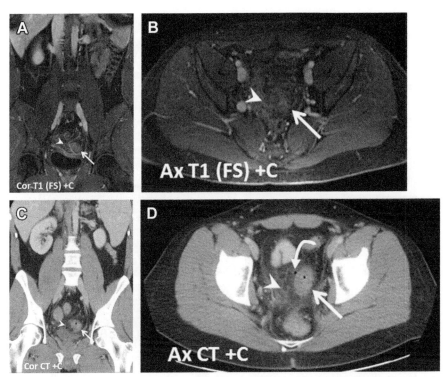

Fig. 3. A 33-year-old man with uncomplicated acute diverticulitis of the sigmoid colon. (*A, B*) Coronal and axial T1-weighted fat-suppressed postcontrast images demonstrate focal thickening and hyperenhancement of the wall of the sigmoid colon (*arrow*), as well as increased enhancement within pericolonic fat (*arrowhead*), indicative of hyperemia. (*C, D*) These findings are confirmed at CT. Note the presence of a small focus of gas within the inflamed diverticulum on CT (*curved arrow*); this is far less conspicuous on MRI.

possibly representing a small contained perforation. Diverticulitis can be complicated by abscess formation or frank perforation with peritonitis.[42] Although often occurring in the sigmoid colon, diverticula anywhere within the large bowel can be affected, including in the proximal colon (**Fig. 4**), where associated right lower quadrant pain can mimic acute appendicitis.[2] Although significantly less common, diverticulitis of small bowel diverticula is also possible, including diverticulitis of a Meckel's diverticulum (**Fig. 5**).[43]

Acute cholecystitis

Acute cholecystitis (**Fig. 6**) classically presents with episodic right upper quadrant pain, but can present with lower abdominal pain.[44] Imaging findings include distension of the gallbladder, thickening of the gallbladder wall, gallbladder wall hyperenhancement, and pericholecystic inflammation and/or fluid. Gallstones are well-visualized with MRI, often lodged within the neck of the gallbladder. Concomitant choledocholithiasis may also be present, manifesting as biliary ductal dilation. Ultrasound examination is generally considered standard of care for the imaging evaluation of the right upper quadrant in cases of suspected acute cholecystitis,[11] but in some cases can be limited owing to patient body habitus, poor acoustic windows, or operator experience. MRI (especially in the form of magnetic resonance

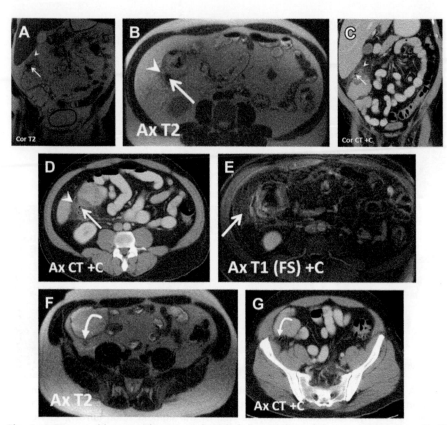

Fig. 4. A 55-year-old man with acute right-sided diverticulitis of the ascending colon. (*A–D*) Coronal and axial T2-weighted images demonstrate focal gas adjacent to the ascending colon, manifesting as a markedly hypointense focus of susceptibility artifact (*arrow*). There is extensive pericolonic inflammation, seen as diffuse, relatively hypointense signal within the T2-weighted hyperintense pericolonic fat (*arrowhead*). These findings are confirmed on coronal and axial CT scans. (*E*) Axial T1-weighted fat-suppressed postcontrast image confirms exuberant inflammation of the ascending colon wall and pericolonic fat (*arrow*). (*F, G*) Axial T2-weighted and computed tomography images at the cecal base show a normal appendix (*curved arrow*).

cholangiopancreatography) often offers excellent visualization of gallbladder disease owing to the inherent high contrast (differences in the MR signal) among the gallbladder wall, intraluminal bile, gallstones, and surrounding tissues.[16] In contrast, evaluation of the gallbladder with CT scanning is often limited owing to little difference in the density among these entities.

Enteritis and colitis
Enteritis and colitis are very common, with foodborne and non–foodborne gastroenteritis alone accounting for more than 200 million cases per year in the United States.[45] Enteritis and colitis commonly present with abdominal pain and may be accompanied by fever, nausea, vomiting, or diarrhea. Presentation and imaging appearance tends to be similar across a wide variety of specific etiologies, including infectious (**Fig. 7**), ischemic (**Fig. 8**), and inflammatory (**Fig. 9**) pathologies. Imaging findings generally include segmental bowel wall thickening, perienteric or pericolonic inflammation surrounding affected bowel segments, bowel wall hyperenhancement, and mesenteric

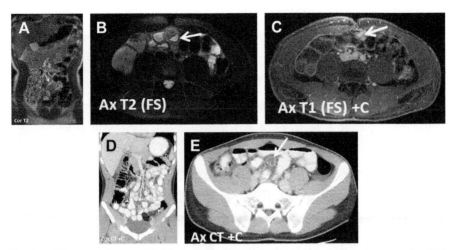

Fig. 5. A 21-year-old man with Meckel's diverticulitis. (*A*, *B*) In a challenging case for MRI, coronal T2-weighted and axial T2-weighted fat-suppressed images demonstrate a small fluid-filled (T2-weighted hyperintense) structure arising from the distal ileum (*arrow*), compatible with a Meckel's diverticulum. (*C*) Axial T1-weighted fat-suppressed postcontrast image shows abnormal enhancement surrounding this structure, consistent with inflammation (*arrow*). (*D*, *E*) The finding is significantly easier to see on computed tomography images as a hypodense fluid-containing structure (*arrow*) among loops of hyperdense small bowel (*arrowheads*), which have been opacified with positive oral contrast.

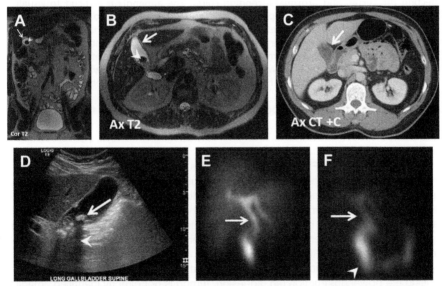

Fig. 6. A 47-year-old man with acute cholecystitis. (*A–C*) Coronal and axial T2-weighted images demonstrate mild gallbladder distension and mild pericholecystic inflammation (*arrow*), which are confirmed on computed tomography (CT) images. Gallstones are seen within the gallbladder neck (*arrowhead*) on MRI, but are not evident on the CT scan. (*D*) Right upper quadrant ultrasound examination confirms gallstones within the gallbladder neck (*arrow*), seen as hyperechoic foci with hypoechoic posterior acoustic shadowing (*arrowhead*). (*E*, *F*) In the same patient, a nuclear medicine hepatobiliary scintigraphy scan shows filling of the common bile duct (*arrow*) and, subsequently, the small bowel (*arrowhead*). The gallbladder never fills, confirming cystic duct obstruction and acute cholecystitis.

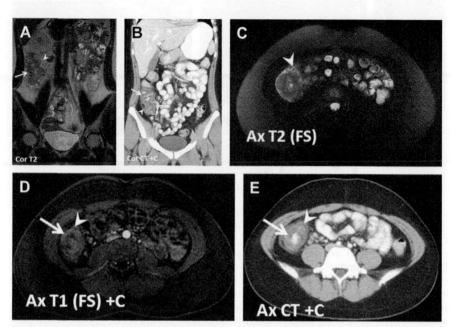

Fig. 7. An 18-year-old woman with infectious colitis. (*A, B*) Coronal T2-weighted images show segmental wall thickening (*arrow*) and pericolonic inflammation (*arrowhead*) affecting the cecum and proximal ascending colon. The appendix is difficult to visualize on MRI, but is normal on a computed tomography scan (CT; *curved arrow*). (*C*) Axial T2-weighted image with fat suppression shows the pericolonic inflammation to better effect, manifesting as a diffuse hyperintense signal surrounding the colon (*arrowhead*). (*D, E*) Axial T1-weighted postcontrast image illustrates hyperenhancement of the thickened colon wall (*arrow*) and again shows pericolonic inflammation (*arrowhead*), which are confirmed on the axial CT image. The patient recovered with only supportive care.

congestion. Mesenteric lymph nodes may be reactively enlarged in the distribution of the affected bowel segments.

Small bowel obstruction

Small bowel obstruction (**Fig. 10**) commonly results in an acute abdomen presentation.[46] In the United States, adhesions related to prior surgery are the most frequent etiology, with other causes including inflammatory bowel disease, cancer, and bowel becoming incarcerated within a hernia.[47] Although CT scanning serves as front-line imaging in cases of suspected small bowel obstruction,[9] some studies have indicated comparably high diagnostic performance for MRI.[48] However, bowel obstruction can be a challenging diagnosis with MRI, especially if the bowel is not well-visualized owing to artifact created by motion and heterogeneous intraluminal contents. Often, the offending agent causing the bowel obstruction (eg, adhesion, tumor) is not directly identified. Imaging diagnosis typically relies on secondary signs of obstruction, including upstream dilated, distended loops of bowel and the identification of a transition point—an abrupt change from dilated to decompressed bowel at the site of the obstruction that can be comparatively difficult to visualize at MRI owing to lower spatial resolution.

Epiploic appendagitis

Epiploic appendages are small, peritoneal-lined protrusions of subserosal fat arising from the surface of the large bowel. Epipolic appendagitis (**Fig. 11**) is a

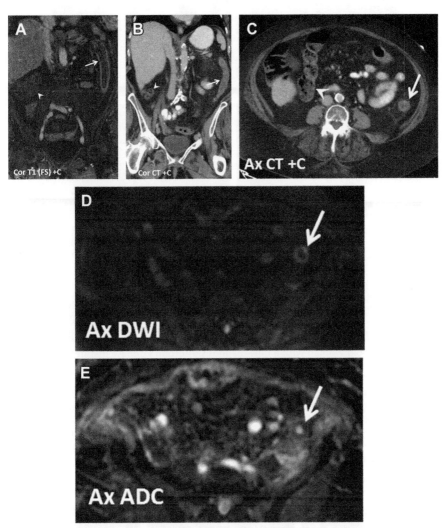

Fig. 8. An 81-year-old woman with self-limiting ischemic colitis. (*A–C*) Coronal T1-weighted fat-suppressed postcontrast images demonstrate wall thickening and hyperenhancement of the descending colon with mild surrounding pericolonic inflammation (*arrow*) and a normal-appearing proximal colon (*arrowhead*); these findings are confirmed on coronal and axial computed tomography images. (*D, E*) In this case, diffusion-weighted imaging shows hyperintensity within the affected descending colon (*arrow*) with a corresponding hypointensity on the apparent diffusion coefficient map (*arrow*), confirming true restricted diffusion. The patient recovered with only supportive care.

benign, self-limiting cause of acute abdominal pain that results from torsion, ischemia, and resultant fat necrosis of an epiploic appendage.[49] Pain results from the corresponding inflammatory reaction. Given that epiploic appendages occur anywhere along the colon, other than the rectum, the pain may mimic acute appendicitis or acute diverticulitis.[50] Laboratory studies are characteristically normal, and patients recover with only supportive care. Imaging findings include focal inflammation (increased T2-weighted signal, increased enhancement) within fat adjacent to the colon, and may be confused with acute diverticulitis.

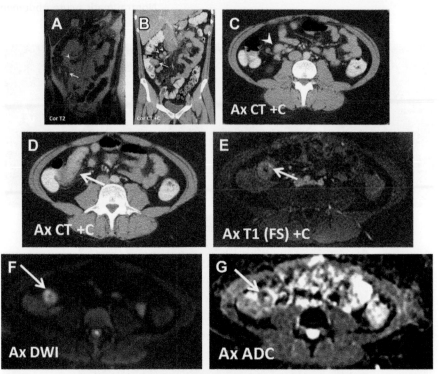

Fig. 9. A 23-year-old woman with a new diagnosis of Crohn's disease manifesting as terminal ileitis. (*A–D*) Coronal T2-weighted image demonstrates marked wall thickening of the terminal ileum with surrounding perienteric inflammation (*arrow*) and enlarged right lower quadrant mesenteric lymph nodes (*arrowheads*), which are confirmed on coronal and axial computed tomography images. (*E*) Axial T1-weighted fat-suppressed postcontrast images show hyperenhancement of the thickened terminal ileum wall (*arrow*). (*F, G*) Diffusion-weighted imaging shows hyperintensity within the affected descending colon (*arrow*) with corresponding hypointensity on the apparent diffusion coefficient map (*arrow*), confirming true restricted diffusion.

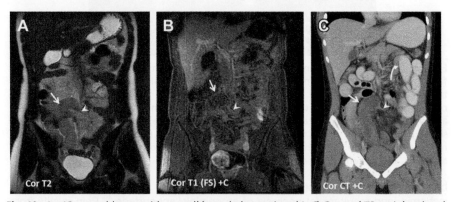

Fig. 10. An 18-year-old man with a small bowel obstruction. (*A–C*) Coronal T2-weighted and coronal T1-weighted fat-suppressed postcontrast images demonstrate a dilated loop of bowel in the midabdomen (*arrows*) in this patient who previously underwent appendectomy. This finding is shown to better effect on the coronal computed tomography (CT) image; note how comparatively hypodense the luminal fluid is just proximal to the site of obstruction when compared with more proximal loops of bowel, which are opacified with positive oral contrast (*curved arrow*). A prominent adhesion (*arrowheads*) is noted at the transition point, also better seen on the CT scan.

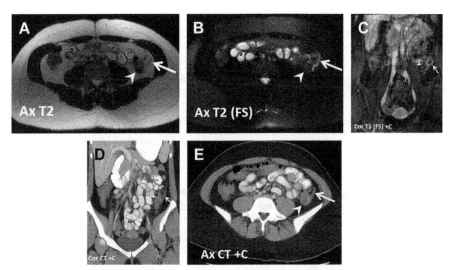

Fig. 11. A 22-year-old woman with epiploic appendagitis. (*A, B*) Axial T2-weighted precontrast images with and without fat suppression demonstrate focal inflammation surrounding a focus of central fat (*arrow*) immediately adjacent to the descending colon (*arrowhead*). The inflammation is seen as a rim of T2-weighted hypointensity against the background of hyperintense fat on the non–fat-suppressed image. When the fat is suppressed, the inflammation stands out as a hyperintense signal. (*C*) Coronal T1-weighted fat-suppressed postcontrast image confirms the inflammation (*arrow*) adjacent to the descending colon (*arrowhead*). (*D, E*) Findings are confirmed on computed tomography images. The patient's symptoms resolved with supportive care.

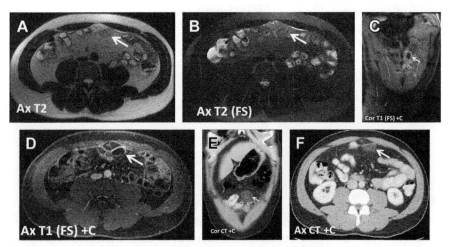

Fig. 12. A 43-year-old man with an omental infarction. (*A, B*) Axial T2-weighted precontrast images with and without fat suppression demonstrate focal inflammation within omental fat adjacent to the anterior abdominal wall; the appearance is similar to that of epiploic appendagitis seen in **Fig. 9**. (*C, D*) Coronal and axial T1-weighted fat-suppressed postcontrast images show enhancement in the region of inflammation (*arrow*). (*E, F*) Findings are confirmed on computed tomography images. The patient's symptoms resolved with supportive care.

Omental infarction

Similar to epiploic appendagitis, omental infarction (**Fig. 12**) is caused by focal fat necrosis within the omentum, and is a benign, self-limiting cause of abdominal pain.[49] Omental infarction may primarily result from mechanical torsion of a portion of the omentum, or may be related to demand ischemia at the periphery of the omental blood supply.[51] Secondary causes include abdominal surgery or trauma. Omental infarction is most commonly reported to occur within the right lower quadrant, but may occur anywhere along the omentum. Imaging features are similar to epiploic appendagitis and include focal inflammation within omental fat. As with epiploic appendagitis, treatment is supportive.

Acute pancreatitis

Most often caused by alcohol abuse or gallstone disease, acute pancreatitis (**Fig. 13**) may present with an acute abdomen.[52] Imaging findings of acute pancreatitis include

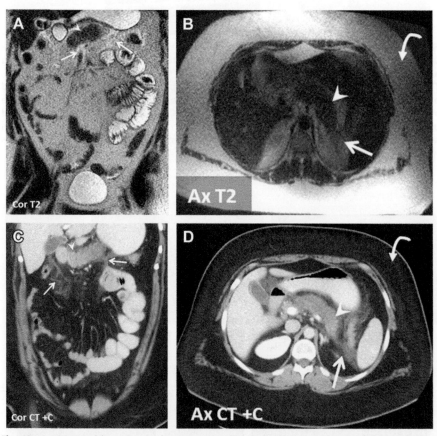

Fig. 13. A 47-year-old woman with acute pancreatitis. (*A–D*) Coronal and axial T2-weighted images demonstrate inflammation and trace free fluid (*arrows*) within the retroperitoneum surrounding the pancreas (*arrowhead*), consistent with acute pancreatitis, confirmed on computed tomography images. Compared with prior examples, the MRI are noisier owing to a decreased signal-to-noise ratio secondary to patient body habitus; note the relatively large amount of subcutaneous adipose tissue (*curved arrow*). This patient was not given intravenous contrast.

pancreatic edema and peripancreatic inflammation and free fluid within the adjacent retroperitoneum. Although acute pancreatitis itself does not rely on imaging for the diagnosis, the usefulness of imaging lies in the evaluation for complications of pancreatitis, including detection of organizing peripancreatic fluid collections, hemorrhage, and identification of regions of pancreatic necrosis,[53] which manifest as hypoenhancing pancreatic parenchyma on both CT scans and MRI. Magnetic resonance cholangiopancreatography in particular offers excellent visualization of the pancreas and pancreatic ducts.[18] Noncontrast T1-weighted MRI is very sensitive to the detection of pancreatic hemorrhage.[54]

Small bowel angioedema

A relatively rare cause of abdominal pain, angioedema of the small bowel (**Fig. 14**) manifests as long segment bowel wall thickening and edema, with or without

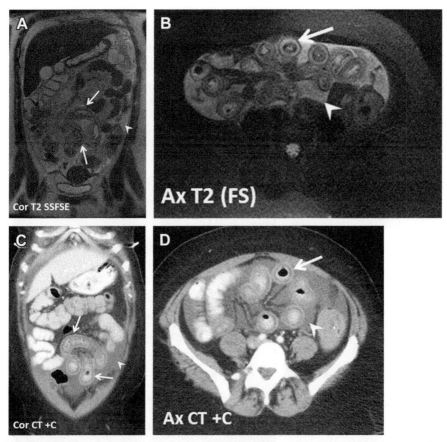

Fig. 14. A 37-year-old woman with small bowel angioedema related to angiotensin-converting enzyme (ACE) inhibitor use. (*A–D*) Coronal T2-weighted and axial T2-weighted fat-suppressed images demonstrate multiple loops of small bowel with diffusely thickened walls and inherent abnormal T2-weighted hyperintensity, consistent with edema (*arrows*). A small amount of abdominal ascites, which appears as T2-weighted hyperintense intraabdominal fluid, is also present (*arrowheads*). Findings are confirmed on coronal and axial computed tomography images. A review of patient medications discovered that she had recently started an ACE inhibitor for hypertension; the medication was discontinued and her symptoms resolved.

secondary signs such as ascites. Although hereditary forms exist,[55] small bowel angioedema is most commonly related to the use of angiotensin-converting enzyme inhibitors.[56] Presenting symptoms may mimic those of bowel obstruction. The condition resolves when the angiotensin-converting enzyme inhibitor is discontinued.

Genitourinary and Female Reproductive Systems

Urolithiasis

Kidney stones are a common cause of pain, and although classically presenting with flank pain, symptomatic urolithiasis (**Fig. 15**) can present with acute abdominal pain as well.[57,58] CT scanning offers excellent detection of kidney stones and the secondary signs of an obstructing stone—upstream hydroureteronephrosis, enlargement or edema of the ipsilateral kidney, and perinephric stranding or free fluid. MRI is relatively poor at direct detection of the relatively anhydrous kidney stones, but is generally

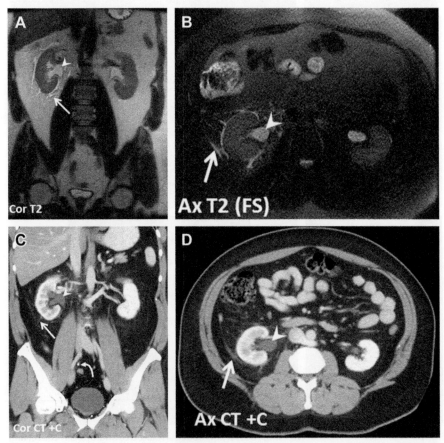

Fig. 15. A 45-year-old man with symptomatic urolithiasis. (*A–D*) Coronal T2-weighted and axial T2-weighted fat-suppressed images demonstrate increased right kidney perinephric fat stranding (*arrows*) and hydronephrosis of the renal collecting system (*arrowheads*). Computed tomography (CT) scanning confirms these findings and reveals the offending 3 mm right distal ureteral stone (*curved arrow*), which is not well-seen on MRI. The CT scan also demonstrates a delayed nephrogram on the right, which was also apparent on the postcontrast MRI (not shown).

comparable with CT scanning at the detection of secondary signs of an obstructing ureteral stone, especially if a designated urography protocol is used.[59,60]

Ovarian torsion

Generally a disease of younger women and adolescents, ovarian torsion (**Fig. 16**) results from twisting of the ovary about its pedicle, causing compromise of blood supply. Irreversible necrosis of the ovary can result if not quickly recognized and treated.[61] Because evaluation of the organs of the female pelvis is often challenging on CT scanning, transvaginal ultrasound examination is the imaging test of choice.[12] Imaging

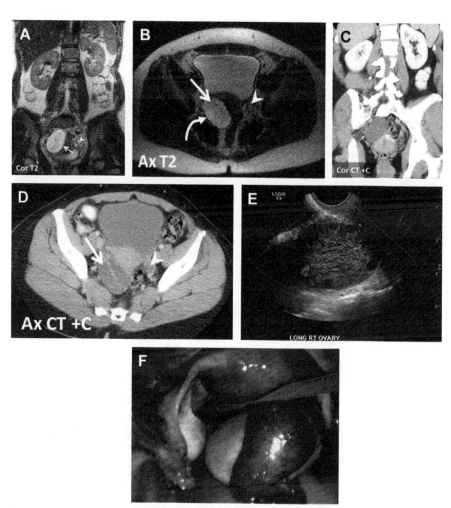

Fig. 16. A 27-year-old woman with ovarian torsion. (*A–D*) Coronal T2-weighted and axial T2-weighted images demonstrate enlargement of the right ovary (*arrows*) compared with the normal left ovary (*arrowheads*). These findings are confirmed on a computed tomography (CT) scan. Note the presence of a prominent ovarian follicle (*curved arrow*), which may have served as a lead point for torsion. (*E*) Power Doppler ultrasound examination shows preservation of blood flow within the enlarged ovary. (*F*) The ovary was salvaged with operative detorsion and ovarian cystectomy.

findings include enlargement (up to 3- or 4-fold) and medialization of the ovary.[62] Doppler ultrasound examination may show a reduced or absent blood flow within the affected ovary, but partially or intermittently torsed ovaries may show some flow preservation. MRI is generally superior to CT scanning for evaluation of the ovaries,[63] and demonstrates ovarian enlargement and edema with decreased contrast enhancement compared with the contralateral ovary.

Pelvic inflammatory disease

Caused by ascending infection within the female reproductive tract, pelvic inflammatory disease (**Fig. 17**) is a clinical diagnosis. Often, no imaging findings are evident. When present, imaging findings include a dilated, fluid-filled fallopian tube (hydrosalpinx/pyosalpinx), inflammation within the adnexa, and an organizing fluid collection (tuboovarian abscess) within the ovary.[64] As with other pathologies of the female pelvis, detection of these findings by CT scanning may be limited, with ultrasound examination and MRI offering better diagnostic usefulness.

Adnexal and uterine masses

Adnexal masses are relatively common findings, and include a wide array of benign and malignant tumors that vary dramatically in imaging presentation and typical age at presentation.[65] Dermoid tumors (mature teratomas) are characteristically benign masses of younger women (**Fig. 18**), although they may be symptomatic.[66] These masses arise from germ cells and may contain cells derived from more than one primary germ layer (ectoderm, mesoderm, endoderm). Consequently, these masses often contain grossly visible fat or calcifications, which are diagnostic when seen. As with any adnexal mass, dermoids may predispose to torsion.

Endometriosis (**Fig. 19**) may present in the form of a discrete adnexal endometrioma. Symptoms may be cyclic, because the ectopic endometrial tissue is hormonally responsive. Pain often results from hemorrhage. Endometriomas may seem similar to other hemorrhagic cysts on ultrasound examination. On MRI,

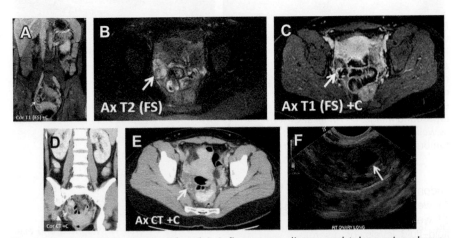

Fig. 17. A 30-year-old woman with pelvic inflammatory disease and tuboovarian abscess. (*A–C*) Axial T2-weighted fat-suppressed and coronal and axial T1-weighted fat-suppressed postcontrast images demonstrate a rim-enhancing fluid collection within the right ovary (*arrow*). (*D, E*) The abscess (*arrow*) is less conspicuous on computed tomography images. (*F*) A complicated fluid collection (*arrow*) with surrounding hyperemia is confirmed at Doppler ultrasound examination. Polymerase chain reaction for chlamydia was positive.

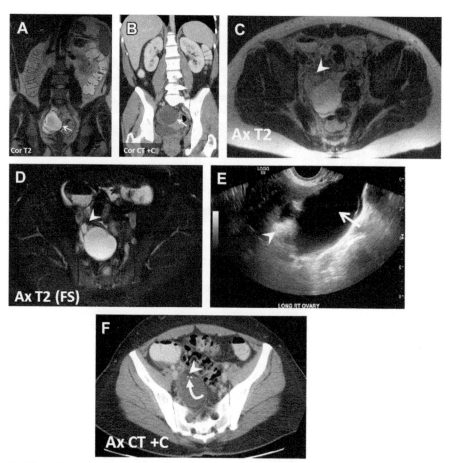

Fig. 18. A 25-year-old woman with right ovarian dermoid (mature teratoma) and ovarian torsion. (*A*, *B*) Coronal T2-weighted image demonstrates a right ovarian mass with a prominent cystic component (*arrows*), confirmed on the coronal computed tomography (CT) image. (*C*, *D*) Careful evaluation on axial T2-weighted images without and with fat suppression reveals a small focus of macroscopic fat within the mass (*arrowheads*), raising suspicion for a dermoid. (*E*) The focus of fat (*arrowhead*), manifesting as an irregularly marginated hyperechoic focus, is noted adjacent to the prominent anechoic cystic component (*arrow*) on the ultrasound image. (*F*) An axial CT scan also shows the focus of macroscopic fat (*arrowhead*) as well as 2 punctate calcifications (*curved arrow*), which are also characteristic of dermoid tumors. The patient underwent right oophorectomy.

endometriomas often present with characteristic hyperintensity on precontrast T1-weighted imaging and T2 shading (appearing darker on T2-weighted than on T1-weighted images owing to the presence of products of hemoglobin degradation), fluid–fluid levels, or discrete foci of marked T2 hypointensity specific for chronic hemorrhage.[67]

Ovarian cancer (**Fig. 20**) typically presents as a heterogeneous adnexal mass with a substantial soft tissue component. Internal blood flow is usually present at ultrasound. MRI is often the imaging test of choice for characterization of ovarian masses when ultrasound examination is equivocal.[68]

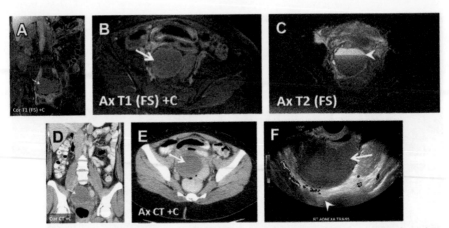

Fig. 19. A 22-year-old woman with hemorrhagic endometrioma. (*A–C*) Coronal and axial T1-weighted fat-suppressed postcontrast images show a nonenhancing mildly T1-weighted hyperintense right adnexal mass (*arrows*) with a fluid–fluid level (*arrowhead*) seen on the axial T2-weighted fat-suppressed image. (*D, E*) Computed tomography findings confirm the mass, but are otherwise nonspecific. (*F*) Doppler ultrasound examination confirms the adnexal mass, showing homogeneous low-level internal echoes (*arrow*) and posterior acoustic enhancement (*arrowhead*), which are often associated with endometrioma. The patient was managed operatively and final pathology yielded endometriosis with hemorrhage.

Although endometrial and cervical cancers are relatively common, these entities present more often with abnormal bleeding rather than acute abdominal pain. Although other primary uterine tumors are relatively rare, uterine fibroids (**Fig. 21**) are very common and may be a cause of lower abdominal or pelvic pain—especially if undergoing spontaneous degeneration—that can mimic other abdominal pathologies. MRI of nondegenerating fibroids typically demonstrates characteristic well-circumscribed mass with decreased T2-weighted signal intensity when compared with the surrounding myometrium.[69] The signal intensity of degenerating fibroids, however, can be highly variable depending on the type of degeneration.

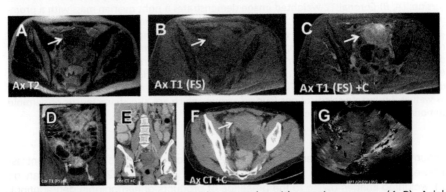

Fig. 20. A 59-year-old woman presenting acutely with ovarian cancer. (*A–D*) Axial T2-weighted and T1-weighted fat-suppressed precontrast images demonstrate a mildly T1-weighted hyperintense, T2-weighted hypointense left adnexal mass (*arrows*) that heterogeneously enhances on coronal and axial T1-weighted fat-suppressed postcontrast images. (*E, F*) The mass seems to be similar on coronal and axial computed tomography images. (*G*) Doppler ultrasound examination confirms a complex soft tissue mass with internal blood flow. Biopsy revealed a high-grade serous epithelial ovarian carcinoma.

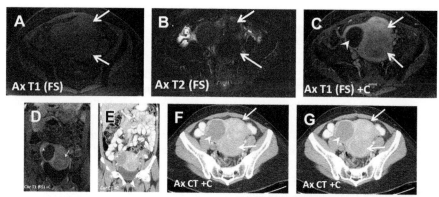

Fig. 21. A 48-year-old woman with a degenerating uterine fibroid. (*A, B*) Axial T1-weighted and T2-weighted fat suppressed precontrast images demonstrate multiple uterine masses (*arrows*), which are both T1-weighted and T2-weighted imaging hypointense, consistent with uterine fibroids. (*C, D*) A single, centrally nonenhancing mass (*arrowheads*) is seen on coronal and axial T1-weighted fat-suppressed postcontrast images, consistent with a degenerating uterine fibroid, whereas the other fibroids demonstrate relatively brisk heterogeneous enhancement (*arrows*). (*E–G*) The fibroids are confirmed on computed tomography images (*arrows*). Note the comparative central hypodensity of the degenerating fibroid (*arrowhead*).

SUMMARY

The acute abdomen encompasses a wide variety of pathologies across multiple organ systems with overlapping clinical presentations, physical examination findings, and laboratory results. The true urgency and prescribed treatment for these disease entities is equally variable, and consequently rapid, accurate diagnosis is essential. Compared with CT scanning, MRI is particularly effective in the imaging of the gallbladder and biliary tree, as well as the female reproductive system.

For the diagnosis of suspected acute appendicitis, emerging data demonstrate equivalent diagnostic performance of MRI and CT. The routine use of MRI as the first-line imaging study for suspected appendicitis, however, has not been established in nonpregnant patients. Given these emerging data, MRI may be appropriate as the first-line imaging for certain patient populations, such as children and young adults in whom avoiding ionizing radiation is desirable, and at institutions where MRI is accessible in the emergency setting.

MRI suffers from other disadvantages, including sensitivity to peristalsis and poor detection of small calcified foci, including urolithiasis, appendicoliths, or other small calcifications. Although CT and ultrasound imaging are likely to remain first-line imaging tests for most indications that require imaging evaluation of the acute abdomen, MRI is an important alternative given its outstanding safety profile. MRI may be appropriate as the first-line imaging study in some circumstances and may also provide timely diagnosis in many cases where other modalities are equivocal, suboptimal, or contraindicated.

REFERENCES

1. Lane MJ, Liu DM, Huynh MD, et al. Suspected acute appendicitis: nonenhanced helical CT in 300 consecutive patients. Radiology 1999;213(2):341–6.

2. Pooler BD, Lawrence EM, Pickhardt PJ. Alternative diagnoses to suspected appendicitis at CT. Radiology 2012;265(3):733–42.

3. Viniol A, Keunecke C, Biroga T, et al. Studies of the symptom abdominal pain–a systematic review and meta-analysis. Fam Pract 2014;31(5):517–29.

4. Ahmed I, Asgeirsson KS, Beckingham IJ, et al. The position of the vermiform appendix at laparoscopy. Surg Radiol Anat 2007;29(2):165–8.

5. Ferzoco LB, Raptopoulos V, Silen W. Acute diverticulitis. N Engl J Med 1998; 338(21):1521–6.

6. Salem TA, Molloy RG, O'Dwyer PJ. Prospective study on the role of C-Reactive Protein (CRP) in patients with an acute abdomen. Ann R Coll Surg Engl 2007; 89(3):233–7.

7. Coursey CA, Casalino DD, Remer EM, et al. ACR appropriateness criteria® acute onset flank pain–suspicion of stone disease. Ultrasound Q 2012;28(3):227–33.

8. Baker ME, Nelson RC, Rosen MP, et al. ACR appropriateness criteria® acute pancreatitis. Ultrasound Q 2014;30(4):267–73.

9. Ros PR, Huprich JE. ACR appropriateness criteria® on suspected small-bowel obstruction. J Am Coll Radiol 2006;3(11):838–41.

10. Smith MP, Katz DS, Lalani T, et al. ACR appropriateness criteria® right lower quadrant pain—suspected appendicitis. Ultrasound Q 2015;31(2):85–91.

11. Yarmish GM, Smith MP, Rosen MP, et al. ACR appropriateness criteria right upper quadrant pain. J Am Coll Radiol 2014;11(3):316–22.

12. Andreotti RF, Lee SI, DeJesus Allison SO, et al. ACR appropriateness criteria® acute pelvic pain in the reproductive age group. Ultrasound Q 2011;27(3): 205–10.

13. Koh DM, Miao Y, Chinn RJS, et al. MR imaging evaluation of the activity of Crohn's disease. AJR Am J Roentgenol 2001;177(6):1325–32.

14. Hammond NA, Miller FH, Yaghmai V, et al. MR imaging of acute bowel pathology: a pictorial review. Emerg Radiol 2008;15(2):99–104.

15. Pedrosa I, Zeikus EA, Levine D, et al. MR imaging of acute right lower quadrant pain in pregnant and nonpregnant patients. Radiographics 2007;27(3):721–43.

16. Catalano OA, Sahani DV, Kalva SP, et al. MR imaging of the gallbladder: a pictorial essay. RadioGraphics 2008;28(1):135–55.

17. Togashi K. MR imaging of the ovaries: normal appearance and benign disease. Radiol Clin North Am 2003;41(4):799–811.

18. O'Neill E, Hammond N, Miller FH. MR imaging of the pancreas. Radiologic Clin North America 2014;52(4):757–77.

19. Masselli G, Gualdi G. MR imaging of the small bowel. Radiology 2012;264(2): 333–48.

20. Bannas P, Pickhardt PJ. MR evaluation of the nontraumatic acute abdomen with CT correlation. Radiologic Clin North America 2015;53(6):1327–39.

21. Repplinger MD, Pickhardt PJ, Robbins JB, et al. Prospective comparison of the diagnostic accuracy of MR imaging versus CT for acute appendicitis. Radiology 2018;171838. [Epub ahead of print].

22. Hastings RS, Powers RD. Abdominal pain in the ED: a 35 year retrospective. Am J Emerg Med 2011;29(7):711–6.

23. Lin E, Alessio A. What are the basic concepts of temporal, contrast, and spatial resolution in cardiac CT? J Cardiovasc Comput Tomogr 2009;3(6):403–8.

24. Feldman MK, Katyal S, Blackwood MS. US artifacts. RadioGraphics 2009;29(4): 1179–89.

25. Sistrom CL, McKay NL. Costs, charges, and revenues for hospital diagnostic imaging procedures: differences by modality and hospital characteristics. J Am Coll Radiol 2005;2(6):511–9.
26. Melendez JC, McCrank E. Anxiety-related reactions associated with magnetic-resonance-imaging examinations. JAMA 1993;270(6):745–7.
27. Dewey M, Schink T, Dewey CF. Claustrophobia during magnetic resonance imaging: cohort study in over 55,000 patients. J Magn Reson Imaging 2007;26(5): 1322–7.
28. Kinner S, Repplinger MD, Pickhardt PJ, et al. Contrast-enhanced abdominal MRI for suspected appendicitis: how we do it. AJR Am J Roentgenol 2016;207(1): 49–57.
29. Ray JG, Vermeulen MJ, Bharatha A, et al. Association between MRI exposure during pregnancy and fetal and childhood outcomes. JAMA 2016;316(9):952–61.
30. Sadowski EA, Bennett LK, Chan MR, et al. Nephrogenic systemic fibrosis: risk factors and incidence estimation. Radiology 2007;243(1):148–57.
31. Bruce R, Wentland AL, Haemel AK, et al. Incidence of nephrogenic systemic fibrosis using gadobenate dimeglumine in 1423 patients with renal insufficiency compared with gadodiamide. Invest Radiol 2016;51(11):701–5.
32. Addiss DG, Shaffer N, Fowler BS, et al. The epidemiology of appendicitis and appendectomy in the United-States. Am J Epidemiol 1990;132(5):910–25.
33. Buckius MT, McGrath B, Monk J, et al. Changing epidemiology of acute appendicitis in the United States: study period 1993–2008. J Surg Res 2012;175(2): 185–90.
34. Humes DJ, Simpson J. Acute appendicitis. BMJ 2006;333(7567):530–4.
35. Pickhardt PJ, Lawrence EM, Pooler B, et al. Diagnostic performance of multidetector computed tomography for suspected acute appendicitis. Ann Intern Med 2011;154(12):789–96.
36. Kinner S, Pickhardt PJ, Riedesel EL, et al. Diagnostic accuracy of MRI versus CT for the evaluation of acute appendicitis in children and young adults. Am J Roentgenology 2017;209(4):911–9.
37. Repplinger MD, Levy JF, Peethumnongsin E, et al. Systematic review and meta-analysis of the accuracy of MRI to diagnose appendicitis in the general population. J Magn Reson Imaging 2016;43(6):1346–54.
38. Dewhurst C, Beddy P, Pedrosa I. MRI evaluation of acute appendicitis in pregnancy. J Magn Reson Imaging 2013;37(3):566–75.
39. Duke E, Kalb B, Arif-Tiwari H, et al. A systematic review and meta-analysis of diagnostic performance of MRI for evaluation of acute appendicitis. AJR Am J Roentgenol 2016;206(3):508–17.
40. Pedrosa I, Levine D, Eyvazzadeh AD, et al. MR imaging evaluation of acute appendicitis in pregnancy. Radiology 2006;238(3):891–9.
41. Jacobs DO. Diverticulitis. New Engl J Med 2007;357(20):2057–66.
42. Kaiser AM, Jiang J-K, Lake JP, et al. The management of complicated diverticulitis and the role of computed tomography. Am J Gastroenterol 2005;100:910.
43. Colvin RW, Al-Katib S, Ebersole J. Perforated Meckel's diverticulitis. J Gastrointest Surg 2017;21(12):2126–8.
44. Strasberg SM. Acute calculous cholecystitis. New Engl J Med 2008;358(26): 2804–11.
45. Sandler RS, Everhart JE, Donowitz M, et al. The burden of selected digestive diseases in the United States. Gastroenterology 2002;122(5):1500–11.
46. Taylor MR, Lalani N. Adult small bowel obstruction. Acad Emerg Med 2013;20(6): 528–44.

47. Miller G, Boman J, Shrier I, et al. Etiology of small bowel obstruction. Am J Surg 2000;180(1):33–6.
48. Beall DP, Fortman BJ, Lawler BC, et al. Imaging bowel obstruction: a comparison between fast magnetic resonance imaging and helical computed tomography. Clin Radiol 2002;57(8):719–24.
49. Vriesman ACV, Lohle PNM, Coerkamp EG, et al. Infarction of omentum and epiploic appendage: diagnosis, epidemiology and natural history. Eur Radiol 1999; 9(9):1886–92.
50. Singh AK, Gervais DA, Hahn PF, et al. Acute epiploic appendagitis and its mimics. RadioGraphics 2005;25(6):1521–34.
51. Kamaya A, Federle MP, Desser TS. Imaging manifestations of abdominal fat necrosis and its mimics. RadioGraphics 2011;31(7):2021–34.
52. Lankisch PG, Apte M, Banks PA. Acute pancreatitis. Lancet 2015;386(9988): 85–96.
53. Miller FH, Keppke AL, Dalal K, et al. MRI of pancreatitis and its complications: part 1, acute pancreatitis. Am J Roentgenology 2004;183(6):1637–44.
54. Sahni VA, Mortelé KJ. The bloody pancreas: MDCT and MRI features of hypervascular and hemorrhagic pancreatic conditions. Am J Roentgenology 2009;192(4): 923–35.
55. Nzeako UC, Frigas E, Tremaine WJ. Hereditary angioedema - A broad review for clinicians. Arch Intern Med 2001;161(20):2417–29.
56. Schmidt TD, McGrath KM. Angiotensin-converting enzyme inhibitor angioedema of the intestine: a case report and review of the literature. Am J Med Sci 2002; 324(2):106–8.
57. Graham A, Luber S, Wolfson AB. Urolithiasis in the emergency department. Emerg Med Clin North Am 2011;29(3):519–38.
58. Hiatt RA, Dales LG, Friedman GD, et al. Frequency of urolithiasis in a prepaid medical care program. Am J Epidemiol 1982;115(2):255–65.
59. Kawashima A, Glockner JF, King BF. CT urography and MR urography. Radiologic Clin North America 2003;41(5):945–61.
60. O'Connor OJ, McLaughlin P, Maher MM. MR urography. Am J Roentgenology 2010;195(3):W201–6.
61. Nair S, Joy S, Nayar J. Five year retrospective case series of adnexal torsion. J Clin Diagn Res 2014;8(12):OC09–13.
62. Duigenan S, Oliva E, Lee SI. Ovarian torsion: diagnostic features on CT and MRI with pathologic correlation. Am J Roentgenology 2012;198(2):W122–31.
63. Ditkofsky NG, Singh A, Avery L, et al. The role of emergency MRI in the setting of acute abdominal pain. Emerg Radiol 2014;21(6):615–24.
64. Thomassin-Naggara I, Fedida B, Haddad S, et al. MR characterization of symptomatic and asymptomatic adnexal masses. Imag Femme 2017;27(4):239–55.
65. Brown DL, Dudiak KM, Laing FC. Adnexal masses: US characterization and reporting. Radiology 2010;254(2):342–54.
66. Outwater EK, Siegelman ES, Hunt JL. Ovarian teratomas: tumor types and imaging characteristics. RadioGraphics 2001;21(2):475–90.
67. Woodward PJ, Sohaey R, Mezzetti TP. Endometriosis: radiologic-pathologic correlation. RadioGraphics 2001;21(1):193–216.
68. Jeong Y-Y, Outwater EK, Kang HK. Imaging evaluation of ovarian masses. RadioGraphics 2000;20(5):1445–70.
69. Murase E, Siegelman ES, Outwater EK, et al. Uterine leiomyomas: histopathologic features, MR imaging findings, differential diagnosis, and treatment. RadioGraphics 1999;19(5):1179–97.

PET/MRI for Gastrointestinal Imaging

Current Clinical Status and Future Prospects

Tyler J. Fraum, MD[a],*, Daniel R. Ludwig, MD[a],
Thomas A. Hope, MD[b], Kathryn J. Fowler, MD[a]

KEYWORDS

- PET/MRI • Colorectal cancer • Hepatocellular carcinoma • Pancreatic cancer
- Neuroendocrine tumor

KEY POINTS

- Integrated PET/MRI scanners acquire PET and MRI data simultaneously, potentially consolidating all the radiologic elements necessary for complete cancer staging into a single imaging session.
- PET/MRI combines the high soft tissue contrast of MRI, which is essential for local tumor staging, with the excellent sensitivity of PET for nodal and distant metastatic disease.
- Colorectal cancer, gastric cancer, hepatic metastatic disease, hepatocellular carcinoma, pancreatic adenocarcinoma, and neuroendocrine tumors are abdominal/gastrointestinal malignancies for which PET/MRI is a promising diagnostic and/or prognostic tool.

INTRODUCTION

Since its introduction, positron emission tomography (PET)/computed tomography (CT) has rapidly revolutionized oncologic imaging.[1] Using the tracer 2-deoxy-2-[^{18}F] fluoro-D-glucose (FDG), a glucose analogue, PET readily identifies hypermetabolic lesions (eg, malignancies) and colocalizes them to specific anatomic sites on CT. Although the primary purpose of the CT component is to provide anatomic correlation, the CT data have the added benefit of facilitating attenuation correction of the PET photons. Attenuation correction is the process of adjusting quantitative measures of tracer uptake, such as the standardized uptake value, on the basis of the relative densities of tissues, improving the accuracy of lesion comparisons both within and between studies. FDG-PET/CT has become the standard of care for the initial staging

Disclosures: T.A. Hope receives grant support from GE Healthcare. The other authors have nothing to disclose.
[a] Mallinckrodt Institute of Radiology, Washington University School of Medicine, 660 South Euclid Avenue, St Louis, MO 63110, USA; [b] Department of Radiology and Biomedical Imaging, University of California, San Francisco, 505 Parnassus Avenue, San Francisco, CA 94143, USA
* Corresponding author.
E-mail address: fraumt@wustl.edu

Gastroenterol Clin N Am 47 (2018) 691–714
https://doi.org/10.1016/j.gtc.2018.04.011
0889-8553/18/© 2018 Elsevier Inc. All rights reserved.

gastro.theclinics.com

and subsequent treatment response assessment of solid neoplasms throughout the body, including the gastrointestinal (GI) tract.[2,3] A particular clinical benefit of PET/CT is whole-body staging, specifically the identification of locoregional and distant metastatic disease. Due to certain intrinsic limitations of CT, PET/CT may be supplemented by magnetic resonance imaging (MRI), which provides the superior soft tissue contrast often needed for local tumor staging. Moreover, some tumor types are not significantly hypermetabolic relative to the tissues in which they arise, due to either high background tracer activity or relatively low tumoral tracer uptake, thereby decreasing the usefulness of FDG-PET imaging for certain indications.

Building on the successes of PET/CT, hybrid PET/MRI scanners were developed to exploit the advantages of simultaneously acquiring and fusing PET and MRI data. PET/MRI provides the potential to streamline oncologic imaging protocols by providing the functional and anatomic information necessary for accurate whole-body and local tumor staging in a single examination. Although MRI data cannot be used as readily as CT data for attenuation correction, this issue is not likely to impact most clinical applications, and further discussion is beyond the scope of this article. Additionally, expanding the number of potential PET/MRI applications, the US Food and Drug Administration has recently approved several new PET tracers targeting distinctive aspects of tumor biology, such as altered receptor expression or elevated amino acid transport.[4] This review article aims to discuss emerging applications of PET/MRI for the evaluation of GI neoplasms while summarizing (when available) the relevant data supporting the clinical utilization of PET/MRI for these indications.

LUMINAL GASTROINTESTINAL NEOPLASMS

Although PET/MRI may eventually prove useful in the assessment of nonneoplastic conditions of the bowel, such as inflammatory bowel disease,[5] there is scant evidence pertaining to these indications. Consequently, we focus on malignant conditions of the luminal GI tract, specifically colorectal cancer and gastric cancers.

Colorectal Cancer

In the United States, colorectal cancer is the third most common cancer and the second most common cause of cancer-related mortality.[6] Imaging is playing an increasingly important role in the management of colorectal cancers, including both initial staging and treatment response assessment.[7] The imaging of colorectal cancer can be separated into locoregional and distant components, with the former focused on the delineation of primary tumor extent (T staging) and the identification of regional lymphadenopathy (N staging), and the latter focused on the detection of metastatic disease (M staging). The role of PET/MRI in assessing for liver metastases is discussed elsewhere in this article. Here, we cover the role of PET/MRI in the locoregional staging of colorectal cancer.

The locoregional treatment of colon cancers typically involves a hemicolectomy with resection of the associated mesentery and regional lymph nodes. Because neoadjuvant therapy for colon cancer has not been shown to improve outcomes compared with surgery alone, preoperative imaging plays a limited role in locoregional staging. By contrast, surgical therapies for rectal cancer are dictated by the spatial relationships of the tumor and involved lymph nodes relative to the mesorectal fascia, anal sphincter complex, pelvic floor musculature, and peritoneal reflection. For example, tumor extension to (or beyond) the mesorectal fascia requires a more extensive surgery and confers a worse prognosis.[8] Neoadjuvant chemoradiation has been shown to reduce the risk of local recurrence and to improve overall survival for patients with high-risk rectal cancers, as reflected in proximity to the mesorectal fascia on pre-operative imaging.[9,10] To this point, pelvic MRI provides essential staging information that informs management decisions related to surgical approach and the need for neoadjuvant therapy.

Potential roles and current evidence

PET/MRI offers potential advantages over PET/CT or MRI alone for the locoregional staging of rectal cancer (see subsequent section for discussion of metastatic staging). Although highly accurate for determining the extramural depth of tumor spread and detecting involvement of the mesorectal fascia (ie, T staging),[11,12] MRI generally relies on size criteria alone for the determination of nodal involvement. For example, one study found that using a short axis diameter of greater than 5 mm to define nodes as suspicious results in an overall accuracy of only 34%.[13] In contradistinction, FDG-PET/CT has been shown to have an overall accuracy of 79% for nodal staging (N staging).[14] Thus, PET/MRI may have the ability to combine the excellent T staging accuracy of MRI with the relatively higher N staging accuracy of FDG-PET/CT (**Fig. 1**).

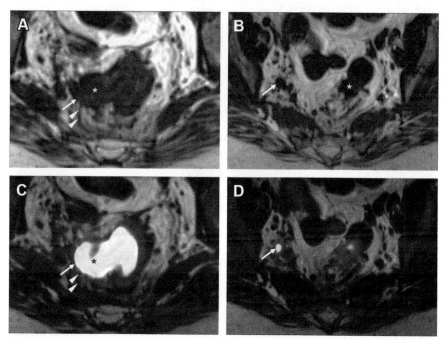

Fig. 1. Usefulness of PET/MRI with 2-deoxy-2-[18F]fluoro-D-glucose (FDG-PET/MRI) for rectal cancer T staging and N staging. A patient with newly diagnosed rectal adenocarcinoma presented for initial staging. Transaxial T2-weighted images of the pelvis (*A, B*) with FDG-PET fusion (*C, D*) demonstrate a markedly FDG-avid rectal mass (*asterisks* in *A–D*) extending through the right lateral rectal wall into the mesorectal fat to abut (*arrows* in *A, C*) the mesorectal fascia (*arrowheads* in *A, C*). These findings are consistent with circumferential resection margin involvement, indicating a higher risk of postoperative disease recurrence. More superiorly, a rounded lymph node in the right internal iliac chain (*arrows* in *B, D*), although suspicious on the MRI alone, is hypermetabolic on FDG-PET, resulting in a more definitive diagnosis of nodal metastatic disease. Based on these imaging findings, the patient was treated with chemoradiation rather than surgical resection. This case demonstrates the ability of FDG-PET/MRI to provide simultaneous rectal cancer T staging and N staging.

This advantage could be particularly valuable to patients with lymph node metastases that would otherwise be outside of the standard surgical/radiation field. Currently, due to limited evidence, PET does not generally play a role in T staging. However, FDG-PET may provide useful adjunctive information in determining local tumor extent (**Fig. 2**) and assessing treatment response (**Fig. 3**).[15–17] Further research is needed to validate PET/MRI for these applications. **Table 1** summarizes current evidence pertaining to the use of PET/MRI in the locoregional staging of colorectal cancer.

Gastric Cancer

Compared with colorectal cancer, gastric cancer is relatively rare in the United States, falling outside of the top 10 for both new cases and deaths,[6] but it remains one of the leading causes of cancer-related mortality worldwide. In the vast majority of cases, surgery offers the only potential for a cure, so the determination of gastric cancer resectability is the primary goal of imaging.[18] After the establishment of a gastric

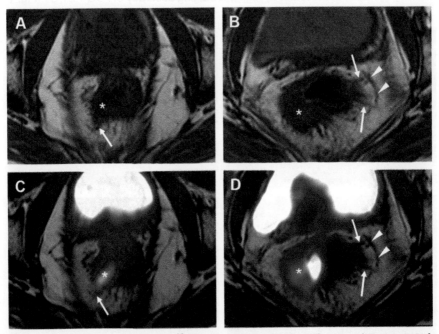

Fig. 2. Value of PET with 2-deoxy-2-[^{18}F]fluoro-D-glucose (FDG-PET) as an adjunct to MRI for T staging. A patient with newly diagnosed rectal adenocarcinoma presented for initial staging. Transaxial T2-weighted images of the pelvis (A, B) with FDG-PET fusion (C, D) demonstrate a right posterolateral hypermetabolic rectal mass (asterisks in A–D) extending through the right posterolateral rectal wall into the mesorectal fat (arrows in A, C) without involvement of the circumferential resection margin. More superiorly, the MRI shows spicules of tissue (arrows in B, D) extending laterally through the mesorectal fat to abut the mesorectal fascia (arrowheads in B, D). Normally, this finding would result in the administration of neoadjuvant chemoradiation before surgical resection. However, there is no corresponding hypermetabolism on the FDG-PET/MRI fusion image (D) in this region to suggest the presence of tumor, raising the possibility of a benign desmoplastic reaction (a known local tissue response to some rectal cancers) at this site. This case demonstrates the potential of MRI for overestimation of tumor extent and highlights a possible advantage of FDG-PET/MRI for the initial staging of rectal cancer.

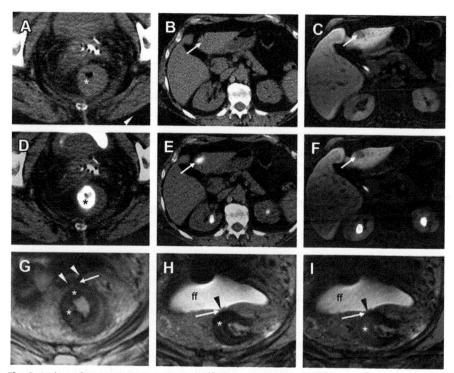

Fig. 3. Value of PET/MRI with 2-deoxy-2-[^{18}F]fluoro-D-glucose (FDG-PET/MRI) for the assessment of response to neoadjuvant therapy. A patient with newly diagnosed rectal cancer presented for an initial staging FDG-PET/computed tomography (CT) (A, D) and MRI (G). Transaxial CT images of the pelvis (A) with FDG-PET fusion (D) show a hypermetabolic right rectal mass (*asterisks*) without definite extramural extension. Transaxial T2-weighted MRIs (G) from the same day suggest tethering (*arrow*) of the peritoneal reflection (*arrowheads*) along the anterior margin of the tumor (*asterisks*). Peritoneal reflection involvement is an indicator of higher risk for local tumor recurrence. Additionally, transaxial CT images of the liver (B) with FDG-PET fusion (E) reveal a vague hypodense mass in segment 3 with marked FDG avidity (*arrows*), consistent with a metastasis. As a result, the patient underwent neoadjuvant chemoradiation, after which a restaging FDG-PET/MRI (C, F, H, I) was performed. Transaxial T1-weighted images of the liver (C) acquired 20 minutes after the intravenous administration of gadoxetate disodium (ie, hepatobiliary phase) with FDG-PET fusion (F) show a persistent mass in segment 3 but no corresponding FDG avidity, suggesting nonviable tumor. From this same imaging session, transaxial T2-weighted images of the pelvis (H) with FDG-PET fusion (I) demonstrate a decrease in the size and FDG avidity of the right rectal mass (*asterisks*). Persistent but mild hypermetabolism within the rectal mass suggests residual viable tumor. However, a fat plane is visible (*arrows*) between the rectal mass (*asterisks*) and the peritoneum (*arrowhead*), which is readily identifiable due to the presence of a small volume of pelvic free fluid (ff). This finding is consistent with local tumor regression related to treatment effect. This case demonstrates the value of FDG-PET/MRI for complete TNM restaging of rectal cancer after neoadjuvant therapy.

cancer diagnosis, the current paradigm involves contrast-enhanced CT of the chest, abdomen, and pelvis to assess for nodal and distant metastatic disease; if no distant metastases are detected by CT, patients may then undergo FDG-PET/CT to assess for CT-occult metastatic disease and endoscopic ultrasound evaluation to complete local tumor staging (T staging).[19] Importantly, FDG-PET can be of limited usefulness

Table 1
Results of studies evaluating the role of PET/MRI in colorectal cancer

Publication	Patients (n)	Findings
Paspulati et al,[101] 2015	12	• Higher colorectal cancer T staging accuracy of FDG-PET/MRI relative to FDG-PET/CT
Brendle et al,[102] 2016	15	• Similar accuracy of FDG-PET/CT and FDG-PET/MRI for N staging and detection of peritoneal spread in colorectal cancer
Kang et al,[103] 2016	51	• Added value of FDG-PET/MRI relative to contrast-enhanced CT for whole-body staging of colorectal cancer

Abbreviation: FDG-PET/CT, PET/computed tomography with 2-deoxy-2-[^{18}F]fluoro-D-glucose.

for the staging of gastric cancers, because the mucinous and diffusely infiltrative tumor types often are not FDG-avid (as for many mucinous colorectal cancers).[20] Patients without evidence of distant metastatic disease or major arterial invasion are considered potentially resectable and subsequently receive neoadjuvant therapy, which has been shown to improve survival relative to gastrectomy alone.[21] Although not standard, MRI may be valuable as a problem solving tool in the setting of gastric cancer staging.[22]

Potential roles and current evidence

As with colorectal cancer, PET/MRI may provide certain benefits over the above-described standard imaging algorithm. Although endoscopic ultrasound evaluation has long been considered the best imaging method for the delineation of local tumor extent, current MRI techniques can now achieve similarly high T staging accuracy.[23] Furthermore, relative to CT alone, FDG-PET/CT confers greater specificity for lymph node involvement[24] and higher sensitivity for distant metastases.[25] Thus, PET/MRI could consolidate the diagnostic strengths of FDG-PET/CT and endoscopic ultrasound evaluation into a single examination, potentially expediting initial staging and improving patient convenience. Finally, MRI with diffusion-weighted imaging (DWI) may be more accurate than FDG-PET/CT for assessing the response of gastric cancer to neoadjuvant therapy, suggesting that PET/MRI might likewise be used for monitoring treatment responses.[26] **Table 2** summarizes current evidence pertaining to the use of PET/MRI in gastric cancer.

Table 2
Results of studies evaluating the role of PET/MRI in gastric cancer

Publication	Patients (n)	Findings
Lee et al,[104] 2016	42	• Better accuracy for gastric cancer M staging with FDG-PET/MRI relative to CT • Similar accuracy of FDG-PET/CT and FDG-PET/MRI for T staging and N staging of gastric cancer • Greater accuracy for determining resectability of gastric cancer with FDG-PET/MRI relative to CT
Lee et al,[105] 2016	11	• FDG-PET/MRI predicts response of advanced unresectable gastric cancers to chemotherapy

Abbreviation: FDG-PET/CT, PET/computed tomography with 2-deoxy-2-[^{18}F]fluoro-D-glucose.

HEPATIC NEOPLASMS

Given its high specificity for characterizing benign and malignant primary liver lesions and its excellent sensitivity for metastatic disease, MRI has become the examination of choice for the evaluation of hepatic neoplasms. Although the role of FDG-PET in liver imaging has been limited, the advent of non–FDG-PET tracers may improve the usefulness of liver PET imaging. Here, we focus on potential roles of PET/MRI in the imaging of hepatic metastases and hepatocellular carcinoma (HCC).

Hepatic Metastases

For many primary GI cancers, the liver is the most common location of distant metastatic disease, the presence versus absence of which can have a dramatic impact on a patient's prognosis and management strategy. New paradigms of resecting metastatic disease have been shown to improve survival and even result in cure for some tumor types, such as colorectal cancer, breast cancer, and melanoma.[27–29] In fact, the primary determinant of mortality in colorectal cancer is the hepatic disease burden.[30] Thus, accurate imaging is key to the identification and treatment of liver metastases and, in turn, critical to achieving optimal outcomes. For patients with widely metastatic disease or comorbidities precluding surgery, locoregional therapies (LRTs) for hepatic metastases (eg, radioembolization, percutaneous ablation, or hepatic artery infusion pumps) or systemic chemotherapy regimens are available. These liver-directed therapies also rely on imaging to select types of treatment and assess responses.

Potential roles and current evidence

Due to its relatively high uptake by normal liver parenchyma, FDG has a limited ability to identify liver metastases. One study found that FDG-PET/CT detects colorectal liver metastases with a sensitivity of only 55%, a rate significantly lower than that of contrast-enhanced CT or MRI.[31] In contradistinction to FDG-PET, MRI is very sensitive for liver metastases, especially when hepatobiliary contrast agents such as gadoxetic acid (Eovist, Bayer, West Haven, CT) are used.[32,33] The addition of DWI to liver MRI protocols may further improve both sensitivity and specificity for liver metastases.[34] Thus, although it may not offer much benefit over MRI alone for the detection of liver metastases, FDG-PET/MRI is almost certainly more sensitive than FDG-PET/CT for this indication (**Fig. 4**).[35]

Given the superb diagnostic accuracy of MRI alone for diagnosing colorectal liver metastases, the main role of FDG-PET in the M staging of colorectal cancer is the detection of extrahepatic metastatic disease. The preoperative identification of extrahepatic metastatic disease has the potential to spare patients from undergoing futile (ie, noncurative) interventions that may be associated with significant morbidity and mortality, such as large liver resections.[36] FDG-PET also plays a secondary role in assessing liver tumor burden, with limitations related to the high background FDG uptake by the liver at the conventional imaging time point of clinical FDG-PET/CT and the relatively low uptake of FDG by small and/or mucinous metastases. In contradistinction, FDG-PET/MRI has the potential to yield better results. In the simultaneous model of hybrid imaging used by the most recent generation of PET/MRI scanners, the PET portion of the examination can be improved by acquiring PET data throughout the entirety of the MRI portion, which is intrinsically longer than a CT acquisition, allowing time for greater tracer accumulation in target lesions. Furthermore, the simultaneity of PET/MRI can improve the registration of the PET data with the anatomic images and facilitates the application of motion correction techniques, such as MRI-based respiratory navigators, that are not available with CT.

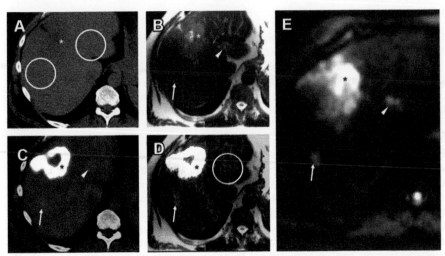

Fig. 4. Value of PET/MRI with 2-deoxy-2-[¹⁸F]fluoro-ᴅ-glucose (FDG-PET/MRI) for the detection of hepatic metastases. A patient with colon cancer presented for initial staging and underwent FDG-PET/ computed tomography (CT) immediately followed by FDG-PET/MRI using the same FDG dose, as part of a PET/MRI optimization protocol at our institution. Transaxial computed tomography (CT) images through the liver (*A*) with FDG-PET fusion (*C*) show vague hypodensity (*asterisk* in *A*) at the junction of segments 8 and 4A, corresponding to a large, hypermetabolic, centrally necrotic metastasis on FDG-PET (*asterisk* in *C*). Other less conspicuous areas of hypermetabolism are visible in the right hemiliver (*arrow* in *C*) and caudate lobe (*arrowhead* in *C*), without definite anatomic correlates on the CT images (*circles* in *A*). These other foci are suspicious for (but not diagnostic of) metastatic disease, in light of the relatively high background FDG uptake and poor soft tissue contrast resolution of noncontrast CT. Obtained roughly 30 minutes later, transaxial T2-weighted MRIs (*B*) with FDG-PET fusion (*D*) and diffusion-weighted images (*E*) show a hypermetabolic, T2-hyperintense, diffusion-restricting segment 8/4A liver mass (*asterisks* in *B*, *D*, *E*). The two additional sites of suspicious FDG uptake seen on PET/CT have clear correlates on the T2-weighted and diffusion-weighted images (*arrows* and *arrowheads* in *B*, *E*), confirming the presence of metastatic disease at these sites. The lesion in the right hemiliver is again apparent as an FDG-avid focus on PET/MRI (*arrow* in *D*), but the caudate lesion is not visible as a discrete FDG-avid focus (*circle* in *D*). This case demonstrates the potential for diagnosing hepatic metastatic disease with greater confidence on FDG-PET/MRI relative to FDG-PET/CT.

Furthermore, as more non–FDG-PET tracers become approved by the US Food and Drug Administration, PET/MRI has the potential to combine the high specificity of a molecular-targeted PET tracer with the high sensitivity of hepatobiliary phase MRI with DWI. For example, as discussed elsewhere in this article, ⁶⁸Ga-DOTATATE-PET has the potential to detect neuroendocrine liver metastases not evident on FDG-PET.[37] Consequently, for certain indications, PET/MRI might offer the greatest diagnostic accuracy for assessment of hepatic metastatic disease. Moreover, for indications such as rectal cancer, PET/MRI with hepatobiliary phase imaging of the liver could be combined with dedicated PET/MRI of the pelvis, thereby providing complete TNM staging in a single imaging examination. **Table 3** summarizes current evidence pertaining to the use of PET/MRI for hepatic metastases.

Hepatocellular Carcinoma

Worldwide, HCC is the fifth most common malignancy and the second most common cause of cancer-related death.[38] Its incidence continues to increase, in conjunction

Table 3
Results of studies evaluating the role of PET/MRI in hepatic metastases

Publication	Patients (n)	Findings
Donati et al,[35] 2010	37	• Higher radiologist confidence for liver metastasis (including colorectal and other primary malignancies) with FDG-PET/MRI than FDG-PET/CT • Higher sensitivity of FDG-PET/MRI than FDG-PET/CT for liver metastases (including colorectal and other primary malignancies)
Beiderwellen et al,[106] 2015	26	• Higher sensitivity and overall accuracy of FDG-PET/MRI than FDG-PET/CT for liver metastases (including colorectal and other primary malignances)
Brendle et al,[102] 2016	15	• Higher accuracy of FDG-PET/MRI with DWI than FDG-PET/CT for detecting colorectal liver metastases
Yong et al,[107] 2011	24	• Greater sensitivity of FDG-PET/MRI for liver metastases than FDG-PET/CT, especially for lesions <1 cm

Abbreviation: FDG-PET/CT, PET/computed tomography with 2-deoxy-2-[^{18}F]fluoro-D-glucose.

with increasing rates of chronic liver disease.[39] Cirrhosis represents the most important risk factor for HCC, and the American Association for the Study of Liver Diseases accordingly recommends routine surveillance imaging in all patient with cirrhosis.[40] Once a diagnosis of HCC is made, patients within the Milan criteria are eligible to receive priority status for orthotopic liver transplantation (OLT), which is often curative.[41] LRTs such as transarterial chemoembolization, radiofrequency ablation, and radioembolization play an important role in the management of patients who are not candidates for OLT or serve as a bridge to OLT for patients who are candidates.[42] Additionally, LRT has proven effective in downstaging patients presenting with disease beyond the Milan criteria, and similar post-OLT outcomes can be achieved for these patients relative to those initially presenting within the Milan criteria.[43] Imaging is vital to detecting and staging HCC, as well as guiding therapeutic decisions. Although MRI has achieved dominance in the realm of HCC imaging, several studies have investigated the use of PET for prognostication and response assessment in HCC, as discussed elsewhere in this article.

Potential roles and current evidence

In patients with established risk factors for HCC, multiphasic contrast-enhanced MRI or CT can establish a definitive diagnosis of HCC without the requirement for tissue sampling.[44] Indeed, the sensitivity and specificity of MRI for the detection of HCC are as high as 82% and 91%, respectively.[40] MRI accurately depicts disease extent, presence of satellite lesions, vascular involvement, and health of the background liver parenchyma.[45] Additionally, DWI may improve the detection rate for smaller lesions,[46] and the degree of diffusion restriction seems to correlate with tumor aggressiveness.[47] In contrast, FDG-PET has limited usefulness in the detection of HCC due to its variable (often low) FDG uptake and the relatively high FDG uptake by background liver parenchyma[48,49] (**Fig. 5**). However, when present, FDG uptake by HCC is associated with higher histopathologic tumor grade, poor tumor differentiation, microvascular invasion, and extrahepatic metastatic disease.[50,51] Accordingly, FDG positivity predicts lower overall survival and greater risk of post-OLT recurrence.[51–54] FDG-PET may also be useful in predicting response to LRT[55] and identifying post-LRT recurrence.[56,57] Thus, FDG-PET/MRI might prove useful for simultaneously diagnosing HCC and predicting its histologic grade.

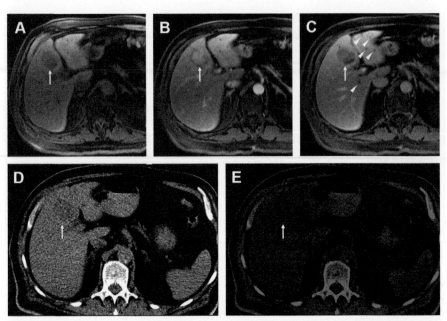

Fig. 5. Limited usefulness of PET with 2-deoxy-2-[^{18}F]fluoro-D-glucose (FDG-PET) for the detection of hepatocellular carcinoma. A patient with an incidentally detected hepatic lesion and no risk factors for chronic liver disease presented for further imaging characterization. Transaxial T1-weighted precontrast (*A*), late arterial phase (*B*), and portal venous phase (*C*) MRIs show a lesion in segment 4B (*arrows* in *A–C*) that demonstrates arterial phase hyperenhancement with delayed phase washout and capsule appearance. These findings are sufficient for an imaging diagnosis of hepatocellular carcinoma (ie, LI-RADS 5 lesion). Incidental note was made of multiple peribiliary cystic lesions (*arrowheads* in *C*), likely biliary hamartomas. Contemporaneous transaxial computed tomography images (*D*) with FDG-PET fusion (*E*) show a hypodense mass with FDG uptake equal to or less than the surrounding liver parenchyma (*arrows* in *D, E*). Percutaneous biopsy revealed moderately differentiated hepatocellular carcinoma, which is known to concentrate FDG poorly owing to expression of glucose-6-phosphatase.

When HCC metastasizes, the most common locations are the lung, lymph nodes, and bone.[58] Despite its limited ability to detect primary HCC, FDG-PET has proven useful for the detection of extrahepatic metastatic disease[59] and post-OLT recurrence.[60] For example, FDG-PET can be helpful in differentiating metastatic from reactive lymphadenopathy, because enlarged periportal lymph nodes are a common finding in cirrhosis[61] (**Fig. 6**). Furthermore, FDG-PET can potentially distinguish benign from malignant portal vein thrombus in HCC patients with equivocal findings on MRI.[62] Several non–FDG-PET radiotracers have also been tested in patients with HCC including [^{11}C]acetate, [^{11}C]choline, and [^{18}F]choline.[63–65] These radiotracers, which are molecular probes for lipid synthesis, have been shown to have a high sensitivity for well-differentiated HCC but a lower sensitivity for poorly differentiated HCC. Accordingly, the optimal detection of HCC occurs when these radiotracers are used in combination with FDG.[63–65] However, these radiotracers are not widely available and thus have a limited role in current clinical practice.

Although no studies have combined PET and MRI for the detection or characterization of HCC, FDG-PET/MRI may prove useful in selected patients. In particular, FDG-PET provides greatest value in the differentiation of high-grade from low-grade

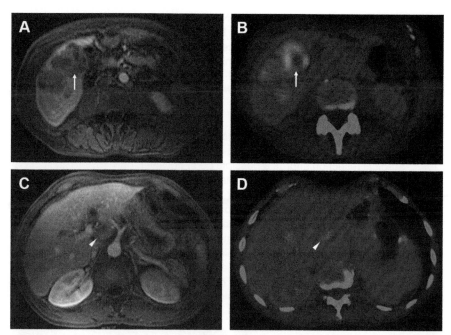

Fig. 6. Usefulness of PET with 2-deoxy-2-[^{18}F]fluoro-D-glucose (FDG-PET) for the differentiation of reactive from metastatic lymphadenopathy in the setting of hepatocellular carcinoma (HCC). A patient with hepatitis C and biopsy-proven HCC presented for a follow-up MRI. Transaxial T1-weighted portal venous phase postcontrast images demonstrate an infiltrative mass involving the right hepatic lobe (*arrow* in *A*), as well as an indeterminate enlarged periportal lymph node (*arrowhead* in *C*). Transaxial fusion images from a subsequent FDG-PET/computed tomography display the HCC as a focal mass that is mildly hypermetabolic relative to the background liver parenchyma (*arrow* in *B*) and reveal moderately increased FDG uptake (*arrowhead* in *D*) by the enlarged periportal lymph node seen on MRI. These findings are suggestive of a nodal metastasis. A follow-up study several months later (not shown) demonstrated progressive nodal enlargement, corroborating the presence of extrahepatic HCC and making the patient ineligible for liver transplantation per the Milan criteria. Thus, by combining the strengths of MRI in assessing hepatic disease extent with the strengths of FDG-PET in assessing nodal metabolism, PET/MRI has the potential to improve the detection of extrahepatic HCC, the knowledge of which is critical for optimizing patient selection for liver transplantation.

disease, identifying extrahepatic metastatic disease, and identifying recurrence after OLT or LRT. For example, in a patient with known HCC, FDG-PET/MRI could simultaneously evaluate for extrahepatic disease and assess the patient's hepatic disease burden, both of which are critical to determining whether a patient is eligible for OLT. Furthermore, PET/MRI can provide tumor-specific dosimetry estimates for HCC (as well as hepatic metastases) treated with [90Y]-labeled microsphere radioembolization, predicting tumor response to this intervention.[66] Overall, further work is needed to define the optimal role for PET/MRI in the evaluation of HCC.

PANCREATIC AND NEUROENDOCRINE NEOPLASMS

Pancreatic adenocarcinomas are challenging to diagnose by imaging at the early stages, when curative treatment is still possible. Similarly, neuroendocrine tumors (NETs), a significant minority of which arise within or adjacent to the pancreas, can be quite difficult to delineate. For example, NETs commonly present as metastatic disease arising from primary tumors that can be occult on conventional imaging protocols. Importantly, several new PET tracers targeting the somatostatin receptor (SSTR) have recently revolutionized the imaging of this unique class of neoplasms. Here, we discuss potential applications of PET/MRI for pancreatic adenocarcinoma and NETs.

Pancreatic Adenocarcinoma

Pancreatic adenocarcinoma is the fourth leading cause of cancer-related death in the United States. Prognosis is typically poor, as evidenced by a 5-year survival of just 8.2%.[67] Surgical resection affords a possible cure; however, only 15% to 20% of patients have resectable disease at the time of presentation.[68] Even when curative resection is performed, the overall 5-year survival improves to only approximately 25%, from less than 5% for patients that do not undergo complete resections.[69] Early diagnosis is essential for achieving maximal survival benefit. Differentiation of malignant from benign pancreatic disease (ie, cancer vs inflammation) is of particular importance, especially after neoadjuvant therapies. Accurate staging determines surgical resectability with key features including the degree of vascular involvement, locoregional nodal involvement, and presence of distant metastatic disease.[70] Accordingly, noninvasive imaging plays a primary role in the management of patients with

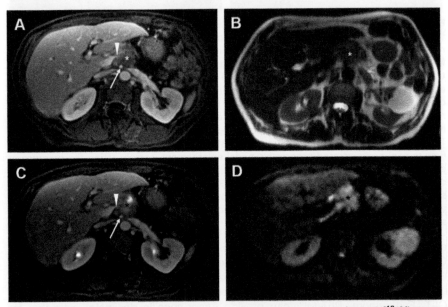

Fig. 7. Staging of pancreatic adenocarcinoma by PET/MRI with 2-deoxy-2-[^{18}F]fluoro-D-glucose (FDG-PET/MRI). Transaxial T1-weighted postcontrast portal venous phase images (A) with FDG-PET fusion (C) and corresponding T2-weighted images (B) demonstrate an ill-defined mass in the body of the pancreas (*asterisks* in A–C). This mass encases the superior mesentery artery (*arrows* in A, C) and encases and severely attenuates the main portal vein (*arrowheads* in A, C). Transaxial diffusion-weighted images (D) also show the tumor (*asterisk*) with excellent conspicuity. There were no suspicious lymph nodes or liver lesions. Overall, these findings are consistent with locally advanced but nonmetastatic pancreatic cancer. This case demonstrates that FDG-PET/MRI clearly depicts local pancreatic tumor extent and provides simultaneous screening for nodal and hepatic metastatic disease.

suspected or confirmed pancreatic cancer. Endoscopic ultrasound imaging and laparoscopy are adjunctive approaches that refine assessment of disease extent and provide a means to establish a tissue diagnosis.[71,72]

Potential roles and current evidence

Multiphasic contrast-enhanced CT, the initial examination of choice in patients with suspected pancreatic cancer, is highly accurate in depicting the degree of vascular involvement owing to its excellent spatial resolution.[72,73] However, it has limited sensitivity for the detection of hepatic and peritoneal metastatic disease.[74] Multiphasic contrast-enhanced MRI has proven equivalent to contrast-enhanced CT for the diagnosis of pancreatic cancer and provides a comparable accuracy for assessing resectability.[75-77] Additionally, MRI is often used when findings on contrast-enhanced CT are equivocal, because MRI can be helpful in differentiating pancreatic adenocarcinoma from focal pancreatitis.[78] As described elsewhere in this article, MRI is also useful for characterizing indeterminate hepatic lesions when metastatic disease is suspected.

The added value of FDG-PET in the diagnosis and staging of pancreatic adenocarcinoma is unclear due to the high degree of accuracy of CT and MRI.[79] FDG-PET/CT does have superior diagnostic performance to CT and MRI in the identification of peritoneal dissemination[80] and distant metastatic disease,[81] which typically preclude candidacy for curative surgery and often eliminate the need for laparotomy. However, the increased sensitivity of FDG-PET occurs at a loss of specificity related to FDG uptake by inflammatory processes; in one series, a false-positive FDG-PET delayed definitive surgical management in an appreciable minority of patients.[82] Furthermore, FDG-PET is a useful problem-solving tool, such as in patients with a suspected malignant biliary stricture but no evidence of malignancy on conventional imaging.[81] Additionally, FDG-PET has proven valuable for identifying malignant transformation within intraductal papillary mucinous neoplasms.[83,84] Finally, FDG-PET performs better than CT or MRI for diagnosing local recurrence in patients with suspected relapse.[85]

Table 4
Results of studies evaluating the role of PET/MRI in pancreatic adenocarcinoma

Publication	Patients (n)	Findings
Joo et al,[108] 2017	37	• Similar diagnostic performance of FDG-PET/MRI relative to PET/CT plus contrast-enhanced CT for determining pancreatic tumor resectability, N staging, and M staging
Chen et al,[109] 2016	60	• Imaging biomarkers derived from FDG-PET/MRI predict clinical tumor stage of pancreatic/ampullary cancers
Nagamachi et al,[110] 2013	119	• *Retrospective fusion* of FDG-PET and noncontrast MRI improves diagnostic accuracy for identifying pancreatic adenocarcinoma, compared with noncontrast FDG-PET/CT
Tatsumi et al,[111] 2011	47	• *Retrospective fusion* of FDG-PET and noncontrast MRI improves diagnostic confidence for identifying pancreatic adenocarcinoma, compared with noncontrast FDG-PET/CT • Slightly higher diagnostic accuracy with FDG-PET/MRI compared with FDG-PET/CT (not statistically significant)
Ruf et al,[112] 2006	32	• *Retrospective fusion* of FDG-PET and contrast-enhanced MRI is feasible and facilitates interpretation of FDG-avid foci, compared with a side-by-side analysis

Abbreviation: FDG-PET/CT, PET/computed tomography with 2-deoxy-2-[^{18}F]fluoro-D-glucose.

FDG-PET/MRI provides the opportunity to combine the diagnostic and locoregional staging performance of MRI with the problem-solving and metastasis detection capabilities of FDG-PET in a single examination (**Fig. 7**). Early clinical experience suggests that PET/MRI may prove most valuable in identifying otherwise occult metastatic disease, potentially altering surgical candidacy. This benefit may, in part, be due the relatively delayed nature of the PET acquisition on PET/MRI relative to PET/CT,[86] along with the added advantage of MRI-based motion correction with PET/MRI.[87] Other areas of potential promise and targets for future research with PET/MRI include the identification of sites of recurrence after treatment in patients with suspected relapse and assessment of surgical candidacy after neoadjuvant therapy in patients initially presenting with locally advanced disease. **Table 4** summarizes the current evidence

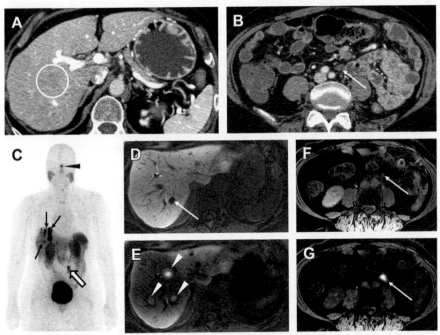

Fig. 8. Staging of carcinoid tumor with DOTATATE-PET/MRI. A patient with a previously resected carcinoid tumor presented for restaging. Transaxial computed tomography (CT) images through the liver (*A*) and lower abdomen (*B*) show a vague area of hypodensity in the right liver (*circle* in *A*) without discrete focal liver lesions, as well as an inconspicuous left retroperitoneal lymph node (*arrow* in *B*). Maximum intensity projection PET images (*C*) from subsequent DOTATATE-PET/MRI show multiple foci of increased tracer uptake in the liver (*short black arrows*), as well as a suspicious lesion in the left abdomen (*white arrow*). Normal tracer uptake is seen in the pituitary gland (*arrowhead*). Transaxial T1-weighted images (*D, F*) acquired 20 minutes after the intravenous administration of gadoxetate disodium (ie, hepatobiliary phase) with DOTATATE-PET fusion (*E, G*) reveal 3 discrete tracer-avid lesions (*arrowheads* in *E*). Note that only one lesion has a correlate on the MRI (*arrow* in *D*) due to misregistration between the PET and MRI. Additionally, the inconspicuous lymph node seen in the left retroperitoneum on prior CT, although still normal in size on the MRI (*arrow* in *F*), is markedly tracer avid (*arrow* in *G*), consistent with an additional site of metastatic disease. This case demonstrates the excellent sensitivity of DOTATATE-PET for neuroendocrine liver metastases. This tracer can also reveal involvement of nodes that would otherwise be deemed normal by size criteria alone.

pertaining to the use of PET/MRI for pancreatic adenocarcinoma. Notably, the majority of available studies involve the retrospective fusion of PET and MRI datasets rather than simultaneous acquisition, although it is reasonable to expect that integrated PET/MRI would offer the same advantages.

Neuroendocrine Tumors

GI and pancreatic NETs are a relatively rare group of neoplasms that arise from the neuroendocrine axis of the GI tract, most commonly within the pancreas, terminal ileum, appendix, or rectum.[88] This heterogeneous group of tumors varies considerably in aggressiveness and the probability of metastasis.[89] Many NETs secrete bioactive substances (ie, functional NETs), such as vasoactive intestinal peptide, insulin, or gastrin, bringing them to clinical attention at an earlier stage due to associated symptoms. Surgical treatment of NETs is often indicated when complete resection of disease can be achieved. Alternatively, patients who have liver metastasis and are not

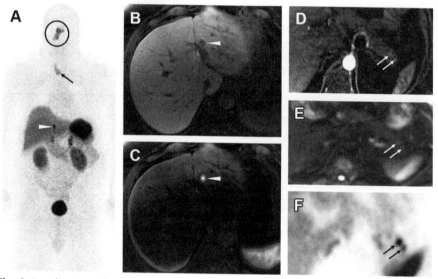

Fig. 9. Localization of small neuroendocrine tumors with DOTATATE-PET/MRI. A patient with multiple endocrine neoplasia type 1 (MEN-1) presented for the workup of a clinically suspected neuroendocrine tumor. Maximum intensity projection (MIP) PET images (*A*) from DOTATATE-PET/MRI show a suspicious focus in the liver (*white arrowhead*). Additionally, in keeping with the patient's known MEN-1 diagnosis, a large pituitary adenoma (*black circle*) and postsurgical changes of hemithyroidectomy (*black arrow* – residual right thyroid gland) as part of a parathyroid adenoma resection are also noted. Transaxial T1-weighted images (*B*) acquired 20 minutes after the intravenous administration of gadoxetate disodium (ie, hepatobiliary phase) with DOTATATE-PET fusion (*C*) reveal a discrete tracer-avid lesion (*arrowhead* in *C*), with a corresponding focal hypointense lesion on the MRIs (*arrowhead* in *B*), suggesting a neuroendocrine tumor metastasis. Transaxial T1-weighted arterial phase postcontrast images (*D*) and transaxial diffusion-weighted images (*E*) of the pancreas reveal 2 subtle hyperenhancing (*arrows* in D), diffusion-restricting (*arrows* in E) lesions in the pancreatic tail that are more conspicuous on the concurrently acquired transaxial DOTATATE-PET images (*arrows* in *F*). These findings confirm the presence of primary pancreatic neuroendocrine tumors, which are the likely source of the liver metastasis. Note that these lesions were obscured on the MIP image (*A*) by normal splenic tracer uptake, highlighting the value of cross-sectional PET reconstructions.

candidates for surgery may undergo LRT, such as chemoembolization or ablation, to reduce the metastatic burden and control symptoms.[88] Finally, patients with widespread metastatic disease may be candidates for radiolabeled somatostatin analogue therapies, such as ^{177}Lu-DOTATATE, provided their disease is detectable on somatosatin receptor imaging studies.[90] Thus, noninvasive imaging plays an important role in the diagnosis and management of these tumors. Endoscopic ultrasound, gastroduodenoscopy, colonoscopy, capsule endoscopy, and laparoscopy are used in a supportive fashion.

Potential roles and current evidence

Imaging of NETs typically includes a contrast-enhanced CT, although protocols vary based on the suspected site of disease.[91] Contrast-enhanced MRI is often used as a problem-solving tool in patients with negative or equivocal findings on CT, as well as a primary modality in younger patients so as to minimize radiation exposure.[92] The detection rate of primary NETs is similar for CT and MRI.[93] However, MRI is more sensitive than CT for the detection of liver metastases, particular when hepatobiliary contrast agents are used.[32,33]

In some circumstances, the primary NET is small and difficult to detect with conventional imaging.[94] SSTR imaging, which takes advantage of SSTR expression by most NETs, is used for primary tumor detection, staging, and assessment of treatment response.[91,95] Although SSTR imaging has been conventionally performed with

---

Table 5
Results of studies evaluating the role of PET/MRI in neuroendocrine tumors

Publication	Patients (n)	Findings
Hope et al,[113] 2015	10	• Higher detection rate of ^{68}Ga-DOTATOC-PET/MRI (including hepatobiliary phase imaging) for NET liver metastasis than ^{68}Ga-DOTATOC-PET/CT
Beiderwellen et al,[114] 2013	8	• Comparable diagnostic performance of ^{68}Ga-DOTATOC-PET/MRI and ^{68}Ga-DOTATOC-PET/CT for identifying malignant NETs • PET/MRI may better characterize abdominal lesions, whereas PET/CT may better detect lung metastases and hypersclerotic osseous metastases
Gaertner et al,[115] 2013	24	• Comparable detection rate of ^{68}Ga-DOTATOC-PET/MRI and ^{68}Ga-DOTATOC-PET/CT for NET on a per-patient and per-lesion basis
Berzaczy et al,[116] 2017	28	• Comparable detection rate of ^{68}Ga-DOTANOC-PET/MRI and ^{68}Ga-DOTANOC-PET/CT for distant metastatic disease in patients with well-differentiated NETs
Sawicki et al,[117] 2017	30	• Higher number of NETs correctly identified, with better lesion conspicuity, for ^{68}Ga-DOTATOC-PET/MRI compared with ^{68}Ga-DOTATOC-PET/CT
Mayerhoefer et al,[118] 2013	18	• *Retrospective fusion* of ^{68}Ga-DOTANOC-PET with contrast-enhanced MRI (hepatobiliary phase) versus DWI alone results in no difference in NET detection rates
Schreiter et al,[119] 2012	22	• *Retrospective fusion* of ^{68}Ga-DOTATOC-PET and contrast-enhanced MRI (hepatobiliary phase) improves detection of NET liver metastasis as compared with ^{68}Ga-DOTATOC-PET/CT or MRI alone

Abbreviations: DWI, diffusion-weighted imaging; FDG-PET/CT, PET/computed tomography with 2-deoxy-2-[^{18}F]fluoro-ᴅ-glucose; ^{68}Ga-DOTATOC-PET/MRI, 68-Gallium-DOTA-D-Phe1-Tyr3-octreotide; NET, neuroendocrine tumor.

[^{111}In]pentetreotide, the introduction of the SSTR PET tracers (eg, [^{68}Ga]DOTATOC, [^{68}Ga]DOTATATE) has substantially improved diagnostic performance and patient convenience.[96,97] Appropriate use criteria for SSTR PET imaging of NETs have recently been published.[98] FDG-PET imaging can also provide prognostic information, because poorly differentiated NETs are less likely to express SSTRs and more likely to exhibit FDG avidity.[99] Additionally, the SSTR PET tracers may be useful for selecting patients likely to benefit from the radiolabeled somatostatin analogue therapies.[100]

PET/MRI combines the high soft tissue contrast of MRI with the sensitivity/specificity of SSTR PET for primary tumor identification and distant metastatic disease detection (**Figs. 8 and 9**). **Table 5** summarizes current evidence pertaining to the use of PET/MRI for NETs. Overall, SSTR PET/MRI is likely more useful in the setting of liver-dominant disease, whereas SSTR PET/CT may be more valuable for disease predominantly involving the bones, lungs, or mesentery. Furthermore, SSTR PET/MRI, when DWI is included, can be helpful for distinguishing between the physiologic and neoplastic etiologies of SSTR uptake in the uncinate process of the pancreas, a location that can be part of the normal biodistribution of these tracers. Additional studies comparing PET/MRI to contrast-enhanced PET/CT are needed, because most available studies have utilized noncontrast PET/CT.

SUMMARY

PET/MRI is a promising hybrid modality for the evaluation of many different GI malignancies, with the potential to provide complete TNM staging in a single imaging examination. Although FDG remains the workhorse of oncologic PET imaging, the recent rapid growth of the tracer armamentarium, as well as improvements in functional MRI techniques (eg, DWI), will further enhance the usefulness of PET/MRI. Despite the vast capabilities of PET/MRI, the majority of studies evaluating PET/MRI in the setting GI malignancies have been retrospective, with small numbers of patients. Large, prospective studies are needed to define the optimal role of PET/MRI in oncologic management algorithms.

REFERENCES

1. Kostakoglu L, Agress H, Goldsmith SJ. Clinical role of FDG PET in evaluation of cancer patients. Radiographics 2003;23(2):315–40.
2. Fletcher JW, Djulbegovic B, Soares HP, et al. Recommendations on the use of 18F-FDG PET in oncology. J Nucl Med 2008;49(3):480–508.
3. Ben-Haim S, Ell P. 18F-FDG PET and PET/CT in the evaluation of cancer treatment response. J Nucl Med 2009;50(1):88–99.
4. Treglia G, Sadeghi R, Del Sole A, et al. Diagnostic performance of PET/CT with tracers other than F-18-FDG in oncology: an evidence-based review. Clin Transl Oncol 2014;16(9):770–5.
5. Maccioni F, Patak MA, Signore A, et al. New frontiers of MRI in Crohn's disease: motility imaging, diffusion-weighted imaging, perfusion MRI, MR spectroscopy, molecular imaging, and hybrid imaging (PET/MRI). Abdom Imaging 2012;37(6): 974–82.
6. Siegel RL, Miller KD, Jemal A. Cancer statistics, 2016. CA Cancer J Clin 2016; 66(1):7–30.
7. Fraum TJ, Owen JW, Fowler KJ. Beyond histologic staging: emerging imaging strategies in colorectal cancer with special focus on magnetic resonance imaging. Clin Colon Rectal Surg 2016;29(3):205–15.

8. Glynne-Jones R, Tan D, Goh V. Pelvic MRI for guiding treatment decisions in rectal cancer. Oncology (Williston Park) 2014;28(8):667–77.

9. Nogué M, Salud A, Vicente P, et al. Addition of bevacizumab to XELOX induction therapy plus concomitant capecitabine-based chemoradiotherapy in magnetic resonance imaging-defined poor-prognosis locally advanced rectal cancer: the AVACROSS study. Oncologist 2011;16(5):614–20.

10. Velenik V, Ocvirk J, Music M, et al. Neoadjuvant capecitabine, radiotherapy, and bevacizumab (CRAB) in locally advanced rectal cancer: results of an open-label phase II study. Radiat Oncol 2011;6:105.

11. MERCURY Study Group. Extramural depth of tumor invasion at thin-section MR in patients with rectal cancer: results of the MERCURY study. Radiology 2007; 243(1):132–9.

12. Kim SH, Lee JM, Park HS, et al. Accuracy of MRI for predicting the circumferential resection margin, mesorectal fascia invasion, and tumor response to neoadjuvant chemoradiotherapy for locally advanced rectal cancer. J Magn Reson Imaging 2009;29(5):1093–101.

13. Doyon F, Attenberger UI, Dinter DJ, et al. Clinical relevance of morphologic MRI criteria for the assessment of lymph nodes in patients with rectal cancer. Int J Colorectal Dis 2015;30(11):1541–6.

14. Mainenti PP, Iodice D, Segreto S, et al. Colorectal cancer and 18FDG-PET/CT: what about adding the T to the N parameter in loco-regional staging? World J Gastroenterol 2011;17(11):1427–33.

15. Patel UB, Taylor F, Blomqvist L, et al. Magnetic resonance imaging-detected tumor response for locally advanced rectal cancer predicts survival outcomes: MERCURY experience. J Clin Oncol 2011;29(28):3753–60.

16. Cascini GL, Avallone A, Delrio P, et al. 18F-FDG PET is an early predictor of pathologic tumor response to preoperative radiochemotherapy in locally advanced rectal cancer. J Nucl Med 2006;47(8):1241–8.

17. Low G, Tho LM, Leen E, et al. The role of imaging in the pre-operative staging and post-operative follow-up of rectal cancer. Surgeon 2008;6(4):222–31.

18. Lim JS, Yun MJ, Kim M-J, et al. CT and PET in stomach cancer: preoperative staging and monitoring of response to therapy. Radiographics 2006;26(1): 143–56.

19. Ajani JA, D'Amico TA, Almhanna K, et al. Gastric cancer, version 3.2016, NCCN clinical practice guidelines in oncology. J Natl Compr Canc Netw 2016;14(10): 1286–312.

20. Stahl A, Ott K, Weber WA, et al. FDG PET imaging of locally advanced gastric carcinomas: correlation with endoscopic and histopathological findings. Eur J Nucl Med Mol Imaging 2003;30(2):288–95.

21. Xiong B-H, Cheng Y, Ma L, et al. An updated meta-analysis of randomized controlled trial assessing the effect of neoadjuvant chemotherapy in advanced gastric cancer. Cancer Invest 2014;32(6):272–84.

22. Sheybani A, Menias CO, Luna A, et al. MRI of the stomach: a pictorial review with a focus on oncological applications and gastric motility. Abdom Imaging 2014;40(4):907–30.

23. Kwee RM, Kwee TC. Imaging in local staging of gastric cancer: a systematic review. J Clin Oncol 2007;25(15):2107–16.

24. Yun M, Lim JS, Noh SH, et al. Lymph node staging of gastric cancer using (18) F-FDG PET: a comparison study with CT. J Nucl Med 2005;46(10):1582–8.

25. Smyth E, Schöder H, Strong VE, et al. A prospective evaluation of the utility of 2-deoxy-2-[(18) F]fluoro-D-glucose positron emission tomography and

computed tomography in staging locally advanced gastric cancer. Cancer 2012;118(22):5481–8.

26. Giganti F, De Cobelli F, Canevari C, et al. Response to chemotherapy in gastric adenocarcinoma with diffusion-weighted MRI and (18) F-FDG-PET/CT: correlation of apparent diffusion coefficient and partial volume corrected standardized uptake value with histological tumor regression grade. J Magn Reson Imaging 2013;0(5):1–11.

27. Simmonds PC, Primrose JN, Colquitt JL, et al. Surgical resection of hepatic metastases from colorectal cancer: a systematic review of published studies. Br J Cancer 2006;94(7):982–99.

28. Selzner M, Morse MA, Vredenburgh JJ, et al. Liver metastases from breast cancer: long-term survival after curative resection. Surgery 2000;127(4):383–9.

29. Rose DM, Essner R, Hughes TM, et al. Surgical resection for metastatic melanoma to the liver: the John Wayne Cancer Institute and Sydney Melanoma Unit experience. Arch Surg 2001;136(8):950–5.

30. Manfredi S, Lepage C, Hatem C, et al. Epidemiology and management of liver metastases from colorectal cancer. Ann Surg 2006;244(2):254–9.

31. Ramos E, Valls C, Martinez L, et al. Preoperative staging of patients with liver metastases of colorectal carcinoma. Does PET/CT really add something to multidetector CT? Ann Surg Oncol 2011;18(9):2654–61.

32. Scharitzer M, Ba-Ssalamah A, Ringl H, et al. Preoperative evaluation of colorectal liver metastases: comparison between gadoxetic acid-enhanced 3.0-T MRI and contrast-enhanced MDCT with histopathological correlation. Eur Radiol 2013;23(8):2187–96.

33. Muhi A, Ichikawa T, Motosugi U, et al. Diagnosis of colorectal hepatic metastases: comparison of contrast-enhanced CT, contrast-enhanced US, superparamagnetic iron oxide-enhanced MRI, and gadoxetic acid-enhanced MRI. J Magn Reson Imaging 2011;34(2):326–35.

34. Parikh T, Drew SJ, Lee VS, et al. Focal liver lesion detection and characterization with diffusion-weighted MR imaging: comparison with standard breath-hold T2-weighted imaging. Radiology 2008;246(3):812–22.

35. Donati OF, Hany TF, Reiner CS, et al. Value of retrospective fusion of PET and MR images in detection of hepatic metastases: comparison with 18F-FDG PET/CT and Gd-EOB-DTPA-enhanced MRI. J Nucl Med 2010;51(5):692–9.

36. Fowler KJ, Linehan DC, Menias CO. Colorectal liver metastases: state of the art imaging. Ann Surg Oncol 2013;20(4):1185–93.

37. Kayani I, Bomanji JB, Groves A, et al. Functional imaging of neuroendocrine tumors with combined PET/CT using 68Ga-DOTATATE (Dota-DPhe1, Tyr3-octreotate) and 18F-FDG. Cancer 2008;112(11):2447–55.

38. Wallace MC, Preen D, Jeffrey GP, et al. The evolving epidemiology of hepatocellular carcinoma: a global perspective. Expert Rev Gastroenterol Hepatol 2015; 9(6):765–79.

39. El-Serag HB. Hepatocellular carcinoma. N Engl J Med 2011;365(12):1118–27.

40. Heimbach J, Kulik LM, Finn R, et al. AASLD guidelines for the treatment of hepatocellular carcinoma. Hepatology 2017. https://doi.org/10.1002/hep.29086.

41. Mazzaferro V, Regalia E, Doci R, et al. Liver transplantation for the treatment of small hepatocellular carcinomas in patients with cirrhosis. N Engl J Med 1996; 334(11):693–9.

42. Lencioni R. Loco-regional treatment of hepatocellular carcinoma. Hepatology 2010;52(2):762–73.

43. Chapman WC, Garcia-Aroz S, Vachharajani N, et al. Liver transplantation for advanced hepatocellular carcinoma after downstaging without up-front stage restrictions. J Am Coll Surg 2017;224:610–21.

44. Elsayes KM, Kielar AZ, Agrons MM, et al. Liver imaging reporting and data system: an expert consensus statement. J Hepatocell Carcinoma 2017;4:29–39.

45. Ayuso C, Rimola J, García-Criado Á. Imaging of HCC. Abdom Imaging 2012; 37(2):215–30.

46. Yu JS, Chung JJ, Kim JH, et al. Detection of small intrahepatic metastases of hepatocellular carcinomas using diffusion-weighted imaging: comparison with conventional dynamic MRI. Magn Reson Imaging 2011;29(7):985–92.

47. Kong E, Chun KA, Cho IH. Quantitative assessment of simultaneous F-18 FDG PET/MRI in patients with various types of hepatic tumors: correlation between glucose metabolism and apparent diffusion coefficient. PLoS One 2017;12(7): e0180184.

48. Teefey SA, Hildeboldt CC, Dehdashti F, et al. Detection of primary hepatic malignancy in liver transplant candidates: prospective comparison of CT, MR imaging, US, and PET. Radiology 2003;226(2):533–42.

49. Khan MA, Combs CS, Brunt EM, et al. Positron emission tomography scanning in the evaluation of hepatocellular carcinoma. J Hepatol 2000;32(5):792–7.

50. Kornberg A, Freesmeyer M, Bärthel E, et al. 18F-FDG-uptake of hepatocellular carcinoma on PET predicts microvascular tumor invasion in liver transplant patients. Am J Transplant 2009;9(3):592–600.

51. Na SJ, Oh JK, Hyun SH, et al. (18)F-FDG PET/CT can predict survival of advanced hepatocellular carcinoma patients: a multicenter retrospective cohort study. J Nucl Med 2017;58(5):730–6.

52. Ye Y-F, Wang W, Wang T, et al. Role of [(18)F] fludeoxyglucose positron emission tomography in the selection of liver transplantation candidates in patients with hepatocellular carcinoma. Hepatobiliary Pancreat Dis Int 2017;16(3):257–63.

53. Lee JW, Paeng JC, Kang KW, et al. Prediction of tumor recurrence by 18F-FDG PET in liver transplantation for hepatocellular carcinoma. J Nucl Med 2009; 50(5):682–7.

54. Yang SH, Suh KS, Lee HW, et al. The role of 18F-FDG-PET imaging for the selection of liver transplantation candidates among hepatocellular carcinoma patients. Liver Transpl 2006;12(11):1655–60.

55. Lee JW, Oh JK, Chung YA, et al. Prognostic significance of 18F-FDG uptake in hepatocellular carcinoma treated with transarterial chemoembolization or concurrent chemoradiotherapy: a multicenter retrospective cohort study. J Nucl Med 2016;57(4):509–16.

56. Ma W, Jia J, Wang S, et al. The prognostic value of 18F-FDG PET/CT for hepatocellular carcinoma treated with transarterial chemoembolization (TACE). Theranostics 2014;4(7):736–44.

57. Dierckx R, Maes A, Peeters M, et al. FDG PET for monitoring response to local and locoregional therapy in HCC and liver metastases. Q J Nucl Med Mol Imaging 2009;53(3):336–42.

58. Katyal S, Oliver JH, Peterson MS, et al. Extrahepatic metastases of hepatocellular carcinoma. Radiology 2000;216(3):698–703.

59. Sugiyama M, Sakahara H, Torizuka T, et al. 18F-FDG PET in the detection of extrahepatic metastases from hepatocellular carcinoma. J Gastroenterol 2004; 39(10):961–8.

60. Lin CY, Chen JH, Liang JA, et al. 18F-FDG PET or PET/CT for detecting extrahepatic metastases or recurrent hepatocellular carcinoma: a systematic review and meta-analysis. Eur J Radiol 2012;81(9):2417–22.

61. Yoon KT, Kim JK, Kim DY, et al. Role of 18F-fluorodeoxyglucose positron emission tomography in detecting extrahepatic metastasis in pretreatment staging of hepatocellular carcinoma. Oncology 2007;72(Suppl. 1):104–10.

62. Sun L, Guan YS, Pan WM, et al. Highly metabolic thrombus of the portal vein: 18F fluorodeoxyglucose positron emission tomography/computer tomography demonstration and clinical significance in hepatocellular carcinoma. World J Gastroenterol 2008;14(8):1212–7.

63. Cheung TT, Ho CL, Lo CM, et al. 11C-acetate and 18F-FDG PET/CT for clinical staging and selection of patients with hepatocellular carcinoma for liver transplantation on the basis of Milan criteria: surgeon's perspective. J Nucl Med 2013;54(2):192–200.

64. Castilla-Lièvre MA, Franco D, Gervais P, et al. Diagnostic value of combining 11C-choline and 18F-FDG PET/CT in hepatocellular carcinoma. Eur J Nucl Med Mol Imaging 2016;43(5):852–9.

65. Talbot J-N, Fartoux L, Balogova S, et al. Detection of hepatocellular carcinoma with PET/CT: a prospective comparison of 18F-fluorocholine and 18F-FDG in patients with cirrhosis or chronic liver disease. J Nucl Med 2010;51(11):1699–706.

66. Fowler KJ, Maughan NM, Laforest R, et al. PET/MRI of hepatic 90Y microsphere Deposition determines individual tumor response. Cardiovasc Intervent Radiol 2016;39(6):855–64.

67. Tempero M, Arnoletti JP, Ben-Josef E, et al. Pancreatic adenocarcinoma. Clinical practice guidelines in oncology. J Natl Compr Canc Netw 2007;5(10):998–1033.

68. Li D, Xie K, Wolff R, et al. Pancreatic cancer. Lancet 2004;363(9414):1049–57.

69. Wagner M, Redaelli C, Lietz M, et al. Curative resection is the single most important factor determining outcome in patients with pancreatic adenocarcinoma. Br J Surg 2004;91(5):586–94.

70. Small WJ, Hayes JP, Suh WW, et al. ACR appropriateness criteria borderline and unresectable pancreas cancer. Oncology 2016;30(7):619–24, 627,632.

71. Katz MH, Savides TJ, Moossa AR, et al. An evidence-based approach to the diagnosis and staging of pancreatic cancer. Pancreatology 2005;5(6):576–90.

72. Tummala P, Junaidi O, Agarwal B. Imaging of pancreatic cancer: an overview. J Gastrointest Oncol 2011;2(3):168–74.

73. Karmazanovsky G, Fedorov V, Kubyshkin V, et al. Pancreatic head cancer: accuracy of CT in determination of resectability. Abdom Imaging 2005;30(4):488–500.

74. Wong JC, Lu DSK. Staging of pancreatic adenocarcinoma by imaging studies. Clin Gastroenterol Hepatol 2008;6(12):1301–8.

75. Koelblinger C, Ba-Ssalamah A, Goetzinger P, et al. Gadobenate dimeglumine-enhanced 3.0-T MR imaging versus multiphasic 64-detector row CT: prospective evaluation in patients suspected of having pancreatic cancer. Radiology 2011;259(3):757–66.

76. Hee SP, Jeong ML, Hei KC, et al. Preoperative evaluation of pancreatic cancer: comparison of gadolinium-enhanced dynamic MRI with MR cholangiopancreatography versus MDCT. J Magn Reson Imaging 2009;30(3):586–95.

77. Shrikhande SV, Barreto SG, Goel M, et al. Multimodality imaging of pancreatic ductal adenocarcinoma: a review of the literature. HPB (Oxford) 2012;14(10):658–68.

78. Kim JK, Altun E, Elias J, et al. Focal pancreatic mass: distinction of pancreatic cancer from chronic pancreatitis using gadolinium-enhanced 3D-gradient-echo MRI. J Magn Reson Imaging 2007;26(2):313–22.

79. Belião S, Ferreira A, Vierasu I, et al. MR imaging versus PET/CT for evaluation of pancreatic lesions. Eur J Radiol 2012;81(10):2527–32.

80. Satoh Y, Ichikawa T, Motosugi U, et al. Diagnosis of peritoneal dissemination: comparison of 18F-FDG PET/CT, diffusion-weighted MRI, and contrast-enhanced MDCT. Am J Roentgenol 2011;196(2):447–53.

81. Kauhanen SP, Komar G, Seppänen MP, et al. A prospective diagnostic accuracy study of 18F-fluorodeoxyglucose positron emission tomography/computed tomography, multidetector row computed tomography, and magnetic resonance imaging in primary diagnosis and staging of pancreatic cancer. Ann Surg 2009;250(6):957–63.

82. Einersen P, Epelboym I, Winner MD, et al. Positron Emission Tomography (PET) has limited utility in the staging of pancreatic adenocarcinoma. J Gastrointest Surg 2014;18(8):1441–4.

83. Sultana A, Jackson R, Tim G, et al. What is the best way to identify malignant transformation within pancreatic IPMN: a systematic review and meta-analyses. Clin Transl Gastroenterol 2015;6(12):e130.

84. Kauhanen S, Rinta-Kiikka I, Kemppainen J, et al. Accuracy of 18F-FDG PET/CT, multidetector CT, and MR imaging in the diagnosis of pancreatic cysts: a prospective single-center study. J Nucl Med 2015;56(8):1163–8.

85. Ruf J, Hänninen EL, Oettle H, et al. Detection of recurrent pancreatic cancer: comparison of FDG-PET with CT/MRI. Pancreatology 2005;5(2–3):266–72.

86. Chen YM, Huang G, Sun XG, et al. Optimizing delayed scan time for FDG PET: comparison of the early and late delayed scan. Nucl Med Commun 2008;29(5): 425–30.

87. Hope TA, Verdin EF, Bergsland EK, et al. Correcting for respiratory motion in liver PET/MRI: preliminary evaluation of the utility of bellows and navigated hepatobiliary phase imaging. EJNMMI Phys 2015;2(1):21.

88. Díez M, Teulé A, Salazar R. Gastroenteropancreatic neuroendocrine tumors: diagnosis and treatment. Ann Gastroenterol 2013;26(1):29–36.

89. Yao JC, Hassan M, Phan A, et al. One hundred years after "carcinoid": epidemiology of and prognostic factors for neuroendocrine tumors in 35,825 cases in the United States. J Clin Oncol 2008;26(18):3063–72.

90. Strosberg J, El-Haddad G, Wolin E, et al. Phase 3 Trial of 177 Lu-Dotatate for Midgut Neuroendocrine tumors. N Engl J Med 2017;376(2):125–35.

91. Sahani DV, Bonaffini PA, Fernández-Del Castillo C, et al. Gastroenteropancreatic neuroendocrine tumors: role of imaging in diagnosis and management. Radiology 2013;266(1):38–61.

92. Sundin A, Vullierme MP, Kaltsas G, et al. ENETS consensus guidelines for the standards of care in neuroendocrine tumors: radiological examinations. Neuroendocrinology 2009;90:167–83.

93. Ichikawa T, Peterson MS, Federle MP, et al. Islet cell tumor of the pancreas: biphasic CT versus MR imaging in tumor detection. Radiology 2000;216(1): 163–71.

94. Polish A, Vergo MT, Agulnik M. Management of neuroendocrine tumors of unknown origin. J Natl Compr Canc Netw 2011;9(12):1397–402.

95. Frilling A, Sotiropoulos GC, Radtke A, et al. The impact of Ga-68-DOTATOC positron emission tomography/computed tomography on the multimodal management of patients with neuroendocrine tumors. Ann Surg 2010;252(5):850–6.

96. Hofmann M, Maecke H, Börner R, et al. Biokinetics and imaging with the somatostatin receptor PET radioligand (68)Ga-DOTATOC: preliminary data. Eur J Nucl Med 2001;28(12):1751–7.

97. Krausz Y, Freedman N, Rubinstein R, et al. 68Ga-DOTA-NOC PET/CT imaging of neuroendocrine tumors: comparison with 111In-DTPA-octreotide (OctreoScan). Mol Imaging Biol 2011;13(3):583–93.

98. Hope TA, Bergsland E, Bozkurt MF, et al. Appropriate use criteria for somatostatin Receptor PET imaging in neuroendocrine tumors. J Nucl Med 2017. https://doi.org/10.2967/jnumed.117.202275.

99. Binderup T, Knigge U, Loft A, et al. Functional imaging of neuroendocrine tumors: a head-to-head comparison of somatostatin receptor scintigraphy, 123 I-MIBG scintigraphy, and 18 F-FDG PET. J Nucl Med 2010;51(5):704–12.

100. Fani M, Nicolas GP, Wild D. Somatostatin receptor antagonists for imaging and therapy. J Nucl Med 2017;58(Supplement 2):61S–6S.

101. Paspulati RM, Partovi S, Herrmann KA, et al. Comparison of hybrid FDG PET/MRI compared with PET/CT in colorectal cancer staging and restaging: a pilot study. Abdom Imaging 2015;40(6):1415–25.

102. Brendle C, Schwenzer NF, Rempp H, et al. Assessment of metastatic colorectal cancer with hybrid imaging: comparison of reading performance using different combinations of anatomical and functional imaging techniques in PET/MRI and PET/CT in a short case series. Eur J Nucl Med Mol Imaging 2016;43(1):123–32.

103. Kang B, Lee JM, Song YS, et al. Added value of integrated whole-body PET/MRI for evaluation of colorectal cancer: comparison with contrast-enhanced MDCT. Am J Roentgenol 2016;206(1):W10–20.

104. Lee DH, Kim SH, Joo I, et al. Comparison between 18F-FDG PET/MRI and MDCT for the assessment of preoperative staging and resectability of gastric cancer. Eur J Radiol 2016;85(6):1085–91.

105. Lee DH, Kim SH, Im SA, et al. Multiparametric fully-integrated 18-FDG PET/MRI of advanced gastric cancer for prediction of chemotherapy response: a preliminary study. Eur Radiol 2016;26(8):2771–8.

106. Beiderwellen K, Geraldo L, Ruhlmann V, et al. Accuracy of [18F]FDG PET/MRI for the detection of liver metastases. In: Lu S-N, editor. PLoS One 2015;10(9): e0137285.

107. Yong TW, Yuan ZZ, Jun Z, et al. Sensitivity of PET/MR images in liver metastases from colorectal carcinoma. Hell J Nucl Med 2011;14(3):264–8.

108. Joo I, Lee JM, Lee DH, et al. Preoperative assessment of pancreatic cancer with FDG PET/MR imaging versus FDG PET/CT plus contrast-enhanced multidetector CT: a prospective preliminary study. Radiology 2017;282(1):149–59.

109. Chen BB, Tien YW, Chang MC, et al. PET/MRI in pancreatic and periampullary cancer: correlating diffusion-weighted imaging, MR spectroscopy and glucose metabolic activity with clinical stage and prognosis. Eur J Nucl Med Mol Imaging 2016;43(10):1753–64.

110. Nagamachi S, Nishii R, Wakamatsu H, et al. The usefulness of (18)F-FDG PET/MRI fusion image in diagnosing pancreatic tumor: comparison with (18)F-FDG PET/CT. Ann Nucl Med 2013;27(6):554–63.

111. Tatsumi M, Isohashi K, Onishi H, et al. 18F-FDG PET/MRI fusion in characterizing pancreatic tumors: comparison to PET/CT. Int J Clin Oncol 2011;16(4):408–15.

112. Ruf J, Lopez Hänninen E, Böhmig M, et al. Impact of FDG-PET/MRI image fusion on the detection of pancreatic cancer. Pancreatology 2006;6(6):512–9.

113. Hope TA, Pampaloni MH, Nakakura E, et al. Simultaneous 68Ga-DOTA-TOC PET/MRI with gadoxetate disodium in patients with neuroendocrine tumor. Abdom Imaging 2015;40(6):1432–40.
114. Beiderwellen KJ, Poeppel TD, Hartung-Knemeyer V, et al. Simultaneous 68Ga-DOTATOC PET/MRI in patients with gastroenteropancreatic neuroendocrine tumors: initial results. Invest Radiol 2013;48(5):273–9.
115. Gaertner FC, Beer AJ, Souvatzoglou M, et al. Evaluation of feasibility and image quality of 68Ga-DOTATOC positron emission tomography/magnetic resonance in comparison with positron emission tomography/computed tomography in patients with neuroendocrine tumors. Invest Radiol 2013;48(5):263–72.
116. Berzaczy D, Giraudo C, Haug AR, et al. Whole-body 68Ga-DOTANOC PET/MRI versus 68Ga-DOTANOC PET/CT in patients with neuroendocrine tumors: a prospective study in 28 patients. Clin Nucl Med 2017;42(9):669–74.
117. Sawicki LM, Deuschl C, Beiderwellen K, et al. Evaluation of ^{68}Ga-DOTATOC PET/MRI for whole-body staging of neuroendocrine tumours in comparison with ^{68}Ga-DOTATOC PET/CT. Eur Radiol 2017;27(10):4091–9.
118. Mayerhoefer ME, Ba-Ssalamah A, Weber M, et al. Gadoxetate-enhanced versus diffusion-weighted MRI for fused Ga-68-DOTANOC PET/MRI in patients with neuroendocrine tumours of the upper abdomen. Eur Radiol 2013;23(7): 1978–85.
119. Schreiter NF, Nogami M, Steffen I, et al. Evaluation of the potential of PET-MRI fusion for detection of liver metastases in patients with neuroendocrine tumours. Eur Radiol 2012;22(2):458–67.

Moving?

Make sure your subscription moves with you!

To notify us of your new address, find your **Clinics Account Number** (located on your mailing label above your name), and contact customer service at:

Email: journalscustomerservice-usa@elsevier.com

800-654-2452 (subscribers in the U.S. & Canada)
314-447-8871 (subscribers outside of the U.S. & Canada)

Fax number: 314-447-8029

Elsevier Health Sciences Division
Subscription Customer Service
3251 Riverport Lane
Maryland Heights, MO 63043

*To ensure uninterrupted delivery of your subscription, please notify us at least 4 weeks in advance of move.

Printed and bound by CPI Group (UK) Ltd, Croydon, CR0 4YY

07/10/2024

01040501-0009